T0289375

Health and British Magazines in the Nineteenth Century

E. M. Palmegiano

The Scarecrow Press, Inc.
Lanham, Md., & London
1998

SCARECROW PRESS, INC.

Published in the United States of America
by Scarecrow Press, Inc.
4720 Boston Way
Lanham, Maryland 20706

4 Pleydell Gardens
Kent CT20 2DN, England

British Library Cataloguing in Publication Information Available

Library of Congress Cataloging-in-Publication Data

Palmegiano, E. M.
    Health and British magazines in the nineteenth century / E. M.
Palmegiano.
        p.   cm.
    Includes bibliographical references and index.
    ISBN 0-8108-3486-3 (alk. paper)
    1. Health—Bibliography. 2. Health—Press coverage—Great Britain—
Bibliography. 3. Medicine, Popular—Bibliography. 4. Medicine,
Popular—Press coverage—Great Britain—Bibliography. 5. British
periodicals—Bibliography.   I. Title.
Z6673.P288   1998
[RA776.5]
016.61—dc21   98-3909

CONTENTS

PREFACE

Health and headlines were serious matters in nineteenth-century Britain. They were significantly linked, although health is essentially individual and headlines are communal. Salubrity spawned a plethora of ideas that the press disseminated. This bibliography offers the spectrum and sequence of those views.

The scope of this book is wellness as science and society understood it at the time. The first reflects the influence of experts, accurate or not; the second, the interests of the government and the governed. While this study draws from many serials whose commentators shaped interpretation or policy authoritatively, all authors spoke with some credibility. For, unlike other areas of opinion, in this one everybody had experience.

From 1824 to 1900, news of health was abundant. This era, when distinguished quarterlies peaked in impact and distinctive magazines appeared, is the timeframe of *The Wellesley Index to Victorian Periodicals*, the chief catalog for serials listed here. Twelve titles from *Poole's Index* have also been included because they had lengthy runs, renowned editors or publishers, a focus otherwise overlooked, and/or known contributors. The reasons for this selection are the multitude of journals, the preeminence of those in the *Wellesley Index* and *Poole's*, and the regularity of their submissions on the subject of health. Such discrimination highlights readers and writers of the middle and upper classes, but their perspectives were neither uniform nor unwavering. Writers' background, bent, and bias sustained discourse different in approach, impact, and importance.

Journalistic coverage was the child of private and public concerns.

Health might be a personal or a public matter, comprehensible to all or only to specialists, valuable to the possessor or as a validator of British success. Always its absence attracted as much as annoyed observers. Tales of illness might reveal the emotions of sufferers or engage the curiosity of readers. The enduring fear of death prompted impatience with medicine, and the escalating faith in technology encouraged optimism about it. Enthusiasm for excellence stimulated demands for vigor and victory over disease as symbols of the social control required for national progress and international paramountcy. Fitness became the goal; illness or disability was excusable but potentially eradicable.

Columnists consequently circulated advice, admonitions, and calls to action. Statutes, official reports, medical treatises, and encounters with ailments or the ailing motivated many to propose models, unique or universal, for subscribers' survival. Epidemics and esoteric maladies, the pregnant and the senile, physicians and charlatans, exercise, diet, and environment engrossed the media. Essays extended the boundaries of the topic in such discussions as the nexus between legislation and longevity, the ethical and intellectual effects of medical research, and the evolution of the hospital. Additionally, commentaries illustrate issues of class, age, and gender, professional status, and personal freedom. By featuring wellness in a prominent and persuasive medium of communication, scribes guaranteed its consideration by citizens.

Creating a checklist of articles on health is hampered by the volume and complexity of the sources. Nineteenth-century papers themselves impede inquiry by altering their mastheads, permitting anonymity and aliases, and masking articles' meanings with arbitrary headings inhospitable to index investigators. Notwithstanding that the aim is to present a sweeping survey, the bulk and barriers of the records make some limitations necessary. Thus, excluded from this register are fiction, poetry, abstracts (as of recent books), and pieces with overseas or military motifs or the consequences of violent crimes.

Emphasis and eloquence, format and formula differed among items. They ranged from dissertations full of statistics to intensely personal reminiscences. Subjects could be theoretical, as "Heredity in Health and Disease" and "Influence of the Mind on the Body," or practical, as "The Purification of Sewage and Water" and "Preventible Accidents." They could compare, as "English and Foreign Spas," expose, as "Quackery and the Quacked," edify, as "The Doctor: His Duties to You," or simplify, as "The Electrical Cure for Cancer." They could express choler, as "The Perils of Industry," confusion, as "Wine Against Physic," complacency, as "The Progress of Medicine," or contempt, as "The Uses and Abuses of Hospitals."

Since contemporaries handled health on many levels, the introduction synopsizes their health concerns, principally using evidence about England, then about Ireland, Scotland, and Wales. Many stories about England discussed the whole of Great Britain, while those on Ireland, Scotland, and Wales typically dealt with local matters. The introduction addresses the following topics: unwellness, the unwell, caregivers and care, being healthy, and health in the kingdom.

The checklist is organized alphabetically by periodical. The opening year of the *Edinburgh Review* and the closing years of the *New Monthly Magazine* and *Tait's Edinburgh Magazine* correspond to those in the *Wellesley Index*. All other publications have been scrutinized from 1824 to 1900 or their dates within those decades. Each has a foreword based on a prospectus, prologue, and/or remarks, internal or in the *Wellesley Index*. The foreword provides supersessions, mergers, patrons, and main points. Title shifts appear as subheadings. Citations, with annotations, are given in chronological order. Signatures are replicated as printed. For unsigned articles, attributions of authorship come primarily from the *Wellesley Index*, with some from *Poole's Index* and the texts themselves, and from Anne Lohrli, *Household Words: A Weekly Journal, 1850-1859, Conducted by Charles Dickens* (Toronto, 1973).

The author index has names and pseudonyms but not initials; the subject index has themes and cross-references. Postings for Ireland, Scotland, and Wales are inclusive. Both indexes refer to entry number.

ACKNOWLEDGMENTS

There is no way to thank all who have contributed to this book, but a few deserve special mention.

The staffs of the British Library, London, the New York Public Library, the Boston Athenaeum, the Chicago Public Library, and the Jersey City Public Library displayed patience and deftness in locating stray serials. I am especially indebted to the personnel at the Newark Public Library where most of the work was done. Their courtesy and efficiency greatly expedited the gathering of evidence.

Christopher DiNardo served as an excellent adviser on computers. Donald Cinotti, M.D., gave generously of his time to talk about medicine.

Saint Peter's College supported this project in several ways. The administration provided funds for the travel necessary to distant collections. The staff of the O'Toole Library responded graciously and rapidly to my many requests. Jerome Gillen made valuable suggestions about style. Larry Thomas and Fadia Joseph assisted with formatting. Eleanor Yelenovsky kept my office running smoothly and my spirits high. Nancy Carbone showed great tolerance of my many moods. David S. Surrey was a colleague in every sense of the word. His technical expertise has been very helpful; his friendship during this writing has been immeasurably more so.

I am grateful to all of these people and to my family, who have always believed in my ability and to whom this book is dedicated.

INTRODUCTION

UNWELLNESS

Unwellness tantalized nineteenth-century columnists. Some of its categories they mastered, some they mistook, and some they missed. Generally, they thought in terms of disease, condition, and accidental or occupational harm. Circumstances leading to ill health, such as those related to industrialism, could catalyze a steady stream of prose, while chance occurrences, such as epidemics, brought banners intermittently.

In the twilight of the reign of George III, the *Edinburgh Review* glanced at gout, diabetes, stones in the gall bladder and kidneys, and brain maladies. Reviewers appraised surgery for hernias, tumors, and cataracts, and vaccination for smallpox. Fevers were even more fascinating. They might be indeterminate in origin or symptoms of influenza and typhus, both publicized for decades. Heat, cold, and water supposedly slowed either type, but quarantine and cleanliness were touted as more effective, especially for typhus. The greatest worry was insanity. Reporters clarified causes, from heredity to insolvency; identified ways to govern the insane, in asylums and by prescription; and delineated genres, such as dementia and melancholia.

By the 1820s, with more serials in circulation and some legislation in place, scribes were less sure about how to identify insanity and therefore how to treat it, medically and legally, notably with respect to property and crime. Insanity shared the limelight with plague and its squabbles about the efficacy of isolation and sanitary statutes and smallpox, with its on inoculation. Other communicable sicknesses that the press noted were yellow and non-specific fevers; typhus; tuberculosis; malaria in Italy; and rabies in Britain, the last an incessant problem. Complaints of dyspepsia, obesity, tooth distress, heatstroke, and colds surfaced in the papers. Readers learned that causes of liver and brain disturbances, aneurisms, and hernias might be fathomed by dissection of the dead and that alcoholism might be considered illness rather than individual weakness. Audiences may have been cheered by the claim that mortality rates were down, though their elation may have been tempered by insurance figures on the incidence of and outlays for sickness. Mishaps were given short shrift as were speech impediments and employment dangers, except for a journalistic decree that mills were not unsalutary.

Work in the 1830s was reputedly very risky for grinders, chimney sweeps, and the young workers in factories where machines and long hours, artificial light and stale air, hastened injuries and infections. Authors who admitted these effects were scattered. The media found ample misfortune elsewhere, in shipwrecks, where crews and passengers drowned allegedly due to faulty construction of vessels, official misclassification of them, and ignorance of officers. This topic apparently touched many in the age as did unintentional ingestion of poison, which the Victorians assumed was too common. They also commenced the century's scrutiny of the hearing impaired and intensified the probe on insanity, possibly to secure in otherwise insecure days the detention of the disorderly. Penmen revisited asylums, scanning everything from cases to committal premises and procedures. They questioned diagnoses, highlighted paranoia, and deliberated the pertinence of hypnosis and phrenology as diagnostic tools. They sketched the behavior of sufferers and blamed insanity on stress, inheritance, physical trauma, and physiology. They looked at local services for those afflicted and literature in which the insane were protagonists. Finally, bystanders asserted that insanity was growing among the poor but did not analyze why this was so. Instead, paragraphs went to ailments momentous and mundane. Cued by an outbreak of cholera, articles plumbed its every aspect. Disagreement about its roots led logically to a variety of curbs and cures, revealing a tension between those who would closet victims and those who would cleanse people and places. The stories on cholera did not drive other contagions from the papers. There were assessments of a Mediterranean station to stop plague; the heating stove, influenza; and salt, the ubiquitous fevers. Rabies and tuberculosis persisted in print as well as in society. Lung ailments, thanks to the use of the stethoscope, snared space as did those of the stomach. Dyspepsia became a refrain because, as more than one person postulated, digestion was the keystone of physical and mental soundness. The interaction of body and mind triggered texts on the bonds between illness and genius, relaxation and hypochondria. Although many surveyors dismissed the mind/body link, they did not other indispositions, from familiar tooth decay, and its corollary false teeth, to exotic epilepsy and cancer. For epilepsy, hypnosis was proposed; for cancer, patent and traditional medicines were deplored.

The 1840s left no time for afflictions that affected the few. Gazettes styled segments on health by class. The pains of the comfortable came from obesity, stress, dyspepsia, toothaches, insects, and the psyche; their comfort, perhaps, from the data of the Registrar-General and the mortality tables of insurers confirming that life expectancy was increasing. Still, even the prosperous may have fretted when reporters converged on the physically and the mentally challenged with confusing advice. Chroniclers showcased hypothetical traits and actual abilities or promoted tutoring for the vision or hearing impaired and pleaded with the public not to exploit these people or others labeled "imbecile." More likely, the wealthy read with anxiety about alcoholism, attributed to leisure or overwork, too many or too few meals, a responsible or a mindless job; and epidemics, charted by researchers or obvious to all as endemic in the new towns. Cholera, arriving abruptly as always, filled pages. There were death counts; divisions in opinion about its spread by air, sewage, food, water, or clothes; and alerts on symptoms and remedies. Ostensibly, vaccination and/or hygiene had harnessed smallpox. Typhus, terrifying in the 1840s, and many fevers were still mysteries despite their links to dirt and dirty water. Sequestering victims proved no parapet against plague and, in fact, begot only foul sites, more expenses, and intrusions on rights. Tuberculosis was professedly so rampant as to require the building of Brompton Hospital. Among the chief candidates for contracting tuberculosis were grinders, although theirs was not considered the only deleterious trade. Contaminations from handling sewage and digging graves, the fumes and fires in collieries, the fierce storms and the rickety crafts in fishing, and the pressures on hand loom weavers and governesses were also in the spotlight. The factory was at the core of contention. Some said that it was debilitating for all and so supported the ten-hour workday and other statutes; many, that it was only bad for females and juveniles and so boosted recreation and schooling; and a few, that it was not detrimental to anyone. Railroad travel, alternatively, was dubbed dangerous for employees and passengers, yet railway observers opined that modern laws would soon lower casualties. Sea journeys were portrayed as equally threatening to voyagers because of hurricanes, conflagrations, and collisions compounded by inept crews and insufficient safety standards. Accounts of these ordinary perils and others more extraordinary, such as spontaneous combustion or premature burial, bare more than inexperience or imagination: their prominence manifests the priorities of social rank. Similarly, the treatises on insanity, but for a nod to governesses, overlooked its incidence among the hired. After the trial of Daniel McNaughton, with its implications for an insanity defense, criminal insanity was the dominant theme. How to penetrate the mysteries of mental illness, however, was not the preoccupation exclusively of criminalists. In a bourgeois world witnessing the social disruptions of industrialism, rationality was regarded as critical for general stability and personal autonomy. Conspicuous consequently were essays on several aspects of insanity and its treatment. Hallucination was supposed to signal it and phrenology, to conquer it. Classification, apart from criminal insanity, seemed simple: curable or incurable. Nonetheless, as certification implied institutionalization, facilities and their activities were in the eye of Parliament and periodicals. Administration was condemned, treatment even more so, except at York where rewards replaced restraints to coax conformity. Inherent in all dialogues were class and class differences in response to insanity. There were hints that the affluent hid their suffering kin and the indigent tolerated theirs.

The resolve to unravel the causes and cures of insanity strengthened in the 1850s when magazines inundated subscribers with language on its antecedents, be they liquor, physiology, strains of the middle class, exhaustion of those below, demon or genius; and on reactions, more humane in proportion to lesser responsibility of the victim for his or her actions. Savants accepted suicide as an unfortunate outcome that reduced the ranks of the unstable. Prison might discourage feigners. Asylums, but for Hanwell, were apparently appalling. From the vantage of visitors, treatment was not kind, quick, or ongoing after release. As petitions advocating better care for the impoverished prevailed, they submerged others on behalf of patients in private havens.

If writers considered neglect a byproduct of insanity, they thought it a determining factor in hearing loss. Filth fostered infections that, through indifference or nostrums, could culminate in permanent damage to the ears of future toilers. Destruction or impairment of vision was likewise disquieting. There were tracts on the abilities and capabilities of the sightless if educated, the merits of eyeglasses for the sight-restricted, and the condition of color blindness.

Narrators agonized about the covert talents of the mentally challenged and about the press's obvious capitalization on gigantism and dwarfism. Editors sensationalized mishaps more directly. Sudden and baffling deaths from poison or tapping a spot between brain and spine might startle, but those from flames claimed more columns. Since blazes in buildings were commonplace, insurance was essential, the fire brigade was a blessing, and safety codes for businesses and residences were imperative. The home held so many harms that handbooks on how to cope with its dangers were reputedly welcome. Outside, railroads, whose cars were also prone to fires, were accused of operating without anti-accident devices and with staffs that did not inform passengers about imminent dangers. As sea travel burgeoned, worry about shipwrecks grew. Critics warned that lifesaving devices were inadequate; authorities reluctant to interfere; captains remiss; and owners, compensated for freight losses, casual about people. Concurrently, tribunes blared, parsimonious entrepreneurs and hesitant parliamentarians winked at the hazards presented by machines and milieu in mills. Gradually, some periodicals exonerated lawmakers by holding laborers culpable for non-compliance with legislation. The mine equaled the factory in entries on labor. Most indicted management and government for underground explosions and aboveground alcoholism but overlooked liability for long-term lung disorders. The press, underlining the insalubrity of overexertion in mill and shaft, pushed private insurance for ensuing ills. Others said to be in jeopardy at their jobs were tailors and needlewomen trapped by seasonal buyers and budding technology; firefighters and police; match and copper workers; maids deprived of sleep and governesses of dignity; rural toilers who tramped miles to fields; and, not satirically, statesmen without enough food and fun. The powerful had other miseries. They tended to fall prey to gout and seasickness, nervous exhaustion and dyspepsia (sometimes related to opium), and to some of the same indispositions as their compatriots.

Cholera defied arrest because its origin remained hidden. Its surge in the 1850s spurred bulletins on sanitation, air, habitation, and quarantine. Conversely, pieces on smallpox estimated the worth of vaccination and those on typhus, of sewerage. Of other afflictions, yellow and generic fevers were briefly absent from print, but rabies endured and syphilis emerged. In addition, respiratory disturbances, such as tuberculosis, bronchitis, pneumonia, influenza, allergies, and the common cold, were important, as was diphtheria. Onlookers ascribed frequent lung complaints to polluted air and uncongenial climate. Alcoholism was by now a refrain, whereas cancer, epilepsy, chorea, and disorders of the eye and ear had a few lines. To discover the origins of malfunctions, contemporaries contemplated such clues as pain, hair and memory loss, blood and temperature fluctuation, fainting, heredity, and mindset.

Study of the roots and types of unwellness widened in the 1860s. Seeking solutions for unhealthiness, some focused on anatomy or heirs, especially of consanguineous marriages. Others branded flies and mosquitoes as universal pests, and dogs as sporadic ones. Essayists tried simultaneously to segregate both the spurious and the psychosomatic and to differentiate between the signs of recovery and of dying. Those sympathetic to the ill cautioned that illness could induce strange conduct.

As for diseases, the communicable were foremost, by title or tether to infant demise and adult grime. Cholera, in the wake of a London episode, was still vexing. Whether searching national and foreign histories, applauding water pumps, or scorning opiates, spectators differed about its etiology and therapy. Typhus, too, remained a puzzle, even with its connections to uncleanliness and malnutrition. Because it flourished in slums, chroniclers concentrated on food, water, atmosphere, and sewage, and prodded doctors toward a ministry in these enclaves. Smallpox was less bothersome. An occasional overseer might grumble that the destitute wore the garments of victims, but the majority of contributors counted on vaccination and a medical corps deputized to overcome resistance to receiving the vaccine. Evaluators were not so sure that the Contagious Diseases Acts could stall venereal diseases, accelerated by urbanism, or that anything could block fevers.

Alongside these chapters were others with old, new, or revised themes. Respiratory conditions were still prominent, now with an accent on the perils of smoking and the parameters of the stethoscope. If the lungs could trouble everyone, scurvy, anemia, trichinosis, and drink were purportedly the curse of those in poverty, in and out of cities. More pages went to stress and heart attacks, gout and malaria, skin rashes and tooth decay, and the perennial dyspepsia, for which baths, spas, sleep, and exercise were advertised. Broken bones, sages confided, could be repaired by grafts. The brain was even more vulnerable and its disorder probably particularly chilling in a world wedded to reason. Blows and high temperatures might yield brain injury, and amnesia, narcolepsy, and coma might confirm a brain lesion. The intersection of brain and insanity was, if somewhat hazy, no less profound to pundits in the 1860s as previously. They catalogued alcoholism and melancholia as species of insanity, inattention and hallucination as indicators of it. The media called experts' ideas of insanity into question. Constantly criticizing certification and asylums, scribes deemed local institutions inferior to those in Belgium and France. Quarterlies lobbied for legislation to relieve the congestion of sanctuaries and for residential care of the poor. Money was certainly a factor in this argument as longevity and the likelihood of commitment increased. Cost was not so crucial for the vision and hearing impaired whose educational potential some recognized or for the physically and mentally challenged whose care several journalists endorsed. There was insensitivity in print, such as the use of the epithet "weakling." Further, monthlies may have aggravated the torment of those with dwarfism or gigantism by turning attention to them, whereas color blindness, another pet subject, was not so susceptible to ridicule.

More voluminous were the logs of accidents. Shipwrecks were the bane of the 1860s, from which shore lights, lifeboat crews, sea buoys, rafts, and navigational improvements could seemingly deliver many. Railroads were the land monsters. Disquisitions, drawing from data, traced often unindemnified injuries and fatalities to labor fatigue, track obstructions, unreliable brakes and wheels, car blazes, crowds, and clumsy porters. The lanes were as terrible for those using them, with carts and people vying for space. Fires, from cavalier strokes of matches, unventilated hearths, or maneuvers in crinolines close to flame, raised the death toll, which safety contrivances and brigades could scarcely slow. If demise from lightning strike or snakebite was unlikely, that from juvenile play with parental guns or tools was deemed ominously possible. Workers might imperil themselves and their families not only by importing diseases from workplaces to domiciles but by cottage industry. Outside employments remained insalubrious. Mining had many titles. Excoriation of other occupations was growing. Columnists coupled match manufacture to jaw maladies; lead smelting, baking, grinding, and printing to skin and lung damage; and sewing, despite the machine, to blindness. Gun making and fire fighting were patently dangerous; farming, not so plainly so. By the decade's close, enactments on the trades had allegedly not addressed their role in unwellness.

Statutes, some speculated in the 1870s, did make toil less detrimental, at least in mills. Interestingly, as talk of economic decline and then cost cutting loudened, sheets echoed earlier motifs: factories were not harmful for women; employees, such as railroaders and boilermakers, were negligent, harming themselves and others. Alternatively, postings on merchant mariners, their diets and drownings in overloaded and undermanned crafts, and on farm hands, wasted and weary, substantiated how employment eroded health. Ruth for people with these and other jobs long decried, mining and sewing, circulated with that for those in the chemical and gunpowder industries. The lung ailments of calico spinners, who breathed clay dust that was adulterating their fiber, reminded readers that respiratory afflictions were significant. Correspondents revisited these complaints, nodded to dyspepsia, seasickness, and toothache, and put eye disorders and cancer in a few paragraphs.

The communicable diseases, however, held the spotlight. Venereal disease legislation sparked a glaringly gendered and raucous debate. Less controversial were other official interventions, such as the recording of outbreaks and the rules for housing. While reporters reckoned that epidemics were eternal and bacteria people's enemies, they credited changes in sewerage and water distribution for a decrease in cholera, typhus, typhoid fever, and smallpox, with a bow to inoculation as efficacious. Outbreaks of measles were apparently down and those of ophthalmia up, notably among the poor. Bewildered but spellbound by rabies, bystanders assessed cases and deterrents, mainly a dog tax, muzzling, and confinement. Inability to crush this and other threats perhaps propelled myriad materials on the brain, as injured, diseased, or diminished by drink or drugs. Addiction could be an ailment, some hypothesized, because it so dramatically interfered with the interdependence of mind and body. Amnesia and narcolepsy could also interfere, as could heredity, unless decoded by surveillance of offspring of consanguineous marriages.

Above all these concerns were the inescapable pressures of modern life to which these moderns imputed mental breakdowns more than heart attacks. Inserts on insanity were regular. Sex, rank, age, religion, family, morality, liquor, mood, shock, and right/left brain dominance were all recruited as causes. The core issue was care, in theory and in law, in infirmary and asylum, by specialist or not. Journals avowed that treatment was cheaper and better than before but bemoaned the suicides and crimes of the insane. Journalists grieved too about the physically and mentally challenged, but their compassion commingled with fears of an inferior populace. Therefore, the hearing impaired should learn signing and the vision impaired, braille. If the first were denominated "dumb," the second were sketched as friendless souls who often survived by begging. Hope was high for the physically challenged, whom surgery and/or prostheses might help, but not so for conjoined twins. Those designated "idiots," incurables, and the comatose should be sheltered, whether for their benefit or relief of others' embarrassment. Since fleeting unconsciousness from a fall or a fright was ostensibly usual, it carried no stigma. Judging from the heralds, transportation misadventures would cause this condition in many readers. According to serials, street carts barreled along; railroads so endangered passengers that public ownership was necessary or private breach of contract might suffice; and ships sank daily. Commentators banked on life rafts and floats, shore groups, even portable inflatable hats for travelers' salvation. Blazes, as theatres multiplied, apparently supplied corrupt builders and panicky audiences with the means to harm. Poisoning by chance ingestion or bite intrigued the press, but gunshot wounds stirred hardly anyone. Since every purchaser of a publication could be a victim of some mishap, publishers recommended insurance for all.

The ever present warnings may have had an effect. By the 1880s, prose on accidents was intermittent but still relevant. Swallowing a rare toxin was remote; poisoning by color-blind chemists and adulterated-food purveyors, not so. Railroad ticketholders had difficulties because of color-blind employees, chiefly signalers. Travelers not so interrupted might be beleaguered in other ways. Dark tunnels invited dangers. Avaricious companies packed too much freight and too many humans on some routes. Profit, largely from insurance, was also the purported motive for mediocre ship maintenance, even as buoys, fog lamps, and lifeboat cadres were lowering the risks at sea. The Red Cross and fire brigades won accolades. Admiration for firefighters did not eliminate counsel on how to escape burning, principally in theatres. Mentors reiterated that faulty construction, gas lamps, and the terror of those caught in fires tipped the scale toward disaster. Alarm was not typically raised in texts on mining with the exception of explosions due to obsolete illumination or novel dynamite. Whether asking for more qualified inspectors or less nonfeasance and malfeasance by miners, organs conventionally concluded that mining was exceedingly hazardous.

Many occupations engrossed the media in the 1880s, the apogee of periodical perusal of deleterious trades. Some had been in the news for years: merchant shipping, with crafts unsuitable for their cargoes and cruel officers; railroads, with exhausted workers; and factories, antiquated structures with antiquated machines. Latterly, sweatshops, trams, and fishing had been singled out as risky for adults and brickyards and theatres, for juniors. Aside from these targets, the trend was toward overall amelioration, from sanitary sites to pensions. Two topics monopolized coverage: employers' liability and employees' hours. Essays on liability, partly because of landmark legislation, plumbed legal definitions and compensatory scope; those on pensions, musing about insalubrities of body and mind, included overwork, liquor, drugs, and tobacco. Essayists of both legislative camps importuned for policies on inspection and access to medical personnel.

Concurrently, other scribes campaigned for the insane. Proprietary asylums and standards of care everywhere were stamped arbitrary, although certifications were less castigated than before. Fewer likewise were the affiliations of insanity with suicide or lawbreaking, whereas paragraphs on heredity as root and hypnosis as remedy persisted. There was more space devoted to consciousness, from hallucination to multiple personality disorder, and, ominously, on the plethora of victims. Some savants translated this census as corroboration of communal infirmity. Eugenics, associating itself with science, thus began to compete with humanitarianism. Dwarfism and congenital conditions were not skipped; hearing and vision impairments were, however, preeminent.

Emphasis was on an education that could focus minds, discipline bodies, and expedite social integration. Not content with local approaches, onlookers imported models from the continent and the United States. This internationalism already applied to sickness. Sea trips, South Atlantic islands, and Swiss refuges were habitually puffed for the tubercular, at least until research on bacteria advanced. Articles also tied bacteria to smallpox, reputedly regular in tenements, but vaccination ignited a quarrel having libertarian, ethical, and medical overtones and a class undertone. The dispute about compulsory vaccination raged just as the one on the venereal disease laws subsided. Cholera was still an enigma. Some hinged it, as they did typhoid fever, to impure water and filth; others concentrated on its pace. To curtail rabies, optimists depended on Louis Pasteur or dog licensing. Scarlet fever, scurvy, and malaria were sobering, but leprosy seemed to be a mere vestige of imperialism. Infectious ailments were eventually displaced by those systemic. According to the monthlies, the companions of progress were anxiety and debility; nervous and heart complaints; alcohol and morphine addiction; obesity and dyspepsia; and irritations of skin, hair, and lungs. What observers could not explain by environment, they charged to blood. Ironically, unlike earlier colleagues, they did not burden their observations with statistics.

Statistics were even fewer, except for those on mortality, in the 1890s when scrutiny of specific disorders was so intense as to suggest universal distress about unwellness. Some penmen recycled communicable diseases as newsworthy, but documenting them conflicted with concerns about privacy. "Germs" was the catchword, a synonym for the perpetrator of fevers or an excuse to pester tramps. Cholera rated many lines but still had no lineage except dirt of any sort. Its reach was said to be too broad and its preventives, too narrow. Smallpox was a close rival in the race for headlines because of the bickering about mandatory inoculation. For infants, opinion was mostly affirmative. For the rest, isolation, purer water and air, hygiene, and sewers were thought to defeat both smallpox and typhoid fever. The origin of tuberculosis was another predilection. For some, cows were culprits; for others, bacteria were, so a vaccine was essential; for still others, sanitation, sanitariums, and specialists were solutions. If tuberculosis resisted remedy, influenza and malaria purportedly fell to salicin. Rabies continued to generate debate about preventive measures. Champions of Pasteur's vaccine warred against those favoring exclusion, licensing, or muzzling of dogs. Dogs so intimidated one soul that he insisted on a department to police rabies, together with typhoid fever, scarlet fever, and diphtheria. Other treatises paired typhoid fever with foul water, diphtheria with antitoxins, tetanus with vivisection. Measles and ringworm seemingly predominated among pauper children, and venereal diseases among prostitutes and their clients irrespective of parliamentary meddling. The state was given the center stage too in passages on alcoholism.

Whether to commit, convert, or constrain from outlawry was at issue. The detriments of smoking soon excited writers as much as those of drink. In a climate where lung maladies were perennial, tobacco was a devil. Culture was more critical according to discourses on headache; nervous, muscular, circulatory, and skin troubles; and digestive indispositions. The brain, one conservative averred, was very susceptible to the pressures of democracy and materialism. Victorians vaunted surgery for eye affliction but not for epilepsy or cancer. On the last, views varied except about reversal. Ostensible cures for cancer were tagged hysteria or hyperbole. As lethal as cancer, if not so absorbing, were diabetes, for which opium was the relief of record, and anemia, for which seaweed was. Not fatal but featured were tooth decay and ear damage. As chroniclers announced ailments, they generally ignored heredity except in the innuendos about class and consanguineous marriages.

At the century's end, analysts of insanity were as uneasy about legal committals, private havens, and public staffs as had been their progenitors. Reacting to the Report of the Commissioners for Lunacy, 1898, scribes resurrected causality and recovery as topics. The crisis of the nineties was whether insanity or institutionalization of the insane was increasing. To verify either claim, entries referred to crime, gambling, and drink. Tracts mentioned that inebriation was likewise a crucial factor in spectator mishaps at football matches, whereas street games were perilous only for participants. Other cautionary tales routinely revealed how precarious health was. At home, poison imbued the wallpaper and some foods; at the theatre, faulty electrical wiring caused incineration. In the roads, there were construction barricades, speeders, but no subway crossings; on the rails, scattered fogmen and whistles, tired signalers, and only red/green signals; at sea, insufficient lifeboats and inefficient officers. As accident victims gained advocates, pages on rescuers, the Red Cross, and ambulance and shore squads multiplied.

Ready for rescue of another sort were employees in old and new trades, from match manufacture to athletics. Miners were, the irate roared, abandoned to stagnant air and successive calamities, and mills were no paradigms of salubrity. Sweatshops, for tailoring, fur pulling, and boot making, but not nail and chain manufacture, supposedly exposed immigrants and women to infections, as did the trades of postal clerks, dustmen, and sewer diggers. Authors clashed about how broad statutes should be. Opponents magnified workers' negligence, private insurance, and the price of an ecumenical short day. Interventionists extolled strict employer liability and the profitability, fiscal and salutary, of the eight-hour day. However, as one dissertation declared, the rules during the reign of the Queen-Empress had improved occupational health. Legislation had also opened, reporters suggested, opportunities for those with impaired vision, hearing, or limbs. While many sermonized that the nation could do better, as Germany had done, they were confident that it would.

THE UNWELL

Study of the unwell deepened in magazines during the nineteenth century when patient conventionally connoted sufferer. If narratives sometimes noticed how the ill molded medical knowledge and practice, they did not limit being a patient to an involvement with a professional or a sojourn in a hospital. The cult of the unwell sometimes reflected distinctions of class, age, and sex; discussion below will reflect these contexts.

In the 1830s, paragraphs on patients traversed two avenues. One recaptured literary deathbed scenes; a second conveyed the emotions of the afflicted in either rapid recovery or near-fatal experience. During the next three decades, banners amplified the sentiments of the sick. These included how excruciating was pain, whether portent or repercussion, as after tooth extraction; how tedious was the sickroom and, more so, the invalid life; how devastating was a diagnosis of incurability; how consoling was religion; and how pleasant were the benevolence of friends and the release from burdens during minor disturbances. Simultaneously, patients became pupils. Penmen advised picking a doctor who was upright and understanding, rejecting hospitals as costly and careless, and clinging to folk cures because faith in, was as important as composition of any therapy. For the convalescent, contributors commended shelters and meal programs, delivered or accessible. For the doomed, they prayed for refuges to help mind if not body.

Mirroring patients' perspectives and articulating their needs were goals after 1870. Nonetheless, although titles blossomed, those from a patient's outlook dwindled. There were some memoirs about examinations, inoculations, or surgeries; hospitals with strange diets, irksome noises, and regimentation; recuperation, primarily from misadventure; the joys of junkets abroad and pampering at home; and the guests who carried gloom with their flowers and gossip. There was also the realization that pain was both a harbinger of disaster and a reminder of how splendid salubrity was. Usually, guides tutored patients on how to deal with sickness and society on how to institutionalize it. The unwell had to be vigilant not aggressive, aware not egotistic. They had to vanquish pain, supposedly stronger for men because of their brains and education in contrast to women who exaggerated every ache. Patients had to discover doctors who were honorable about clients and fees. The rich might be cheated, their rehabilitation extended exclusively for money, or be the cheaters, utilizing free facilities so driving up imposts. The poor, with much attention synopsized below, had incomplete physical histories that hindered treatment and few options for care other than bad hospitals and worse infirmaries. Status notwithstanding, everyone might be prey to the incompetents who prescribed or administered wrong doses; the nurses who tyrannized; the doctors who tyrannized more; the medical students who were ignorant; the chaplains who ignored; and the swindlers to whom people resorted from disgust or pride or for solace. To stem the tide of charlatanism, milieu and science must improve. Meantime, the poor, the young, and women, each a symbol of rebellion or regression, were in the limelight.

The Poor

The poor were a cohort at once plain and profound whose membership messengers presumed but whose circumstances they explicated. Until the 1820s, the impoverished ill were not news and then, only occasionally. Humanitarianism, possibly the incentive for ideas about the elderly in pieces on the poor law, was invisible in those on anatomists' dissection of paupers' bodies. The privileges of the aged and anatomists coexisted, in the 1830s, in articles on nutrition, habitation, recreation, and hygiene. Without voluntary or statutory assistance, workers might be candidates for many maladies, resulting in unrelenting poverty and ultimately insanity.

By the 1840s, death eventualities were less pivotal than life's realities. Some papers nudged Parliament to shield the destitute infirm and elderly but acknowledged that these persons were neither foremost for nor always amenable to state action. Other organs, impelled by self-help and the fisc, glorified benefit groups that might not defray the total tariff of ailing but would guarantee initial treatment if layoffs did not interrupt or temporary hirings preclude payments. Conversely, suspicion of and distance from professionals apparently elevated the panaceas offered by kith and kin. Texts were unanimous that for lengthy indispositions, havens for the underclasses were few, unfortuitously located, and foolishly managed. Beyond this unanimity, spectators recited a litany of reasons for the troubles of the masses. Dirt was the villain in chapters on bigger towns where slums, without sun or tubs but with throngs, abetted the morbidity of dwellers and their affluent neighbors. Nevertheless, local governments, peopled by those who paid taxes and might own such nuisance properties, purportedly would not authorize sewerage or water supply. If the itinerant bachelors who toted contagions from one region to another were cast as culprits, the mother and children consigned to the workhouse were judged the least culpable. Albeit captivated by commissions and statistics, reporters were disheartened that the Registrar-General's data on death confirmed their hypotheses.

Segments in the 1850s did not surprise with their ideas. The domestic, occupational, and atmospheric evils of the metropolis were prominent. Some columnists clamored for legislation. In the spirit of the decade, others, even under labor mastheads, backed individual insurance. Pessimists immediately retorted that jobs were fundamental to pay for insurance, yet such funds procured neither more expertise than of humble healers nor more remediation than of popular potions, most notably opiates. Hospitals and workhouse infirmaries reputedly had paltry supplies and opprobrious staffs, but even the best could do little for those decimated by years of destitution. The insane, featured in the bulk of articles, evoked much empathy because the "incurable" were permanently shuttered and the "cured" were returned without reenforcement to the very milieu from which their condition had emanated.

Interest in the insanity of the indigent did not dissipate in the 1860s, but it did wane. As a minority avouched that incidence was up and therapy inappropriate, the majority incorporated this concern into a larger one about the poor law. Because its establishments did not aid the afflicted and augmented afflictions, the law, according to foes, betrayed its beneficiaries. Reformers preached that benefit clubs and charities, though laudable, were no substitute for the state. The authorities were urged to act because frail females betokened like offspring. If one pundit advanced a French scheme because it was better and cheaper, most peers underlined native wants. There must be doctors in each district, reasonably remunerated, who earned the trust of their patients by dedication and skill and thus routed superstition and insalubrious tonics. There must be reserves, medicinal and nutritional, and able personnel in workhouse infirmaries. There must be sanctuaries and meals for invalids and convalescents in the city and the country. Above all, there must be keen inspectors instead of perfunctory bureaucrats. Watchdogs must not only oversee but also teach the dangers of alcohol and the merits of habitual hygiene. In issuing edicts, few advisers apprehended the contradictions, such as that stipulations on slaughterhouses might raise the price of meat or that hospitals and infirmaries might wrestle for the same purses.

In the 1870s, those in hospitals were lionized. Monthlies muttered that paupers were relegated to incompetent students or to inconsistent outpatient departments. The infirmary, not so featured, was not less damned. There were disclosures of miserly boards, fumbling doctors, extortionist nurses, and horrid rooms and fare. Patients' prudence, not their arrogance, averred the acerbic, kept them out of such an abyss. Thus, the press revived former formulas, namely public in-home assistance, private munificence, and benefit societies. The services offered by societies, some reiterated, did not offset charges. Unless nationalized, insurance was beyond the reach of many, irrespective of rumors about supplementing family income by neglecting the insured, typically babies, until they died. Gazettes prized abodes that would stall epidemics and doctors who would trek to tenements. Saluted too were rural and urban nurses who tended those in poverty and tutored wives about disinfectants and menus. The conviction that women would transform households was naive but no more so than the reliance on mineral water, red meat, and leisure to cure a class whose wages fluctuated.

Dependence on district nurses to help the poor remain healthy was obvious in the 1880s when Londoners were celebrated. Attendants in workhouses were not. Nonetheless, contemporaries believed that laxity and malevolence had become less common and management and treatment, less retrogressive in workhouses. Enemies of infirmaries liked hospitals for their cheap and ready access to specialists, ironic because surgery, as earlier pathology, could victimize the impoverished. Choices for the sick poor were few. Smaller sick clubs and insurance companies with affordable rates bordered on bankruptcy. Urban missions, however heroic, were unsophisticated and village ones, random. Government allowed protracted poverty that bred generations of physically and mentally unwell. Thus, seers projected state indemnity and sanctuary for accident, illness, and aging, customarily synonymous with decrepitude.

The notion that the poor were perpetually ailing was preponderant in the 1890s. Scribes bewailed the statistics on measles and insanity but now celebrated parliamentary zeal. Stories paraphrased the Royal Commission on Agricultural Labourers as proof of the care for rural constituents or assured readers that the poor law, with scrutiny, could be thorough. Women, a plurality voted, were the best inspectors because of an instinct for nursing and an affinity for their sisters, the young, and the old. Those who opposed workhouses, especially for the elderly, opted for subsidized separate dwellings and stipends, likewise advocated for paupers during epidemics. Even without a catastrophe, the astute comprehended, the needy had needs. Visiting nurses were readily available but not always accurate in their care. Dispensaries sometimes contested with general practitioners for business. Hospitals portended a condition so serious as to convulse many patients' previously precarious existence. Boycotters simply succumbed in lodgings that, but in Birmingham, hurried demise. Even those who would dedicate free places only to the "respectable" doomed, the tubercular, and the cancerous, envisioned philanthropy as ancillary to state support. The Salvation Army, medical missions, and peoples' kitchens, thrift and dues, were commendable, but, according to the media, minimally available. In 1900, as for decades before, serials stood for the principle that the welfare of the sick poor should be a matter of public policy.

The Young

The young were an amorphous guild, enrolling everyone from the neonate to the teen, so formats of stories were more fluid than in the headings anchored by status. As with the impoverished, youths except in industry did not initially appeal to adult readers. In the 1820s fleetingly and the 1830s more fully, fulminations about factories appeared. Even essayists unimpressed by the detriment of mills conceded that legislation was occasionally obligatory. By the 1830s, abstracts assigned disability from injuries and debility, gauged by height and weight and mirrored by drugs and disease, to overwork. If junior operatives were unwell, chimney sweeps were presumably fitter because of stoves, not statutes. A few entries stereotyped scions as frail or flabby.

In the 1840s and 1850s, journalistic voices on unwell youth loudened. Babies' menus were inappropriate, their muscles unflexed, and their cleanliness in question. Many of those under five perished from narcotics, famine or fattening, or overstimulated brains. Survivors did not ineluctably bloom, as treatises on children's hospitals testified. Descendants of the destitute and of the wealthy suffered because of diet, dress, parental delinquency, and diphtheria. Schools, without effective ventilation and drainage and with indoor and sedentary routines, compounded ills. The curriculum, sages lectured, slighted physiology and hygiene, although pupils might eat at some institutions. Jobs in mills and collieries exacerbated any propensity for insalubrity by robbing adolescents of sleep and of breathable air. Among the prescriptions for ailing juveniles were red meat and cold water, bucolic sojourns, and health instruction.

Tidings of infirm heirs did not abate in the 1860s. The state, savants chanted, should impose inoculation, ban laudanum, combat smoke and sewage that killed progeny first, and monitor meals to prevent malnutrition or overfeeding. The asthenia of the masses was perceived as erosion of the polity. Editors, who passed over the gangs of displaced casual workers in the countryside, bruited city folk. Infant mortality, cited in official records and by the National Association for the Promotion of Social Science, was stunning, with some forty percent of those under the age of one seemingly falling to contagions or malnourishment. The other sixty percent ate badly, drank vile water, wore on dirty bodies the discards of the deceased, and frolicked in traffic or with parental tools. Quoting from the Children's Employment Commission, 1866, and other evidence, articles unearthed more young patients. Farm youths walked to distant fields before beginning long days; needle and straw workers had equal hours but in foul air and dim light; match, lace, and nail toilers and paper stainers were also destroyed by their environments. When minors were stricken, the workhouse was no haven and special hospitals, scarce. Chronic cases and convalescents had recourse to alms, which some applauded but most admitted were no surrogate for public money.

By the 1870s, with enactments for infants and juvenile employees, tribunes trumpeted less about Westminster and more about current public facilities and coming private ones. Poor law infirmaries hastened ophthalmia. Children's hospitals did not serve the terminal or the recuperating, address the needs of the child as patient, or appoint enough female nurses. By contrast, language on establishments for the vision or hearing impaired and for the physically or mentally challenged demonstrates greater sensitivity for children than for adults. Village boarding homes were the panacea for the puny, the pallid, and the despondent. Whether as refuges for the orphaned and the indigent or an opportunity funded by family, the rural boarding home, allies proclaimed, had triumphed in locales as different as Scotland and Germany. The class bias of this discourse permeated other accounts of unwell youths. Reviewers who acknowledged starving and dehydrated babies as the norm for pregnant workers espoused Nestle's milk powder and much scrubbing and lamented maternal laxity or murder to collect death insurance. Other pieces, on toddlers poisoned by nibbling on wallpaper and preteens, by smoking, intimated that rank was irrelevant when identifying dangers to the young.

The disquisitions on motherhood muted in the 1880s though not without some space on how factory tasks altered the fetus. In myriad words, penmen etched patterns of parents' disinterest in or damage to their progeny. Descriptions of baby farming; beatings at home, on the streets, or in school; and abandonment proliferated next to paens to the Society for the Prevention of Cruelty to Children. Reports of abuse animated anthems for the shelters of charities and orders to Parliament for more. Spectacular though brutality seemed, it was recognized as less likely to father young patients than was indeliberate but inexorable debilitation from other causes. Descendants of such preventible problems, some fumed, were candidates for sicknesses of all sorts. This thesis produced a plethora of projects. Emigration was loved and loathed. Feeding slum waifs at school, selling food at cost, and clothing the ragged would, gazettes guessed, be less expensive than supporting the ill. The pastoral interlude for children was a favorite; without it, city playgrounds would have to do. Protective legislation for juvenile laborers in theatre, mill, and brickyard was another goal. A cluster of proposals dealt with medicine. Heralds countenanced removal of contagious pupils by a health deputy. They encouraged urban dispensaries, ecumenical youth hospitals outside London, and ones for the vision impaired and the physically and mentally challenged. Among this torrent of titles were sporadic ones on satisfactory growth and the impact of illegitimacy on it.

In the 1890s, there were fewer lines on children, but any inference that they were less unwell was belied by entries on government responsibility for the health of the young. Parroting former concepts, those at century's finish were on official willingness or unwillingness to quell minors' maladies. Some were particular: the formidable measles; tooth decay, said to be soaring because babies were without milk; and smallpox, field for a battle over infant vaccination. Some were familiar: physical impairments about which the powers that be were reputedly apathetic; occupational fatigue not halted by statutes on straw, paper, and laundry drudgery; harms inflicted by parents in towns and hamlets with or without the incentive of insurance rewards, harms that refuges assuaged but could not terminate; and city respiratory, dietary, and muscular curses and road mishaps that rural holidays and urban playgrounds were supposed to reduce. These motifs were by now banal. What was not was the conviction that any school was more useful than any hospital. Special facilities were no longer justified, but more diligence for convalescents and outpatients was. Writers would have schools propagate doctrines of cleanliness, redress nutritional deficiencies so severe that urchins searched bakery refuse for bread, invigorate with gymnastics, detect by teacher-agents physical and mental problems, and exile those with ringworm and ophthalmia. The last two, blights of the workhouse, underscored the slant of banners with audiences not poor. The gospels on the ailing lower classes were nonetheless significant because they highlighted the ailments of the majority of the young.

Women

Women, unlike the poor or the young, were not a vague coterie. Before the 1840s, chapters about females were on hysteria, hypochondria, and hidden insanity, all of which hypnosis might alleviate. This prose was prologue to Victorian endeavors to reconcile female passivity and sexuality by configuring them medically, then accusing patients and occasionally their physicians of chicanery. In the 1840s, articles adjusted their vista somewhat. Their predilections were the hazards of birthing with or without ether and chloroform and of labor in shafts and factories, though the insanity of governesses continued as a thread. Inmates in insalubrious infirmaries were a mere filament, and contraception, with its implications for power, class, eugenics, ethics, and gender paradigms, was absent altogether, notwithstanding that it might have dampened abortions and infanticide. Conspicuous, possibly because men followed them, were insurance tables wherein wives outlived husbands.

The 1850s had more coverage of women's health. In these and future years, rank was somewhat blurred. For instance, diets and beatings might jeopardize all women for different reasons. Similarly, characteristics fastened to femininity, such as modesty, humility, and passivity, professedly discouraged dialogues with doctors even when knowledge of anatomy allowed. Monthlies moored a host of adult troubles, from spinal deformities to psychic distresses, to background. Thus, advisers recommended refurnishing girls' schools, requiring exercises for brain and body, and redesigning corsets for better respiration and circulation. Additionally, authors viewed jobs as detrimental. Prostitutes contracted venereal diseases from buyers, field hands starved themselves to feed their families, needlewomen lost their sight, maids became dyspeptic, and governesses broke mentally as maidens or struggled with indigency as seniors. Concurrently, wives were pummeled, and mothers, with chloroform or without midwives, died in delivery. If women were behind some of their own and their sisters' misfortunes, so, quarterlies murmured, might they be the therapies. The wealthy, presumedly puppets of ennui, might be social reformers, nurses, or doctors, bringing expertise and empathy to gendered cases. Men would not be idle since they would have to authorize women as professionals and sustain the hospitals for the sex.

Women attending women, as doctors or nurses, was one theme of the 1860s. Another was the uninspiring lessons and unrelenting languor of girl-pupils. A third was fashion. Flammable crinolines were in the spotlight. Corsets that cramped the limbs and punctured the lungs were next in disrepute. Eye shadow deceived diagnosticians. Dieting devastated the body. Toil topped numerous inventories of insalubrity. Rheumatism and alcoholism beset the governess; eye and lung woes, the needlewoman; venereal diseases, which intrusive law did not stay, the prostitute; and enervation, every worker. Essays on the perils of pregnancy and birthing, especially in workhouses and slums, were salient; the companions of maternity, namely anemia, varicose veins, and dental, spinal, and digestive disorders, and the dangers of abortion were not. For the bored, none had mercy because they fancied that volunteering would dissolve unhealthy stress and specters.

This hypothesis was disguised in the 1870s in the accolades to activists for sanitary, dietary, and nursing improvements. Simultaneously, tracts returned to prior theses. When young, women ate improperly from necessity or preference, moved muscles scarcely at school or wrongly at jobs, and risked their health in unsafe factories and filthy quarters or with tainted cosmetics and tight bodices. Among workhouse residents, there was too much ophthalmia and among belles, too much fainting. For the first, the sincere dictated rustic retreats that would end that epidemic and retard another by reorienting future prostitutes, and for the second, a regimen of walking, rowing, swimming, and calisthenics. All women should learn physiology and nutrition to lessen unwellness for themselves and their progeny. To embolden women to divulge indisposition, they must have doctors of their own sex. Dissertations corroborated that male doctors were aloof and medical students disdained the pregnant poor. Most tales on birthing, however, were on painkillers, chiefly chloroform. Pregnancy problems, subscribers saw, might not be the outcome of inattention but of occupation. Farming was still said to be deleterious but mill work not for either mother or fetus. Two jobs, however, overshadowed others in danger to women. Sewing persisted as the bane of the genteel, and prostitution, as the crux of the crusade against the Contagious Diseases Acts.

The furor about this legislation stopped in the 1880s with repeal. Words on other labors did not mushroom. Narrators hailed statutes on overwork, tuberculosis, and accidents in factories that hurt both women and men, but the heroine of articles was the gentlewoman. In childhood, she might go with a nanny to a park, though she habitually had as little fresh air as her impoverished sisters. In adolescence, her clothes, cosmetics, and recently intense education were harmful. As an adult, she was betrayed by doctors who misdiagnosed and humiliated her.

Convinced by the 1890s that women were disserved by medicine, one mentor wished for female inspectors for hospitals, poor law and prison infirmaries, insane asylums, and work sites. Others would have women supervise all health care facilities because of their purportedly caring nature. If the nail trade was not necessarily hazardous, that of glove manufacture was still synonymous with neuralgia and tuberculosis, and prostitution, with syphilis. Mills might be better than in the 1820s, but sewing was perennially bad and sweatshops lately so. Likewise, the destitute gentlewoman should not have to die because her savings or others' gifts could not pay the price of treating a serious illness. Instead, the state should inaugurate pensions for her and others and should either mimic private efforts to coach poor females in villages and tenements on how to deter disease or divest mothers of their offspring. Laws had to embrace more than work. Schools had to train girls physically yet not rigorously and mentally, in ways suitable for their smaller brains. The precariousness of pregnancy and then puerperal fever prefaced entreaties for the education and certification of midwives. Alternatively, some magazines would not leave everything to government. Manufacturers had to modify the corset and the crinoline. If fashion might have a fatal result, breast cancer most certainly did. While there had been inserts on cancer before, breast malignancies, or their diagnosis may have soared, enough that one person categorized miracle cures as part of the "hysteria" about the disease. Demoting women's legitimate desperation about an incurable illness simply to delusion was not the only published disparagement of sick women. Other bulletins depicted women as less aware of pain than men with the same maladies. Consequently, the pampering appropriate for male patients would reputedly stir nervous disorders in female patients. This line of analysis may explain, for example, men's derision of women's complaints about dyspepsia. Such language embodies a disturbing trend in print by 1900, one that did not bode well for unwell women.

CAREGIVERS AND CARE

The nineteenth-century media category of caregiving encompassed people and places. In the first, doctors and nurses were principals, then administrators and auxiliaries, such as pharmacists, midwives, and ambulance squads; in the second, facilities, other than those for the insane (which were illness-specific), were featured.

Starting in the 1820s, sections on doctors were initially trifling and invariably on squelching sickness rather than preserving wellness. Tribunes publicized the quarrel over dissection, measuring its worth in medical training against its dependence on the capricious even criminal acquisition of bodies, with undercurrents about the class of the dissected. Status of another sort was an issue in the far more perennial discussions about the professional rank of surgeons.

In the 1830s, the inconsistencies in standards among the Court of Examiners of the Apothecaries' Company, the College of Physicians, and the College of Surgeons were downplayed. What nettled the press was the seeming inclination of each to enroll bunglers. Reformers sought uniform education and qualification for each group, suggesting that surgeons have solid intellectual and clinical backgrounds and physicians, the serial stars, genuine proficiency. Memorials to past practitioners did not dissuade some commentators that the present were superior. They were eager to set benchmarks for judging success. From dress to demeanor, office station to patient interaction, every aspect of a doctor's life had its counselor. As before, covertly in these counsels and overtly in those on "burking," (from William Burke, executed in 1829 for smothering people to sell their bodies for dissection), notions about class obtained.

Ideas about class and medicine were far clearer in the 1840s when caregiving to the poor, with its import for doctors and insurers, emerged as another topic in the papers. They pushed too for standards of instruction, accreditation, and practice for all in medicine. Penmen endorsed either self-regulation or legislation. Both sides sanctioned testing to eliminate the "quack," connoting both the criminal and the nonconformist, one beyond the boundaries of the state and the other, of the brotherhood of doctors. The heretic might manifest how rules crushed creativity and stratified colleagues. Yet, compromise was not forthcoming. Writers dogmatized about science lectures and field experiences or belittled courses and counted on apprenticing for facts, judgment, humor, and fellowship. Whereas the future preoccupied most, a few toasted the famous, a Charles Bell or a T. Southwood Smith, and the anonymous, the country doctors and city-dwelling soldiers against cholera.

Biographies were more collective in the 1850s. Although the careers of such doctors as Thomas Watson or Henry Clutterbuck were not deemed trivial, those of their forgotten confederates were characterized as more typical. Paragraphs portrayed the skeptic and the czar, the chatty and the silent, the morbid and the jolly. Correspondents, exhorting audiences to grade common sense and skill much higher than looks and charm, assumed that readers had the resources to select and commingled economics and ethics by putting relations among doctors, still in flux, ahead of those with their patients. Skipping over these concepts, mastheads, not with unanimity, contemplated how skill could be validated. Friends of statutes formed a minority. For the majority, internally formulated conventions would permit experts to fix expertise; resolve disputes among physicians, surgeons, and apothecaries; and daunt the unorthodox, translated usually as male activists but also applied to female aspirants. Discussion of standards resuscitated the matter of a degree, entailing tariffs and apparently without purpose, and launched proposals for alternatives. Some would keep students in laboratories dissecting corpses, while others would dispatch them to hospitals. In any scenario, the biases of the notary, the discontented muttered, might vitiate notarization. Whether persuaded by educational costs or uneasiness, occasional reviewers rejected a caregiver role for doctors, consigning them to prophylaxis, as scholar or bureaucrat, and to pedagogy, as witness in criminal trials.

The opinion that doctors were inept did not evaporate in the 1860s. Again and again organs rallied for better education, intellectual and experiential. They delineated the aims and ambit of a university program, footnoted by recollections of burking and approbation for training in the kingdom. They urged government to be scrupulous about those guarding insanity and public health, from which guardianship slim income deflected the best. Nevertheless, contributors knew that considering the array of illnesses, some asymptomatic, others imitative, and an army of casualties looking for care, some dissemblers were to be expected. The press thus forgave the mistaken and the diffident as doing less mischief than the promises and placebos of patent vendors. Sure that science and those who commanded it would finally win, its disciples beseeched professionals to be decent and dutiful. Integrity could displace the doubt that thwarted recovery and could reap rewards for the agent. Otherwise, the sick would turn to amateur healers. Perhaps to evade this eventuality, there were plaudits for renowned physicians, rural surgeons, and urban hospital staffs. Older heroes appeared in print next to younger heroines whose arrival, some whined, would unsettle the medical fraternity.

The female doctor had champions, nonetheless, in the 1870s. They denounced legal impediments to her accreditation and defended her right to practice if properly credentialed, even as male professionals, motivated by status, were campaigning against midwives. Since the curriculum for either sex was not firm, tracts called for official norms for it, in hospitals or not, and for licensing. Enemies dismissed the hospitals for training because they attracted inferior students whose education took from charitable endowments. A few disclosed that hospital doctors could substitute administrative pay when wealthy patients renounced residential care or could gain from referrals by past students. Stories on qualifications passed over the generalist who ministered to the middling rank but accentuated the specialist. Items celebrated experts for their expertise. Their feats, in plastic and other surgeries, ophthalmology, pediatrics, and mental maladies, were praised. By contrast, those who thought that a doctor's obligations were to aid the unwell and to promote their siblings' wellness treasured London Medical Missionaries more than London consultants.

Such pieces remained rare in the 1880s when specialization stole the limelight. Partisans rhapsodized about progress; their opposites hoped that generalists would emulate the South London Medical Institute, which served the poor. With respect to women doctors, heralds recommended their exclusion from all but the practice of gynecology, despite enjoining that their training be the same as that of men. Indeed, several aspects of education were in print. Sages, after comparing courses in England, Ireland, and Scotland, concluded that curricular revision and faculty research had been inadequate. Associates saluted hospitals, in the capital and away, for grooming stellar candidates and fostering scientific inquiry. In 1881, Frances Power Cobbe sparked an outcry when she announced in the *Modern Review* that students were unprepared and undedicated and that doctors, dedicated to the rich and each other, mistreated females and animals. Rebuttals, for doctors and against state meddling as demeaning to practitioners and detrimental to patients, filled pages. The apolitical withdrew from the fray, concentrating on stalwart physicians since the sixteenth century and the color-blind of the nineteenth.

The last disability might have underlain some of the blundering showcased in the 1890s. By this date, training was a stale topic, though hospital tutelage was again controversial. Reputedly, specialized hospitals had funds for top teachers and resources, whereas general ones were worthless for both science and alliance. Students learned either the latest methods or merely the field with the highest fees. Either research was fundamental for recovery or care was its keystone. Competition, not collaboration, was inherent in many essays. The monopoly of the College of Surgeons in certification, for example, carried patronage to a handful and penury to the uninvited. Specialists, with their books and bulging rates, were cast as rivals of generalists with average skills; the latter, of dispensaries; and males, of females, mainly in obstetrics. Women were directed toward marginal groups, either in gynecology or the empire. Lastly, doctors had nurses as contestants. Journalists intermittently interrupted this script to chide themselves, mentioning that doctors might be dissuaded from broadcasting medical ideas when journals concurrently censured them for their breach of confidentiality, cool manner, or laxity toward patients. For one writer, equilibrium between the laboratory and the bedside was essential. This notion of balance, the linchpin of life for so many mid-Victorians, did not seem to calm most of their successors.

Nurses were never as newsworthy as doctors. Indeed, until the 1860s, they were almost invisible. Remarkable therefore is a chapter of the 1820s that placed test-authenticated Protestant sisters supervised by doctors ahead of less skilled apothecaries or nurses animated by salary, science, or "humanity." Words about the lack of adept nurses were few in the 1840s and early 1850s. Thereafter, the endeavors of Florence Nightingale, Mary Pickard, and Catherine Mompesson, the concomitant theory that women made outstanding nurses, and the multiplication of hospitals fueled publicity about nursing.

The 1860s profiled Nightingale, and her *Notes on Nursing*, and less famous nurses, such as the founder of the Liverpool Nursing Home. Although authors glanced at workhouse personnel, they converged on hospital staffs. In specialized metropolitan establishments and generic village ones, on day and night shifts, nursing was assayed. Discourses profoundly gendered decided that Parliament must supervise nursing and that lady volunteers could serve patients, themselves, and their sex as models. As reporters espoused better patient care and greater opportunity for the middle class woman, they either missed or misinterpreted how women's paramountcy in nursing foreclosed the field of doctoring for females.

So absolute was the acceptance of nursing as women's domain that a lone voice mustered men to the occupation in the 1870s. In most texts, purportedly feminine traits were inextricably interwoven with nursing tasks. Nurses of all types were apotheosized in the press, from the fabled Sister Dora, Dorothy Pattison, to her anonymous companion district nurses. Ever vigilant, even in retirement, the nurse supposedly stood ready to succor anyone in need. Nonetheless, contemporaries complained about the training and professionalism of nurses. Not contradicting their words on the nurse's value but seeking to underpin it, they graded the education of hospital and private personnel in Britain below its German counterpart and argued for higher wages and status.

Efforts in the 1880s to enhance the prestige of nurses, coeval with a bid for their registration, catalyzed more biography, notably of those who roamed the Black Country and of nuns who ranged further. Their fans would promote nurses to physicians' adjuncts and parish infirmary supervisors. As in the 1870s, trust in nurses' talents did not preclude pages on their faults, chiefly in tending the poor in and out of hospitals. Most scribes agreed that training was thorough, but they lamented that district nursing did not attract the best graduates and that workhouses retained the worst, from the color blind to the extortionist. Hospital staffs, some conjectured, had better academic and moral backgrounds, though a brouhaha at Guy's about the scope of the nurses' role demonstrated that this assessment was not accurate. Boosters blamed long hours, crowded wards, and female superintendents for the flaws of duty nurses. More foreboding was the insinuation that nurses were not auxiliaries but adversaries of doctors, interlopers between patient and male professional.

This particular theory did not flourish in the 1890s but resentment of women did, documented by propaganda for masculine recruits and against women without proper deference. Critics declared that nurses had been overly flattered and that nursing by giddy girls reared to be bored could be slipshod at best. Defenders reiterated the argument that women were natural nurses because they were serene, alert, and able around the sick. Mediators admitted that nursing was not without difficulties but contended that it was novice nannies and private duty autocrats who disgraced the profession. If poor-law attendants displayed little aptitude and district nurses distributed too many drugs, these people were available and might improve by copying Sister Dora. Hospitals could appoint superior employees if they extended accommodations, salaries, and opportunities for advancement. Until then, nursing would not intrigue those with options for other work, suggestive not only for nurses but for all women.

As with nursing, dialogue about hospitals was infrequent until after mid-century. In the 1840s and 1850s, however, columnists introduced motifs that would recur, such as the circumstances of nursing and the price of treating the poor, notably in London, Liverpool, and Manchester. Another thread in the early accounts was the unhealthiness of health facilities. Unlike French hospitals, British establishments allegedly did not disinfect but rather adhered to a minimal level of care. More than once did observers summon Parliament to act on this health threat. A third theme was special hospitals, designated by the age, occupation, disorder, or likelihood of death of patients.

This focus on special hospitals did not blur in the 1860s when establishments for juveniles, orphaned or not, predominated. Other hospitals, for the feverish, the paralyzed, and the recuperating, were in the headlines as were the London Royals, estimated as excellent for teaching and exploitation by pauper outpatients for trivial ills. National dispensaries apparently did not approximate the services of their Gallic analogues, whereas hospitals did surpass workhouse infirmaries. Pilgrims to pastoral sites thought that they were adequate but underutilized and visitors to provincial places, that they were exorbitant, disorganized, and staffed by the unqualified. Nursing might be superb or so dreadful as to warrant laws to make its practitioners adequate. Investigators of hospitals tracked routines, and sporadic inserts abridged surgery and anesthetics.

Papers of the 1870s were somewhat more aware of hospital patients. Commentators ranted about the rich who bought beds for trivial aches, malingering outpatients, doctors who diagnosed incorrectly, and nurses who doled out wrong dosages. If the hospital milieu did not expedite recuperation, it was, most imagined, above the infirmary, where even meals conspired with maladies. Some votaries solicited donations for care of the destitute; others exposed the channeling of charity from the indigent to medical students who showed ineptitude and incivility toward these same clients. Outpatient departments spawned debates about dispensaries, their cost and scope of responsibility. Queries rose about the merits of the free hospital against the provident and the exclusion or admission of contagious patients. Columnists also studied how hospitals administered and staffed clinics and other wings. Women predominated in nursing, but their pay and responsibilities were not monolithic. Evaluators, who appreciated volunteers, realized their limitations. The female legions were very visible in excerpts on special hospitals for youths, the terminally ill, convalescents, and the physically challenged. Titles also targeted special facilities for victims of accidents and of ear and throat disorders. Of the general establishments, the rustic were disapproved of less often than the urban, except for those in London. The Great Northern garnered many laurels and other London hospitals, some.

The medical institutions of the capital continued to snare space in the 1880s. One arbiter nominated the twelve best for medical training and patient care; another singled out those that had specialists at bargain rates; and a third drew on the perspectives of nurses, students, and young and poor sufferers. East End venues were pictured as sanctuaries for those in recovery, the pregnant, and ailing children. If the contrarian bellowed about swarming wards, others parried with platitudes about havens for physically challenged children and for all with fevers. Out of London, hospitals cataloged by their patients' diseases, employments, or sex and those of no discernible faction were more in vogue. Appraisals were mixed, albeit heedfulness of patients' dietary demands seemed positive. Equally so was the burgeoning of outpatient departments, which, serials summarized, diagnosed, dealt with injuries and indispositions, and dispensed remedies and rules for wellness. Penmen admired the hospital as a vehicle for sharing research and skills that surely benefited the sick but acknowledged its limitations. Nurses, even dexterous and virtuous paragons of the profession, ruffled doctor-patient relationships. Doctors exhibited no genius for administration and lay administrators, none for medicine. Philanthrophy was precious to or perverted by hospital directors.

Revenue issues resurfaced in the 1890s. Watchers wondered why endowments went to laboratories and students rather than to patient treatment. Inventories of personnel training were common. In London, food and lodging for apprentices won accolades. Everywhere, the preparation and practices of nurses failed journalistic muster, and those of doctors just passed. Supplies and management received low marks because, for example, oxygen was not always accessible in emergencies, and staffs were not adroit in handling trauma cases. Disquisitions decreed restructuring of medical establishments by males and monitoring by females. As one pundit proclaimed and others intimated, general hospitals were futile for cure or education. Specialized institutions might serve as either surrogates or supplements to general ones, might afford experts not otherwise available, and could harbor those near health or death. The workhouse, in fewer sentences, was ostensibly too outmoded to offer quality care in the future. Yet, retrospectives on humanitarianism and on legislation confirmed a belief that care of the ill was substantially better for everyone by 1900 than in former years.

BEING HEALTHY

Nineteenth-century media versions of being healthy comprised concepts of restoration and maintenance. The first subsumed studies of anatomy, physiology, and psyche and assessments of amateur and professional remedies. Ideas on preservation of salubrity, more voluminous, interpreted illness as negative. Extirpation of its roots, individual and communal, made prevention positive and longevity a logical corollary.

Restoration

Chroniclers assumed that healing came from understanding, so pages on research proliferated. Until the 1850s, treatises on the eye, ear, and skin, circulation, and respiration were prominent, but those on the brain and the nervous system were more so. According to magazines, the brain not only coordinated physiology and psychology but also transformed data into the discovery of cures. Thus, the brain, and with it phrenology, were popular subjects.

The brain was again in the news in the 1850s and 1860s. Sheets capsulized its size and shape; memory and emotions; the ramifications of sleep, dreams, and drugs for its well-being; and its impact on heart, nerves, muscles, and hearing. Muscles suddenly became a theme, from a probe of cell differentiation to a peek at laughter. Regular headlines on the eye, its structure and capabilities, and on vision loss communicate how much Victorians treasured sight. They pirated from predecessors thinking on respiration and circulation but not on temperature and sensation.

The senses, possibly because of a perceived nexus with psychology, were important subjects in the 1870s and after. Vision was another cornerstone of abstracts until 1900 and hearing, almost as long. Muscles were more frequently juxtaposed with exercise. Heart and lungs, which might have been similarly yoked, were instead banded with stress and climate. As before, the bulk of prose went to the brain and nerves. Phrenology reappeared abruptly and with scant proselytes. Dreams were less crucial to this generation than right brain/left brain functions and the aftermath of alcohol and anesthetics. Secure that consciousness and subsequent wellness were the sprouts of a healthy brain and nerves, periodicals ultimately blessed the mating of physiology and psychology.

From the outset of talk about treatment, it was tethered to specific complaints. Nevertheless, from the 1820s, such dissertations ran next to those on more catholic restoratives. The earliest was homeopathy, then, in the 1830s, hypnosis. German spas and French researchers were always honored, while traditional curatives and commercial tonics were not. Diatribes on sham elixirs were steady throughout the century.

Reporters of the 1840s confessed some culpability for the success of fraud, which, they ruminated, thrived partly because of publicity. Additionally, they faulted ignorant patients, incompetent doctors, fees, and false promises for the resort to folk or trendy therapies. Conventional correctives that writers sponsored were alcohol, primarily wines; coffee, tea, and cocoa; and change of climate, local or foreign. Allies of self-help spurned homeopathy, suspected hypnosis, and squabbled about hydropathy. Admirers of science promulgated its achievements, chiefly chloroform and ether but, significantly, pitted expert against individual knowledge as a basis for decisionmaking.

Chloroform and ether were topics again in the 1850s. Allaying pain in childbirth or from burns eclipsed for most writers the fatalities that sometimes ensued. Drugs, such as the omnipresent opium, were more worrisome because of alleged adulteration and assault on the body. Hypnosis was controversial but had potential for diagnosis and recovery. Hydropathy and homeopathy were fading in print. Adversaries of the second labeled it quackery; they assured readers that either nature cured homeopathic patients or they died having delayed appropriate treatment. Qualms about homeopathy and other methods precipitated partiality for non-intervention or folkways from herbal to spiritual. A clique counted on professional medicine for survival.

The clique became a chorus by the 1860s. Putting vivisection in the spotlight, journalists struggled with questions about human and animal welfare. On other fronts, opinions were firmer. Nature was reputedly at least as good as patent brews. Research was more certain to yield benefits, to which anesthetics reputedly attested. Guides looked to baths, in the kingdom and the German realms, to liquor over laudanum, and even to lightning. Narrators raved more about neighbors who healed by faith and poultices than about professionals whose prescriptions could hurt or bankrupt a sufferer. Attitudes toward homeopathy and hypnosis were less prejudiced and toward hydropathy, almost ardent.

The zest for the "water cure" slackened in the 1870s, although baths garnered some attention. Seaweed, voyages, and alcohol, principally light wines, were the idols of independents. Scribes esteemed surgery but warned that post-surgical medication might reach the wrong person or be dispensed in the wrong dosage. Notwithstanding these risks, respect for science was swelling except where it entailed vivisection. The altercation about animals for research coincided with parliamentary notice of the technique. Apologists, with Darwinian nuances, mocked the hypocrisy of antagonists who ate meat and engaged in a blood sport. Antivivisectionists replied that experiments, conducted by the unskilled, the unkind, or the vainglorious, were morally regressive and nationally demeaning.

Wrangling continued shrilly in the 1880s, even with use certification in place. While the neutral balanced animal agony and human mortality, most observers were obdurate. Friends locked the technique to learning, as about rabies. Foes detested the technicians who devised painful and futile tests that undermined community ethics. Conversely, reckoning that failure in a laboratory disheartened doctors or success in practice diverted them from research, everyone encouraged more medical investigation. Still, as editors eulogized the development of anesthetics and vaccines, they did not repudiate homeopathy and hypnosis. Customary cures, domestic and alien, and refuges, on the coast or overseas, were fancied over narcotics and tonics. Drink remained soothing for some.

By the 1890s, the furor about vivisection had receded, replaced by ratifications of research. Frequently with forewords on Louis Pasteur, sheets underlined advances in vaccines and bacteriology. Gazettes pressured Westminster to fund and doctors to concentrate on intensive studies. There was applause for advances in surgery, antiseptics, and the ubiquitous anesthetics, but not for medications too commonly tainted or shared. Hypnosis, ticketed as probative, therapeutic, perilous, or fraudulent, symbolized an ongoing battle in the tribunes between professional and home remedies. Uncertainty renewed reverence for nature and reliable restoratives. Sunshine would halt bacteria; herbs would heal quicker than manufactured chemicals; and a little liquor or laudanum would dull aches. Above all, several saw then, as others had for decades, that prevention was the best antidote for ailments.

Maintenance

Columnists expected citizens to guard their own health, at least initially, and the state to step in when they could or would not. Deluged by cues from the monthlies, the reader was to discern the distinction between the need for individual and public action in such matters as food, drink, and drugs; cleanliness in residence and of person; and air quality, recreation, and rest. In all, the baseline was balance as greater faith in experts coexisted with greater forebodings of over government.

Food perennially headed the agenda on wellness, but water, for drinking, washing of all sorts, and sewage disposal, was invariably next. Two tones that sounded very early echoed in later orations on nutrition. One was adulteration of food; the other was dyspepsia. Both bespoke bad eating, by default or deliberation.

In the 1810s, the *Edinburgh Review* lectured on the preservation of food and the hazards of alcohol and tobacco. However, in the 1820s, alcohol stock rose as quarterlies bemoaned the pollution of previously potable water. The 1830s brought more grumbling, about London's tainted Thames and humans' peculiar habits. Correspondents castigated the prosperous for indulging in feasts that fathered gastric distress and workers for taking drugs to dilute factory horrors and to swallow sullied food. The fare of the masses, a prerequisite for labor, did not yet seem important. Nutritionists talked softly; connoisseurs of French cuisine and overseas tobacco did not.

The ingestion of deleterious substances was more bothersome in the 1840s. The rush to feed urbanites was unfettered by bureaucracy but not by the urgency that bolstered shoddy commodities. Liquor had many assailants, although its advocates insisted that it was a tonic, a painkiller, and a beverage in towns with contaminated water. Adversaries retorted that drink damaged already undernourished bodies and diverted pennies from the purchase of food. As in other contexts, this one had a class orientation. How the indigent, even without this expense, could buy quality comestibles from slum street peddlers eluded most prophets. Those who sermonized ceaselessly about food as the linchpin of wellness seldom joined its deprivation to low wages. Some thinkers did concede that those who could afford choice chose unwisely, shunning nutrition and precipitating dyspepsia and obesity. Disquisitions denominated as salubrious, grains, fish, potatoes, sugar, and bread, and disdained coffee, tea, and bathing after meals. Segments traced menus from infancy through maturity and, borrowing from Justus von Liebig, studied food chemistry.

By the 1850s, nutrition was news. Savants literally located it: the homeless dropped from starvation; urbanites declined from malnourishment; suburbanites had erratic meals; and rustics had insufficient fare unless the entire family tilled. Extremes, particularly obesity and emaciation, though explicable, were undesirable; critiques of criteria for healthy diets were incessant. There were articles on the merits or not of vegetarianism and of vegetables. Fish, perhaps because familiar, was absent from the discussion aside from cautions about catches from lethal water and raves for those farm-bred. Meat was the order for young and old despite its defects. There were banners on the breeding and feeding of cattle, the nuisance of the Smithfield market, and the contamination of tinned meat. Taint was not confined to the canned but was, to many, frequent and frequently intentional in fresh meat. Sloppy handling, therefore, was less forgivable in merchants than in shoppers. Tea, beer, wine, penny sweets, and preeminently bread were purportedly the most menacing to health. Of other wares, minerals were the least controversial and alcohol, the most, followed by opium and tobacco. There were sentences on the physiological and psychological repercussions of cannabis and on the value of stimulants from thorn apple to coffee. Potable water, the conventional core of wellness, was problematic because seepage from cemeteries and waste from habitations, hospitals, and workhouses allegedly defiled sources. How to reconcile metropolitan industrialism and imminent poisoning was obviously a dilemma, so recommendations were rampant. Most were on how to purify water; some, on how to dispose of pollutants; a few, on how to induce national officials to authorize taxes for and local governments to effectuate transmission of water; and one, on the advantages of public fountains in pauper lanes.

An emphasis on water persisted in the 1860s. Convinced that London's was scarce and spoiled, publications soon intensified their onslaught on the capital and elsewhere. Attributing typhus particularly and epidemics universally to water, the press proffered few means to alter reserves or content. Alcohol was not so broadly condemned. A minority embraced it as sustenance or anesthetic. Opponents termed it the sire of insanity and idiocy but absolved the lower ranks who emulated the upper. Tobacco, to chew, sniff, and smoke, was said to be less harmful. Judges, tabbing food as dreadful, ordained wider legislation to curb ongoing malefaction, though not chemical preservatives. Bread, sugar, pepper, and milk were principal perils and mushrooms, permanent ones. Candy, but not meat, seemed safer than before. The sale of diseased carcasses and decaying joints appalled those who bound vigor to beef. Realists could not square consumer and slaughterhouse supervision costs. Pretending that the impoverished could have both enough and excellent meat, sages paraded it as a diet essential in their perpetual inventories of food as a preventive. As before, city and country dwellers faced obstacles to eating well and eating for wellness. Towns had few cheap restaurants with wholesome menus; hamlets had more food, albeit of no variety. Prone to sickness, the needy supposedly survived on charity meals. The comfortable had other, ordinarily self-inflicted disturbances. Recorders hinted that "banting" (named for William Banting, a proponent of planned weight loss) was killing women and overweight was killing men. Prudence should dictate what to buy and how to store and prepare it. The rule was that eating should comport with lifestyle and check dyspepsia.

Dyspepsia as a correlative of diet was the lesser evil in the 1870s when adulteration of food was the star. Irrespective of decades of parliamentary hostility, adulteration purportedly had not abated. Flour, beer, and narcotics were the colonels of the battalions of impure products destined for the realm and the empire. To stifle swindling, audiences must be wary of meat not from cold storage and all fish and mushrooms. Water defied individual wariness. From the Thames to the towns, tales tagged it unpotable because of dumping by sewers and factories and disinclination to cremate. Indicting local boards for inviting epidemics, commentators turned to Westminster but for one eccentric who wanted mineral water for all. The temperance cadre conflicted with those who either drank or doubted that statutes could repress drink. Routinely, alcohol was affirmed as remedy; tobacco, as relaxant except for youths; coffee and tea, as animating for all. Optimists cheered because native drinking customs were apparently no worse than foreign imbibing of wine. Besides, the sanguine swore that nutrition could cancel any subsequent calamity and, not incidentally, stress. Concordance that vegetables, primarily potatoes and legumes, were vital did not mean that everyone endorsed vegetarianism. It did mean that how animal fat affected the body was of some interest. Indicative of more interest was the litany on laborers' fare wherein farm hands ate better than previously, mill workers did not, and those in workhouses or on the roads bordered on starvation.

Alarms about the poor and their access to drinkable water and untainted food waxed in the 1880s. The water in most towns and in the country, writers fulminated, was so full of human and technological waste as to justify a system solely for drinking. Urbanites had other complaints. City life severely strained digestion, and city prices prohibited purchase of uncontaminated viands. Some authors synchronized the eating of tinned goods and thrift. Colleagues banked on schools and subsidies as food sources that cost less than infirmaries and hospitals and were more secure than alms. Impurity did not prey just on paupers. If laws had stemmed reprehensible adulteration of meat and dairy products, polluted rivers still begot poisonous fish. Mooring robustness to meat, Victorians were not receptive to vegetarianism. They did comprehend that bread, the eternal staple, varied in value according to ingredients. Liquor was food to a few, restorative for stomach and nerves to most devotees. They were pro-choice against a rising tide of teetotalers. Some dodged the debate by denouncing opium, cannabis, and tobacco to ease fatigue or dispel depression because these substances could destroy users and their heirs, and coffee, tea, cocoa, vinegar, and mineral water because they could disrupt digestion. Partisans of mineral water responded that it and lighter ales were the only beverages that could diminish dyspepsia. Overall, pieces pontificated that excess was the enemy. Alongside this discussion, another on bacteria in food preparation and preservation developed, portent of the coming outcry.

Opinionmakers devoted scores of lines in the 1890s to bacteria. Sponsors of pasteurization fretted about milk and the milk container; their disciples, about all dairy goods. Then, mineral water was suspect and finally, all consumables. Rejoinders, far fewer, claimed that some bacteria were benign, as in cheese ripening. The war on dairy wares was bold and vexing at a moment when more arbiters were substituting milk and eggs for mediocre meat from the sick cow or the healthy horse, both befouled in filthy abattoirs. Fans of flesh did not waver. Other sources of protein, mainly peanuts and seaweed, were never more than a whisper. Vegetarianism was more popular than previously but hardly a fashion. Searching for norms, journalists retreated to the late-sixteenth and early-nineteenth centuries. From the former, they extrapolated evidence that overeating was always baneful; from the latter, that metropolitan menus were improving. Confronted by fasting women and feeble laborers, catalogers converged on the toilers. Vulnerability to illness was the precursor of lower profits and higher taxes, both of which the consumption of cheap nourishing food and instructions on its handling would offset. Paens to the Salvation Army and its confederates insinuated that preparing meals was better done for than by the destitute. More explicitly about class was the avowal that donations to children did not strengthen workers but subverted the work ethic. Water was a glaring peril. Faced with rivers of refuse, bottles of bacteria, expensive and arbitrary supplies, and negligent local councils, control over water, tirades thundered, ought to be centralized. London was conventionally the symbol of bad and badly distributed water. Birmingham was much better, but no community was the paradigm for purification. Predictably, some seized on alcohol to foil indisposition and to reduce stress. As wets prattled about moderation, teetotalers promulgated liquor's menace directly and indirectly. Most stimulants were forgotten in print: one account advertised mescal for the sturdy, and a few, tobacco until the voice vanished. Coverage of adulteration decreased and of dyspepsia reversed it from a male to a female trouble. What endured was a trite regimen for wellness in which food, water, and other ingestibles were as dominant as they had been for decades.

Water had another role in health maintenance, that of cleanliness. This word enveloped personal action and public policy, but talk of sewers and housing had far more columns than hygiene. Sanitation was the goal for streets and homes; the "sanitary question" was an exegesis on class wherein the lodgings and alleys of the poor were conspicuous.

Postings in the 1820s averred that London was dirty. By the 1830s, heralds were vociferous. They worried about disease spontaneously formed from filth, then disseminated by subsequent gases, and reacted to statutes meant to stifle cholera. London, onlookers snapped, was a morass and its officials paralyzed. Manchester was a sinkhole, but other towns too were engulfed in waste because humans, obliviously or deceitfully, obstructed reform. If optimists regarded the present as innovative, their opposites dissented saying that sewage and housing combined to beckon ills that curtailed capitalism. Without municipal baths, the masses brought maladies beyond their quarters.

In the 1840s, titles on cleanliness multiplied. Quoting the Census of 1841 and the Health of Towns Association, tribunes petitioned for sewerage, dwellings, and hygiene. Chapters construed public health laws as precedents for more legislation and as signs of parliamentary concern. The vigilant, determined to waken local boards, knew that members owned nuisances or owed their appointments, such as the London Sewer Commissioners, to patronage. Local empowerment was hardly novel, but now language was unequivocal: proper disposal was pivotal lest fevers last forever. The propertied must connect to mains and sewers, price and privacy aside, and waste handlers must have disinfectants. Such edicts exhibit a conceptual link between science and sanitation to fortify wellness yet a slighting of such specifics as the scale of and tolls for engineering and the availability of engineers. Housing was ancillary to this dialogue. Denigration of slums boomed though not demands for their demolition. Lodging houses were either abysmal or adequate in London. For bathing, municipal facilities akin to Liverpool's were deemed obligatory as companies reputedly restricted access to canals. Both the needy and their cousins were warned about immersion after "profligacy." Other barriers to cleanliness that mastheads memorialized were interment, also within Parliament's purview, and slaughterhouses that blighted already littered paths.

With thanks to Edwin Chadwick, the famous proponent of sanitation, texts of the 1850s had more words on the subject. Sewage in water sources was the chief concern. Proposed alternatives were treating waste with chemical solvents and sending it to rural areas as fertilizer, but most mentors urged local councils to invest in sewerage and impeached townsmen who procrastinated, unlike those in oft-cited Barnard Castle. City abodes were in bold print. Positive that they fostered epidemics, essays welcomed laws, as on lodging houses. Essayists ordered government to guarantee residences resistant to fire and with reasonable space, drainage, and water. Only one mused that, as dark, dank, and tumultuous as tenements were, they were superior to homelessness. Even those excited about new building preached other cautions. Authorities must erect more baths and laundries and must enlighten the uninformed about disinfectants and washing. The theory that the state could coordinate individual cleanliness seems strange in a culture that supposedly treasured individualism. An arena more susceptible to control was the nuisance presented by interment. As pundits promoted cremation, boosters of burial conceded that cemetery statutes should be strict and sanitary acts should encompass coroners' dissection sites.

Sanitation was a less popular theme in the 1860s compared to the frenzy of the previous two decades, although sewers were as significant as before. Treatises on typhus, cholera, and other contagions, from infancy to senility, were laden with statistics on waste mismanagement as a barrier to health. As legal improvements accelerated, there was a shift from prompting Westminster to move to prompting it to move efficiently. Narrators expected their engineers to design sewerage that eradicated, not exacerbated, water contamination and their government to implement that outcome. To encourage it, they praised air valves for domestic waste disposal. Slaughterhouses continued to be irritating and slums, fascinating. Congested, choked by garbage from living and laboring, rooms were so unsalutary to investigators that they mandated regular inspection. For inhabitants without stations for washing and familiarity with disinfectants, the sanguine asked women of the upper ranks to teach their lower class siblings. To dull the dangers from the dead and their interment, quarterlies advised amending public health law to require cooperation between doctors and health officers.

Tracts of the 1870s were not dramatic. Public policy, after new legislation, was characterized as too weak or too strong. Stories clamored that government studies were not broadcast, so they were duplicated as seasons passed. Sewerage was still irksome, just as amelioration of water had been sluggish. No longer exuberant about wider parliamentary involvement, and with a bow to community efforts, some assessors were amenable to downsizing by disbursing revenue only to extend or revamp existing systems. If those of towns were notoriously bad, those of older village and recent suburb were apparently little better. Housing drew more diatribes. London's, namely in the East End and Irish sections, scandalized observers. Outside the capital, law and local endeavors were tagged equally ineffective because epidemics persisted. Farm workers, current journalistic pets, were said to slumber in shacks surrounded by undrained marshes as toxic as metropolitan abattoirs and cemeteries. Horrendous as were these habitations, a cabal brooded that coercive health statutes had converted police and sanitary officers into spies and had culminated in less stability as citizens constantly disobeyed the laws. Preferable to legislation were common sense, medical guidance, and private enterprise, such as that of Octavia Hill. Hill, who did not attempt sweeping ouster of tenants without provision for the displaced, was something of a heroine. She stood for a cadre that contributors applauded, one of responsible females who campaigned for the health of the poor and thereby affirmed, in ways traditionally feminine, the social worth of their sex.

Individual initiative was not a motif in the 1880s, and testimony was not unique. Too much sewage was in rivers. Too few homes, of rich and poor, had efficient waste disposal. Chagrin about housing was greater as exasperation succeeded expectation. The crowded, gray, grimy tenements and lodging houses blotted too many towns as acts went unenforced or enforced in waves of evictions that only created new congestion. Model dwellings supervised by sanitary troops and dwellers indoctrinated in bourgeois ideas were the ideal. After 1888, there was hope that a centralized London government would organize sewerage, residential sanitation, and removal of the dead. Cremation, more bruited from the 1870s as an antidote for water pollution, and hygiene, mundane but not habitual, were other topics.

Pages in the 1890s praised victories and shouted for more. Exaltations underscored how deeds, public and voluntary, of peers and those prior, had substantially diminished dirt. There was enthusiasm for Birmingham housing but objection to the Salvation Army plan for the state to build more. The skeptical thought that change was slow, partly because plumbing standards were not scrupulously set by government. Slums, realists reaffirmed, spread bacteria, which thrived in refuse recurrent without water to flush abodes and avenues. The sweatshops of London and the lodging houses throughout the land proved the pervasiveness of disease in foul surroundings. Parliament had not only to construct habitations but to certify habitability. Burial was less debated, but cremation kept its adherents. Finally, and perhaps fittingly, one writer reminded readers that cleanliness of any type was trifling for health maintenance without accompanying temperance in life.

Savants saw a nexus between one aspect of cleanliness, hygiene, and clothing. Eventually, types of attire would appear as separate hindrances to wellness. Until the 1860s, dress was subordinate to detergent. Especially during the 1840s and 1850s, prose paired bathing and laundering as checks to contagions not class-bound. Abstracts gradually transformed the theme, recognizing that paupers in rags, without washing venues, could not make cleanliness a motto.

From the 1860s onward, categories of apparel were more important.

Children of the destitute allegedly wore castoffs of the dead; of the wealthy, copies of adult garments, equally unsuitable. Women's corsets, crinolines, cosmetics, and even slickers were under siege. So were men's underwear and beards, and the shoes of both sexes. Chroniclers thus did not foresake clothes but shifted their vantage from the soiled to the silly as deleterious.

Air quality, which could hamper humans at the most fundamental level, was one of the earliest entries on health maintenance. From the beginning, essays were cluttered with allusions to status. The *Edinburgh Review*, in its first volume, bared the peril of "infected air," a phrase considerably inflated as industrialism and urbanism broadened. In the 1830s, spectators hinged salubrity in towns to green spaces where townspeople could run or relax. By the 1840s, air was not merely a section of the sermons on wellness. Impurity connoted, as before, transmittal of disease and now also denoted pollution by technology. Smoke, bulletins blared, was everywhere, offending the eyes, nose, and lungs and screening light. Pessimists blamed the climate; reformers proposed country sojourns and environmental laws.

Smoke, whether from factories or hearths, was the chief culprit of the 1850s. Everyone apparently persevered in a permanent haze with minimal sunshine and ventilation. Compounding the harm was the crush of people, at the Great Exhibition or in tiny rooms, who breathed tainted air and simultaneously defiled it. Rural reassignment, except for juveniles, was not feasible, although the railroad did permit day junkets for their parents. Parks, as did those in London, could provide respiratory relief in cities. They could hypothetically supersede the pub as communal hub, a premise that by focusing only on workers' drinking confirms the class perspective of some pieces. This faith reverberated in the 1860s when paragraphs pledged that urban open areas would revivify the urbanite. They offered light and color to those accustomed to dusky dens, respite from mobs stealing or corrupting oxygen, and districts to play or doze. These oases would reinvigorate the mature and sire a sturdier generation.

The smells of foul air were secondary to pollutants in the 1870s. Manufacturing, without watchdogs in government, was the consummate criminal, but inappropriate interments and inescapable germs were accessories. Impurities were supposedly so rampant that the bucolic outings commanded for adults and the seaside holidays for children might be futile. Mediterranean trips, usually undertaken by affluent invalids, might save a few. However, most crusaders, unwilling to rescue a handful, resumed the philippic against towns. The program of the timid was plants inside, trees out; of the aggressive, illuminated, ventilated homes for all. The mansions of the rich entered the lists of insalubrious dwellings in the

1880s. Smoke and fogs, filled with dust and bacteria, penetrated indiscriminately. Analysts tagged sojourns to country or coast as nonsense in an inhospitable climate. Rather, playgrounds and parks would rehabilitate. Adjacent to this hackneyed projection were specific projects to alleviate the smog and the smells that devastated the lungs. London should be in the forefront. Instead, messages divulged, its East End was an embarrassment, and its officials were lax about environmental matters.

London was still astonishing journalists in the 1890s. Its residences and recreational regions were ostensibly better than before but still not equal to Birmingham places, or so that city's allies chanted. Nevertheless, the press celebrated as lung ailments decreased. Houses had fresh air and fewer persons, parks promised strong adults, and rural enclaves restored the frail. Accounts advertised how to remove bacteria and debris from air. Some methods, such as hosing streets and replicating parks of the United States, were rudimentary enough for any reader to understand; others were complex, accompanied by illustrations for those without a technical bent. Both anticipated that fogs would evaporate. Carrying contaminants that haunted observers, these shrouds bespoke the failure of technology, the failure of Victorians.

Stories about the effects of exercise on health, by contrast, concluded the century differently. In the 1820s, exercise was not high on serials' dockets for health. By the 1830s, inserts were less muted but not booming. They resounded, in the 1840s and 1850s, primarily in prayers for municipal parks. Oracles predicted that if the masses could exercise, they would not drink so much to relax. Their masters should swim or walk but not race to relieve stress. For juveniles, advice was not class-bound. Infants and toddlers should be mobile. Children should romp outdoors in urban playgrounds or rustic gardens. Schools should have athletic programs, certainly for boys and probably for girls. Activity should, for offspring and parent alike, parallel food and rest in order to sustain wellness.

In the 1860s and 1870s, exercise received more coverage. Organs tagged it positive for health, a recreation with physical and mental rewards, against negative overindulgence in food and liquor. Cognoscenti hailed athletics, notably cycling, for abetting respiration and digestion and loosening life's burdens. Only a few doubted the merits of any metropolitan regimen or labeled some sports and strenuous gymnastics ruinous for minors and the mature. This view prevailed more in lines on females but was quickly contradicted by two others, both gendered. One blamed apparel, not anatomy, for injuries to women; the other, superficially asexual, ascribed national vigor, and therefore lower taxes, to vigorous heirs.

Repetition of the connection between Albion's paramountcy and a healthy citizenry was a refrain of the 1880s and 1890s. Fields for recreation and rural treks, abstracts apprised audiences, would create a robust and well-adjusted population. Exercise, followed by massage and sleep, could energize the body and tranquilize the brain, but it was not for neophytes. The aghast decried arduous exercise for females and excessive athletics for all pupils. Football was fraught with risks for a few. Cycling was a craze classified as either exhilarating or destructive, mainly for women. To contend with injuries, volumes recommended food, clothing, and schedules by age and sex. This propaganda might not have extended or safeguarded activity but surely made subscribers more conversant with the assets of exercise and cautious in its undertaking.

Sleep too was no simple boon. While it was routinely recognized from the 1820s as cardinal for salubrity, the effects of interrupted slumber were not investigated until the 1850s. As dreams and somnambulism betokened nervous exhaustion, sleep as therapy metamorphosed into sleep as symptom. Titles of the 1860s and 1870s, when dialogue on sleep peaked, underlined both concepts. Authors scrutinized its stages and milieu, whether at home or on holiday. Sleep, probers asserted, neutralized daily pressures and aided digestion. Dreams continued as omens of physiological and psychological disorders, but somnambulism and narcolepsy switched from signs of unwellness to illnesses complete with treatments.

Analysis and advice about sleep lingered into the 1880s and 1890s. Recorders returned to dreams and started to scan the states of consciousness between sleeping and waking. There were reiterations of the worth of restful vacations and of domestic repose. Alert to urban noises and occupational strains, segments suggested ways to sleep at home. Counselors eschewed drugs in favor of atmosphere and awareness of the causes of insomnia, but some realized that the sounds of civilization were the central obstacle to revivifying rest.

Longevity

Papers did not immediately identify a bond between wellness and longevity. Except for an aside on behavior or family, they were strangely silent until the 1830s. Even then, they merely mentioned that mortality figures were down and measured life spans against those of the French, Swiss, and Russians. Once census statistics and insurance tables spread, so did assessments. They pondered the physiology and psychology of aging and declared that marital and economic status, responsibilities and recreations were central. From the grey to the decrepit, elders validated the theories of those who would distinguish nature or nurture as factors for health and those who pursued restoratives and preventives. Seniors also set precedents. Statutes and services that they spurred would redound to their heirs.

By the 1860s and 1870s, when information on morbidity was increasing, attitude and erudition joined lineage and ambiance as causes for longevity. If more survivors furnished more chances to penetrate the secrets of long life, the aging of large numbers centered finance in their memorials. In the twilight of the era, poverty was the linchpin of articles on ancients, infirm or not. There were schemes for pensions and boarding homes, for thrift and the poor law. If disquisitions did not laud medicine, they did not deny that science, and even pseudo-science, had had a role in prolonging life. Gazing besides at eugenics and stress, editions outlined the expansion of elder law and envied a former generation's moderation, morality, and energy. As one wag in the *Fortnightly Review* (1889) reckoned, it was "better to wear out than to rust out," a judgment still valid.

HEALTH IN THE KINGDOM

The bulk of British magazines, published in and out of England, devoted disproportionate space to that country, either alone or alongside the other components of the kingdom. This preponderance sprang from an interest in London, as the capital and therefore a model, and in urbanism, with its potential for undermining wellness. Narrators noticed Ireland, Scotland, and Wales but neither steadily nor equally.

The health of the Irish was not a subject until the 1830s. Copying from government inquiries on the ills and ill treatment of the peasantry, quarterlies highlighted improper food and inadequate medical care. They pictured the young and the old as most vulnerable but the hungry of any age as prone to disease and perpetually with fever. Prodding Westminster, publications demanded a poor law. This solution had no ordinary test once the 1840s ushered in years of extraordinary famine. The occasional ostrich might negate the starvation, but the majority tabbed it the last blow to an ailing cohort. Portrayed as dirty souls, living in hovels, and cloaked in rags, the Irish had purportedly fallen to epidemics long before the potato blight. That catastrophe merely hurried the onset of maladies. As some spectators prattled that adult alcoholism hastened death, most regretted that child fatalities did not speed state assistance without which none would be robust.

The 1850s and the score after were seasons of ongoing assessment and reorientation. Remembrances of the Famine's typhus and cholera and synopses of recent infirmities circulated. Workhouses were allegedly warrens of ophthalmia; Dublin's hospitals, curiously funded; London's Irish enclaves, like others, filthy and full of people. The evils may have defied elimination because gazettes slighted Irish health in the 1860s and scarcely glanced at it in the 1870s. By then, the tales were trite and, more telling, about Gaels in England.

Headlines in the 1880s reminded the reading public that insufficient and insubstantial fare were precursors of dysentery and other disorders. Training of doctors elated one evaluator and, by the 1890s, colleagues were crediting diets and domiciles for greater vitality. The gloomy did not vanish, although their vantage narrowed. Insanity, they averred, was escalating and ignorance, the nemesis of salubrity, not declining. Until knowledge triumphed, they predicted, the unhealthiness of the Irish would continue.

Scotland likewise had no serious coverage until the 1830s. Then, as with Ireland, there was a plea for a poor law at least for the sick and seniors. By the 1840s, when stories were more numerous, the impoverished were in the spotlight. Akin to their southern compatriots, they arrived racked by typhus and by insanity induced by alcohol or need. Whatever their pain, they had few medical resources, to which the death rate of Glasgow youths was said to attest. Fervor for prophylactics was pointless, the righteous raged, when town sanitation and housing were worse than in England.

For the next three decades, opinions about health in Scotland were uninspired and sporadic. In the 1850s, messages about poverty mentioned a mining disaster, heavy drinking, and ongoing insanity and, in the 1860s, the care under and costs of legislation. Rare honors went to the Edinburgh Hospital for Sick Children and a Glasgow eatery, cheap, spotless, and with a nutritious menu, for laborers. By the 1870s, a glimpse of this city's convalescent care accompanied puffery on the virtues of boarding homes over workhouses to rear sturdy youths.

Bulletins of the 1880s and 1890s were not very inventive. Those on the destitute, often in Glasgow, repeated how their meals and accommodations amplified afflictions and how their progeny drooped because of parental cruelty or neglect. Doctors were stars in biographies, individual or group, and in explorations of medical education, past and present, Scottish compared to English and Irish. There was even a retrospective on sixteenth-century remedies. As about Ireland in the 1890s, there was an impression that the march toward health had stalled in Scotland.

Wales was the silent partner in the kingdom. If statistical tables and tenuous surveys did not omit it, contemporaries did not conventionally flag it. Its burgs and jobs, principally coal mining, were incorporated in generic sweeps. Only rarely did journals feature the land, but accounts were neither amazing nor abundant. In the 1850s, talk was of copperworkers and the insane. In the 1870s, tracking colliers' seemingly incessant injuries, one onlooker discovered the dimensions of harm when coalfields had no infirmaries. A confrere toured with a local doctor. These notices demonstrate the importance of coal and the unimportance of the Welsh to nineteenth-century editors.

Any intellectual imbalance between industry and citizenry, which periodicals in part shaped, they in part redressed. By 1900, the press had contributed in no small measure to public consciousness, not only of the scope of sickness, but of its deterrence, perhaps the more valuable legacy.

CHECKLIST OF ARTICLES

AINSWORTH'S MAGAZINE, 1842-1854

Designed as recreational by William Ainsworth, who also directed the *New Monthly Magazine* after 1845, *Ainsworth's* rarely reported on wellness.

1   Ainsworth, W. Francis. "The Cholera in Ireland." 2 (1842): 438-43, 530-35.
     Reminisces about cholera outbreak in Ireland.
2   Raymond, George. " 'Run for the Doctor!' " 8 (1845): 25-32.
     Satirizes doctors in various times and cultures.
3   "Pestilence and the Great Exhibition for 1851." 18 (1850): 519-21.
     Anticipates epidemics due to crowds at the Great Exhibition.
4   Rowsell, E.P., Esq. "A Few Chapters on the Working Classes." 25 (1854): 537-42; 26 (1854): 24-27, 136-40, 262-64, 297-302, 432-34.
     Overview of workers recommends rest for well-being and insurance for debts from illness.

ALL THE YEAR ROUND, 1859-1895

Supplanting *Household Words*, *All the Year Round* retained the format and crusading focus of its forerunner. Captained by Charles Dickens, father and then son, the serial adapted its coverage as dimensions of health developed. Recurrent themes were hospitals and hospices, youthful vigor, and accidents in employment and elsewhere.

5   "Good Qualities of Gout." 1 (1859): 102-05.
Explains physical and psychological reactions of gout victims.
6   "Buying a Practice." 1 (1859): 416-19.
Cautions that some medical practices are not remunerative.
7   "Good Samaritans." 2 (1859-60): 74-76.
Salutes London's Samaritan Free Hospital for Women and Children. Believes that both groups require special treatment.
8   "Poisonous Mushrooms." 2 (1859-60): 175-76.
Distinguishes poisonous from edible mushrooms.
9   "Without a Name." 2 (1859-60): 291-92.
Discusses Bethlehem Hospital from a former patient's vantage.
10   "Infallible Physic." 2 (1859-60): 448-52.
Scoffs at those who promise quick cures for cancer and other afflictions.
11   "Life in Danger." 2 (1859-60): 506-08.
Urges dredging London's Serpentine because its mud traps many bathers.
12   "Good Water." 2 (1859-60): 530-32.
Lists methods, such as boiling, to ensure that water is potable.
13   "Bedside Experiments." 2 (1859-60): 537-42.
Outlines duties and styles of nursing.
14   "Paying the Doctor." 2 (1859-60): 566-68.
Would pay doctors an annual fee to maintain health by preventive advice, as on sanitation.
15   "A Plea for Coal-Miners." 3 (1860): 102-05.
Promotes safety lamps to reduce mine accidents.
16   "An Important Matter." 3 (1860): 270-74.
Endorses smallpox vaccination.
17   "Shipwrecks." 3 (1860): 342-46.
Applauds skills and courage of lifeboat crews after shipwrecks.
18   "Of Right Mind." 3 (1860): 557-59.
Considers insanity in relation to crime.
19   "Sanitary Science." 4 (1860-61): 29-31.
Calls for London sewer improvements.
20   "Poor Law Doctors." 4 (1860-61): 210-11.
Favors higher salaries for poor law doctors if in every district.
21   "Registration of Sickness." 4 (1860-61): 227-28.
Posits that compiling data on illnesses would be useful to combat them.

22   "The Frozen-Out Poor Law." 4 (1860-61): 446-49.
Grumbles that the poor law does not protect any destitute sick.

23   "A New Chamber of Horrors." 4 (1860-61): 500-01.
Deplores that many penniless die from starvation.

24   "The Sick Pauper." 5 (1861): 44-45.
Seeks more comforts in workhouses for all seriously ill, not just those chronically so.

25   "In Peril Underground." 5 (1861): 61-64.
Recites dangers of floods in collieries.

26   "Fire in a Coal-Mine." 5 (1861): 107-10.
Reports on mine explosion.

27   "Children of All Work." 5 (1861): 254-58.
Focuses on health hazards to youths in non-factory jobs, such as lace or nail making.

28   "Dials for the Sea." 5 (1861): 304-06.
Celebrates the invention, by Captain Charles James C. Perry, of navigational device to diminish ship collisions.

29   "Medical Nuts to Crack." 5 (1861): 358-60.
Highlights doctors' difficulties in differentiating between real and feigned symptoms.

30   "Underground London." 5 (1861): 390-94, 413-17, 453-56, 470-73, 486-89.
Opines about London's sewer system.

31   "Growth of a Hospital." 5 (1861): 475-80.
Traces the history of London Fever Hospital, especially its typhus cases. See #52.

32   "Rather Interested in Railways." 6 (1861-62): 17-19.
Reviews laws of compensation in railroad accidents.

33   "London Water." 6 (1861-62): 137-40, 150-53.
Details sources of London water.

34   "A New Disease?" 6 (1861-62): 164-68.
Presents instances of females who, having blackened their eyelids, are thought, or wish to be thought diseased.

35   "The Good Servant: The Bad Master." 6 (1861-62): 323-26.
Suggests ways to prevent injuries from fires, such as dress "fenders" near fireplaces and chimneys for lamps. See #36.

36   "Ladies' Lives." 6 (1861-62): 441-42.
Proposes means to fireproof women's clothes. See #35.

37   "Between the Cradle and the Grave." 6 (1861-62): 454-56.
Lauds hospitals for the young sick. See #1229.

38   "Two Cures for a Pinch." 6 (1861-62): 462-67.
Records the relevance of benefit societies for the sick poor.

39   "The Cost of Coal." 6 (1861-62): 492-96.
        Points out perils of mining.
40   "M.D. and M.A.D." 6 (1861-62): 510-13.
        Questions how doctors determine insanity.
41   "A Mortal Struggle." 6 (1861-62): 542-43.
        Frets about new typhus episode.
42   "Pinchbeck's Cottage." 7 (1862): 31-34.
        Mutters that laborers' cottages are old and unhealthy.
43   "Fanciful Insanity." 7 (1862): 154-55.
        Specifies some signs of insanity.
44   "Bone-Making." 8 (1862-63): 209-11.
        Describes grafting procedures.
45   "Illiberal Doctors." 8 (1862-63): 519-21.
        Opposes attempts by doctors to categorize alternatives, such as
        hypnosis and homeopathy, as quackery.
46   "The Point of the Needle." 10 (1863-64): 36-41.
        Emphasizes seasonal overwork of needlewomen.
47   "Happy Idiots." 11 (1864): 564-69.
        Visitor to an asylum at Earlswood relates impressions of care of
        the mentally challenged.
48   "A Touch of the Gout." 11 (1864): 583-85.
        Ponders symptoms and causes of gout.
49   "The Lives and Deaths of the People." 12 (1864-65): 198-205.
        Approves smallpox vaccination, nutritious diet, and good job
        conditions for wellness.
50   "Workmen's Diseases." 12 (1864-65): 272-75.
        Concentrates on scurvy and skin and lung ailments of printers and
        producers of lead and mirrors.
51   "Number Seven, Brown's-Lane." 12 (1864-65): 304-08.
        Praises London charity that assists the indigent infirm.
52   "A Fight with Fever." 13 (1865): 16-18.
        Honors doctors and nurses of London Fever Hospital. See #31.
53   "Dry Meat." 13 (1865): 79-82.
        Encourages meat preservation so as to increase its intake.
54   "Milk." 13 (1865): 126-31.
        Stresses the importance of milk to health, and condemns its
        adulteration.
55   "The Chemistry of Washing." 13 (1865): 248-53.
        Regards clean apparel as essential to salubrity.
56   "Circumlocutional Vaccination." 13 (1865): 377-78.
        Since other Europeans are adopting smallpox vaccination, wishes
        the British to continue it.

57   "To Smoke, or Not to Smoke?" 13 (1865): 413-18.
      Assesses effects of tobacco on health.
58   "Wine Against Physic." 13 (1865): 521-23.
      Prefers alcohol to drugs as a remedy.
59   "Lightning-Struck." 14 (1865-66): 6-9.
      Notices recent deaths by lightning.
60   "The Fire Brigade." 14 (1865-66): 126-29.
      Links fires to chimney congestion and improper use of matches.
61   "Ill in a Workhouse." 14 (1865-66): 176-79.
      Deprecates facilities, food, and staff in workhouse infirmaries.
62   "Every Man's Poison." 14 (1865-66): 372-76.
      Observes that widespread unsanitary housing contributes to the
      spread of fevers affecting the entire population. See #68.
63   "Village Hospitals." 14 (1865-66): 474-75.
      Asserts that village hospitals are adequate but underutilized by
      ignorant locals.
64   "The Pleasures of Illness." 14 (1865-66): 560-62.
      Cites advantages, such as leisure, reading, and drinking, of being
      a patient.
65   "Children's Dinner-Parties." 15 (1866): 130-34.
      Exhorts readers to support charities for the juvenile sick poor.
66   "A New Humane Society." 15 (1866): 177-80.
      Objects to the ambiance and personnel in workhouse infirmaries,
      particularly practices by men and women attendants.
67   "Inhumane Humanity." 15 (1866): 238-40.
      Argues that vivisection is unjustified to satisfy scientific curiosity
      or to lessen human suffering.
68   "Home, Sweet Home." 15 (1866): 303-06.
      Sanctions the construction of more sanitary housing in order to
      contain disease. See #62.
69   "Touching Englishmen's Lives." 15 (1866): 582-85.
      Avers that London and other large cities have high death rates
      because of substandard sanitation.
70   "The Hole in the Wall." 16 (1866-67): 325-29.
      Broods about railroad accidents because one signalman, on an
      eight-hour shift, controls all traffic at Victoria Station.
71   "In Praise of a Rotten Board." 16 (1866-67): 342-46.
      Satirizes conditions in workhouse infirmaries.
72   "French Treatment of the Drowned." 16 (1866): 475-76.
      Catalogs French methods of resuscitation.
73   "M.D." 16 (1866): 514-16.
      Profiles Dr. Mary Walker as representative of female doctors.

74   "Superstition Dies Hard." 17 (1866-67): 29-31.
        Shows how superstitions can harm health.
75   "London Preserved." 17 (1866-67): 61-66.
        Extols fire brigades in London.
76   "London Fires." 17 (1866-67): 84-88.
        Deals with fire brigades in London.
77   "What Is Sensational?" 17 (1866-67): 221-24.
        Insists that the press does not exaggerate deficiencies of
        workhouse infirmaries.
78   "Lucifer-Box Making." 17 (1866-67): 352-56.
        Alleges that this occupation results in unsanitary habitations but
        not always unhealthy inhabitants.
79   "Licensed to Kill." 18 (1867): 255-58.
        Denounces doctors who buy degrees from foreign schools.
80   "Two Plagues." 18 (1867): 367-69.
        Expects sanitary improvements to slow cholera and tuberculosis.
81   "A Workhouse Probe." 18 (1867): 541-45.
        Faults health care, among other things, in workhouses. See #82.
82   "Another Workhouse Probe." 18 (1867): 558-64.
        Reiterates ideas of #81.
83   "A Country Workhouse." 19 (1867-68): 16-20.
        Declares that the female sick are treated better than are the male
        in some workhouses.
84   "The Butcher." 19 (1867-68): 54-58.
        Posits that the cost of sanitary restrictions on slaughterhouses
        limits the diet of the poor.
85   "Flies." 19 (1867-68): 88-92.
        Includes maladies transmitted by the mosquito.
86   "Called over the Coals." 19 (1867-68): 112-16, 327-31.
        Headlines risks to miners.
87   "The Rack in the Nineteenth Century." 19 (1867-68): 202-04.
        Supposes that excessive gymnastics are detrimental.
88   "Saved from the Sea." 19 (1867-68): 227-28.
        Commends lifeboat groups who rescue the shipwrecked.
89   "Locomotion in London." 19 (1867-68): 295-98.
        Claims that London street accidents, as from carts, injure more
        people than do railroad accidents.
90   "A Discreet Report." 19 (1867-68): 350-54.
        Quotes Dr. Edward Smith, who pressed for competent doctors and
        nurses and effective sanitation in workhouses.
91   "Poison of the Rattlesnake." 19 (1867-68): 372-78.
        Delineates how to counter bites by the rattlesnake.

92   "Pit Accidents." 19 (1867-68): 568-72.
      Covers statistics on and causes of mining injuries and deaths.
93   "Ague and Its Cause." 19 (1867-68): 606-10.
      Associates malaria with marshes.
94   "Foolish Fashions." 20 (1868): 65-68.
      Warns that some fashions, as corsets, are deleterious.
95   "Lightning." 20 (1868): 274-76.
      Says that both cures and fatalities follow lightning strikes.
96   "Painless Operations." 20 (1868): 298-300.
      Elucidates effects of nitrous oxide, ether, and chloroform.
97   "No Communication." 20 (1868): 522-23.
      Tells of railroad car fire.
98   "Canker in the Bud." 20 (1868): 540-44.
      Reveals private efforts to help the ill and abandoned young.
99   Dickens, Charles. "Uncommercial Samples: A Small Star in the
      East." n.s., 1 (1868-69): 61-66.
      Credits East London Children's Hospital for offering good food,
      ventilated rooms, and hygiene to poor youths. See #158.
100   "Good Company for New Year's Day." n.s., 1 (1868-69): 204-08.
      Essay, on children's diseases treated at King's College Hospital,
      London, recognizes medical students' increasing interest in and
      knowledge of ailments and nurses' skills.
101   Dickens, Charles. "New Uncommercial Samples: On an Amateur
      Boat." n.s., 1 (1868-69): 300-03.
      States that lead production is safer for producers.
102   "Sewing Machines." n.s., 1 (1868-69): 394-97.
      Alerts that sewing machines generate overwork for women
      operators whose diets should be adjusted accordingly.
103   "A Plea for Bare Feet." n.s., 1 (1868-69): 402-03.
      Affirms shoelessness as salubrious.
104   "Apparent Death." n.s., 2 (1869): 109-14.
      From French cases, demonstrates that symptoms of death may
      mislead.
105   "Mr. Chaffinch to Mr. Childers." n.s., 2 (1869): 349-52.
      Would move seamen's hospital from ship to land in order to
      expand care.
106   "Fasting Girls." n.s., 2 (1869): 442-44.
      Doubts those who purport to remain well while fasting.
107   "Riding for Health." n.s., 2 (1869): 444-50.
      Advertises the bicycle as good exercise.
108   "Light-Ships." n.s., 2 (1869): 473-75.
      Clarifies the function of titled ships along coasts. See #110.

109   "Getting Better." n.s., 3 (1869-70): 204-08.
        Hails Mrs. [?George] Gladstone whose convalescent homes, with
        volunteers, tend orphans of cholera, then victims of accidents and
        others, such as needy governesses with rheumatism.
110   "Light for Lighthouses." n.s., 3 (1869-70): 282-85.
        Evaluates means to make lighthouses more effective. See #108.
111   "Blind Leaders of the Blind." n.s., 3 (1869-70): 550-52.
        Bases the education of the vision impaired on their experiences.
112   "Parental Rights." n.s., 4 (1870): 348-52.
        Demands aid for abused or neglected children.
113   "Pilots and Pilotage." n.s., 4 (1870): 426-29.
        Would mandate pilot service at all ports to stall accidents.
114   "How the 'Captain' Was Lost." n.s., 4 (1870): 493-97.
        Classifies turret ships as unsafe.
115   "Poisonous Fishes." n.s., 5 (1870-71): 366-72.
        Depicts fish, not exclusively British, that poison on ingestion or
        by bite.
116   "Sleepers and Somnambulists." n.s., 6 (1871): 6-10.
        Tracks somnambulists' activities.
117   "Double People." n.s., 6 (1871): 103-05.
        Explicates the physiology and appearance of joined twins.
118   "Alcoholic Drinks." n.s., 8 (1872): 88-92.
        Defends moderate consumption of alcohol, chiefly wine, beer, and
        cider, as healthful.
119   "A Foggy Subject." n.s., 8 (1872): 175-81.
        Chronicles fog signals along coasts.
120   "Shoddy, Chalk, and Jonathan." n.s., 8 (1872): 246-49.
        Protests the adulteration of flour by sawdust (Jonathan) and of
        calico by used wool and clay, the last harming spinners' lungs.
121   "Mad Dogs." n.s., 8 (1872): 300-04.
        Enumerates signs of rabies. Would check it by a dog tax rather
        than by muzzling.
122   "Sea-Sickness." n.s., 8 (1872): 342-46.
        Surveys origins of and remedies for seasickness.
123   "Seaweeds." n.s., 8 (1872): 366-70.
        Relays curative power of some types of seaweed.
124   "Overwork? Or Overworry?" n.s., 8 (1872): 605-07.
        Postulates that stress is more likely to cause death than is
        overwork.
125   "Remedies for Hydrophobia." n.s., 9 (1872-73): 17-20.
        Because of the failure of researchers to find an antidote for rabies,
        counsels fewer contacts with dogs.

126 "Wallsend Coals." n.s., 9 (1872-73): 154-57.
Publicizes risks of mining, such as explosions and floods.

127 "A Lunatic Ball." n.s., 9 (1872-73): 349-52.
Sketches a dance at Hanwell Lunatic Asylum.

128 "Old Edinburgh Doctors." n.s., 9 (1872-73): 389-93.
Admires late eighteenth-century Scottish doctors.

129 "A Day in a London Hospital." n.s., 9 (1872-73): 437-43.
Tour of London insititution has some asides on youthful patients, as those who have had plastic surgery.

130 "Health in Town and Country." n.s., 10 (1873): 388-93.
Based on data of Registrar-General, concludes that suburbs are not healthier than towns.

131 "My Friend the Mad-Doctor." n.s., 10 (1873): 469-76.
Interview with a specialist encompasses causes and forms of and treatments for insanity.

132 "Imaginative Medicine." n.s., 10 (1873): 520-24.
Itemizes numerous folk therapies.

133 "Mushroom Gossip." n.s., 11 (1873-74): 437-40.
Measures the jeopardy from mushroom poisoning.

134 "Forgetting a Language." n.s., 11 (1873-74): 464-67.
Avows that a variety of afflictions and accidents can spawn amnesia.

135 "From Gay to Grave." n.s., 11 (1873-74): 488-92.
Contrasts Valentine festivities and patient life in French Hospital, London.

136 "An Inside View." n.s., 12 (1874): 340-44.
Recounts throat examination at Central London Throat and Ear Hospital.

137 "Railway Suicides." n.s., 12 (1874): 400-04.
Propounds reasons for railroad mishaps and suicides.

138 "Winter Resorts for Invalids." n.s., 13 (1874-75): 270-74.
Predicts that winter at the seaside or in some milder climate (Mediterranean or Madeira) will forestall or abate lung diseases.

139 "Scientific Aspects of Nutrition." n.s., 13 (1874-75): 414-20.
Analyzes the worth of alcohol and drugs, as cocaine, and the nutritiousness of several nations' diets.

140 "South Wales Colliers." n.s., 14 (1875): 52-58.
Biography of Welsh miners mentions that, notwithstanding their history of job injuries, no hospital exists in the coalfields.

141 "Left-Handed People." n.s., 14 (1875): 136-40.
Spotlights left and right brain activities in relation to brain disorders.

142   "Legs: Wooden and Otherwise." n.s., 14 (1875): 463-67.
        Remarks on the utility and design of prostheses.
143   "The Royal College of Surgeons." n.s., 14 (1875): 496-501.
        Proceeds from the College's early days to its current actions with
        respect to certification.
144   "A Kitchen for the Sick." n.s., 15 (1875-76): 15-19.
        Features St. Mary's Kitchen, London, which prepares, on doctors'
        orders, meals for convalescents.
145   "What We Drink." n.s., 15 (1875-76): 77-80.
        Judges merits of sundry wines and coffee and tea.
146   "Human Longevity." n.s., 15 (1875-76): 366-70.
        Attributes longevity to heredity and avoidance of doctors.
147   "Hygienic Precepts." n.s., 16 (1876): 224-29.
        Identifies common sense as the root of wellness.
148   "The Rule of the Road." n.s., 16 (1876): 413-16.
        Studies anti-collision regulations for ships.
149   "Blind Guy Fawkes." n.s., 17 (1876-77): 255-58.
        Concentrates on training the vision impaired to read braille and to
        write.
150   "Fresh Meat Ahead." n.s., 17 (1876-77): 495-98.
        Fixes on cold storage to protect foreign meat from spoilage.
151   "At Sea with the Doctor." n.s., 17 (1876-77): 514-19.
        Reminds doctors of their responsibilities for health maintainence
        and attendance to the ailing.
152   "Weighed in the Balance." n.s., 18 (1877): 12-17.
        Accuses overseas dependencies of exporting adulterated food.
153   "Unintended Blazes of Triumph." n.s., 18 (1877): 199-203.
        Fears fires in badly constructed theatres. See #159.
154   "Early Workers at Vestas." n.s., 18 (1877): 352-57.
        Despises working conditions of juveniles who manufacture
        matches.
155   "In the Silent World." n.s., 18 (1877): 515-21.
        Expounds on the teaching, by lip and sign, of the hearing
        impaired.
156   "Whimsical Ideas, Sanitary and Otherwise." n.s., 19 (1877-78):
        566-68.
        Refers to ideas, in unnamed study by a 'Social Improver,' on how
        to stay well.
157   "The Seaside in Spring." n.s., 20 (1878): 415-20.
        Has a few words on the salubriousness of coastal locations.
158   "A Small Star in the West." n.s., 21 (1878): 11-15.
        Esteems London hospitals for impoverished children. See #99.

159 "Panic and Panics." n.s., 21 (1878): 512-16.
Recalls that sounds of fire could so panic a crowd as to end in fatalities. See #153.

160 "Some Popular Cures." n.s., 22 (1878-79): 250-54.
Glances at diverse folk restoratives.

161 "About Teeth." n.s., 22 (1878-79): 320-24.
Probes some popular correctives for toothache.

162 "The Young Deaf and Dumb at Lessons." n.s., 22 (1878-79): 371-77.
Portrays learning programs for the hearing impaired who are children under the age of nine and do not speak.

163 "Cremation." n.s., 23 (1879): 127-31.
Repeats the notion of proponents of cremation, among them doctors, that it advances public health.

164 "The Visitor's Hour." n.s., 23 (1879): 350-56.
Juxtaposes hospital visitors' news, food, and anxiety and patients' depression after departure. Additionally, pushes for donations to hospitals.

165 "A Deaf and Dumb Debate." n.s., 24 (1879-80): 20-24.
Apprises audience of how the hearing impaired communicate in sign language.

166 "Very Cruel Beer." n.s., 24 (1879-80): 271-74.
Discloses the danger of drinking adulterated beer.

167 "Convalescent Hospitals." n.s., 24 (1879-80): 325-31.
Article on the growth of convalescent institutions opts for cottage rather than large hospitals.

168 "Hospital Sketches." n.s., 24 (1879-80): 516-21.
Ruminates about wrongly-taken medications, unsick patients, and the need for better nurses in hospitals and some dreaded diseases, such as rabies and tetanus.

169 "A Home Hospital." n.s., 25 (1880): 175-81.
Discovers a hospital for the well-to-do middle class heretofore apparently deprived of such ministration.

170 "Domesticated Moonshine." n.s., 25 (1880): 326-31.
Envisions that illuminated paint in mines and railroad tunnels and on buoys would decrease land and sea accidents. See #175.

171 "Hospital Out-Patients: Their Waiting-Time." n.s., 26 (1880-81): 223-28.
Picture of waiting rooms for outpatients underlines that they are treated without fee.

172 "The Blind at Gymnastics." n.s., 27 (1881): 201-06.
Respects the skills in various exercises of the vision impaired.

173   "Hospital Work." n.s., 27 (1881): 497-99.
       Contends that because London hospitals are overcrowded, long-
       term patients do not have bed rest and good nursing. Appeals for
       improvement of workhouse infirmaries and for sick clubs for the
       "respectable poor."
174   "Among the Mines and Miners." n.s., 28 (1881-82): 179-83.
       Documents colliers' unhealthy living and working situations.
175   "Saving Life at Sea." n.s., 29 (1882): 512-14.
       Inventories maritime lifesaving devices, among them lifeboats and
       buoys. See #170.
176   "Christmas at Brompton." n.s., 31 (1883): 28-33.
       Journeys to a hospital for those with tuberculosis.
177   "Surveying and Inspecting of Old and To-Day." n.s., 31 (1883):
       101-06.
       Ratifies new sanitation, principally sewers.
178   "Before the Hospital Fire." n.s., 31 (1883): 509-13.
       Characterizes cooking for special diets in University College
       Hospital, London.
179   "Letters to a Country Doctor." n.s., 32 (1883): 161-63.
       Reprints show common ailments and medications of the poor.
180   "Davos am Platz." n.s., 32 (1883): 377-79.
       Would send tuberculosis sufferers to Davos because of its air.
181   "Little Sisters." n.s., 33 (1883-84): 156-59.
       Reveres Little Sisters of the Poor because they succor the aged and
       ill poor.
182   "Our Playgrounds." n.s., 35 (1884-85): 341-46.
       Backs projects of Playground Association for juvenile health.
183   "The Terrors of the School." n.s., 36 (1885): 438-41.
       Decries beatings of students by peers and teachers.
184   "Some Famous Doctors." n.s., 37 (1885-86): 444-50.
       Commemorates British doctors from the sixteenth through the
       nineteenth centuries. See #187.
185   "Diet and Dyspepsia." n.s., 37 (1885-86): 545-48.
       Indicates how to have a wholesome diet and how to avoid
       dyspepsia.
186   "The Children's Holiday." n.s., 38 (1886): 418-20.
       Sponsors groups that brought sickly urban youths to the country
       for holidays.
187   "Some More about Doctors." n.s., 38 (1886): 470-75.
       Echoes #184.
188   "Living out of Tins." n.s., 39 (1886-87): 565-68.
       Assumes that tinned food could supply nutrition cheaply.

189   "Knights of the Wheel." n.s., 40 (1887): 34-36.
Boosts tricycling as good exercise that also carries people to places with cleaner air.

190   "Fire!" n.s., 40 (1887): 297-300.
Guides escapes from burning buildings by using chutes or crawling close to the floor. Acclaims fire brigades.

191   "Lifeboat Work." n.s., 40 (1887): 394-98.
Prizes lifeboat crews, but regrets that some seamen still die because of inadequate communication between stations.

192   "Hospital Life in East London." n.s., 41 (1887): 9-14.
Silhouettes the ailing, rich and poor, young, and outpatient, and their nurses and doctors.

193   "An Invalid's Grievance." n.s., 41 (1887): 442-44.
Imagines that in novels sickness magnifies invalids' talents.

194   "Brewers and Others." n.s., 41 (1887): 466-68.
Detects that citizens are drinking lighter ales and mineral water.

195   "The Outcasts' Havens." n.s., 42 (1888): 30-33.
Appreciates homes that feed and clothe abandoned waifs.

196   "The Gordon Boys' Home." n.s., 42 (1888): 225-30.
Talks about Chobham institution where boys thrive on hearty meals and country air.

197   "A Night's Lodging." n.s., 42 (1888): 364-67.
Investigates conditions in lodging houses.

198   "A Chat about Clothes." n.s., 42 (1888): 389-92.
Connects well-being to attire.

199   "Curiosities of Suicide." n.s., 43 (1888): 546-48.
Reflects on some ways to commit suicide in London.

200   "The Somers Town Blind Aid Society." n.s., 43 (1888): 615-16.
Stars a society that befriends the vision impaired, some of whom also are hearing impaired or have epilepsy.

201   "The Children's Bread." 3d ser., 1 (1889): 58-61.
Champions day industrial schools that, with some parental money, nourish and train youths. Would have the state give food to the offspring of "worthy poor" temporarily unable to feed them.

202   "Some Fogs." 3d ser., 1 (1889): 78-81.
Underscores how fogs, from industry and climate, are baneful.

203   "Vegetarian Dinners." 3d ser., 1 (1889): 174-77.
Irrespective of the abundance of vegetables and vegetarian recipes, rules that vegetarianism is deleterious for most persons except occasionally.

204   "Somnambulism." 3d ser., 2 (1889): 6-9.
Confirms, by cases, how somnabulism alters memory. See #205.

205   "Some Phenomena of Memory." 3d ser., 2 (1889): 78-82.
       Seconds the theme of #204.
206   "Pigmies." 3d ser., 2 (1889): 82-86.
       Essay on dwarfism does not equate it with disability.
207   "Alternate Consciousness." 3d ser., 2 (1889): 153-56.
       Concerns consciousness between sleeping and waking, in the
       seasons, and of the insane.
208   "Oddities of Eating and Drinking." 3d ser., 2 (1889): 420-26.
       Chooses ingenious diets over ordinary, often adulterated foods.
209   "Noise." 3d ser., 2 (1889): 474-76.
       Whines that London noises disturb the sleep crucial for fitness.
210   "Rest and Unrest." 3d ser., 2 (1889): 569-73.
       Proposes restful vacations for vitality.
211   "The Romance of a Vegetable." 3d ser., 2 (1889): 605-09.
       Proclaims onion juice a remedy for scurvy, skin diseases, and hair
       loss.
212   "On Professional Irresponsibility." 3d. ser., 3 (1890): 257-61.
       Censures, among others, bungling doctors and manufacturers of
       poisonous goods.
213   "Giantology." 3d ser., 3 (1890): 415-19.
       Compared to those with dwarfism, those with gigantism are
       purportedly "sickly, knock-kneed," and even mentally challenged.
214   "Longevity." 3d ser., 4 (1890): 202-05.
       Realizes that reasons for long life are unknown.
215   "The Career of Invalid." 3d ser., 5 (1891): 175-79.
       Spotlights those who travel because they are victims of some
       malady.
216   "Sunday in Hospital." 3d ser., 6 (1891): 91-93.
       Converses about hospitals and their visitors.
217   "A Real Free Hospital." 3d ser., 6 (1891): 301-06.
       Compliments Royal Free Hospital, London, for its patient care and
       its instruction of doctors and nurses. Accepts female doctors for
       practice in India.
218   "Historic Epidemics." 3d ser., 7 (1892): 228-32.
       Admits that influenza is a serious threat to health but not cholera
       because many British cities have pure water.
219   "Street Accidents." 3d ser., 8 (1892): 496-500.
       Announces that ambulance services are multiplying in proportion
       to injuries due to road construction, bad weather, and speeding, so
       calls for subways at dangerous crossings.
220   "A Visit to a London Eye Hospital." 3d ser., 9 (1893): 251-56.
       Summarizes some cases at Royal Eye Hospital.

221 "Municipal and Other Lodgings." 3d ser., 9 (1893): 276-79.
Fosters the trend toward cleanliness in modern housing.
222 "Professional Football." 3d ser., 10 (1893): 558-62.
Text on the game does not omit injuries to players.
223 "A New Food-Material." 3d ser., 12 (1894): 346-48.
Lectures about nutritional value of peanuts.
224 "Notes on Familiar Food." 3d ser., 13 (1895): 7-13.
Incorporates numerous topics, such as the merits of ingesting eggs and alcohol.
225 "Dust and Hygiene." 3d ser., 13 (1895): 154-58.
Ties bacteria in dust to skin, respiratory, and digestive ailments. Would flush homes and streets with water.
226 "In the Land of Nails and Chains." 3d ser., 13 (1895): 179-81.
Accents noxious circumstances in nail and chain fabrication.
227 "Health." 3d ser., 13 (1895): 250-55.
Defines health as being moral and sound of body and mind. Joins most disorders to digestion. Holds that doctors, their medicines, and sanitation are no more helpful than living in moderation.

BENTLEY'S MISCELLANY, 1837-1868

Started by Richard Bentley for the diversion of subscribers of some wealth and learning, and held by William Ainsworth from 1854 to 1857, *Bentley's* offered occasional pieces on salubrity.

228 Poyntz, Albany [Catherine Gore]. "The Children of the Mobility versus the Children of the Nobility." 9 (1841): 164-67.
Suspects that heirs of the wealthy are victims of improper clothing and insufficient exercise.
229 [Forrester, C.R.]. "The Philosophy of Physic." 11 (1842): 335-44.
Ridicules remedies of doctors and others.
230 Smith, Albert. "Popular Zoology." 19 (1846): 316-32, 404-12, 512-19, 574-81; 20 (1846), 76-82.
Scrutinizes various occupations, among them the country doctor.
231 [Boissier, G.R.]. "The Proper Food of Man." 28 (1850): 428-29.
Mulls over books by John Smith on nutrition, and Spencer Thompson, M.D., on the hazards of liquor.
232 "Cretins and Their Benefactors." 31 (1852): 405-12.
Contemplates, in an international context, the occurrence and treatment of a syndrome of dwarfism.

233   [Cooper, William White]. "Chloroform." 34 (1853): 33-42.
       Elucidates effects of chloroform and its uses in surgery.
234   "The Water Cure." 36 (1854): 640-42.
       Recapitulates notions of James Watson, M.D., on hydropathy.
235   *"Sudden Death."* 36 (1854): 642.
       Parrots a book by A.B. Granville, M.D., on the frequency of
       sudden deaths with no known causes.
236   [Jacox, Francis]. "Mingle-Mangle by Monkshood: Mal de Mer."
       48 (1860): 52-65.
       Copes with seasickness.
237   Andrews, Alexander. "A Town Full of Mad People." 55 (1864):
       179-92.
       Ruminates about the insane in asylums.
238   "Mushrooms." 60 (1866): 412-22.
       Alludes to perils of eating some mushroom types.
239   "Watercresses." 60 (1866): 485-93.
       Assures that watercress is nutritious.

BLACKWOOD'S EDINBURGH MAGAZINE, 1824-1900

Created by William Blackwood, this Tory organ had no slant toward
Scotland on matters of vitality. Common columns dealt with anatomy and
alcohol.

240   "Notice Respecting Mr. Broster's Newly Discovered System for
       the Removal of Impediments of Speech and Defective
       Articulation." 17 (1825): 46-47.
       Introduces John Broster, of Chester, who explores problems of the
       speech impaired.
241   [Gooch, Robert]. "Protestant Sisters of Charity." 18 (1825): 732-
       35.
       Advocates Protestant nurses, supervised by doctors, with books
       on how to practice and knowledge tested by frequent quizzes, as
       alternatives to apothecaries in counties. Distrusts sisters motivated
       only by money, "scientific zeal," or humanity.
242   [Gooch, Robert]. *"The Quarterly Review* of Dr. Macmichael on
       Contagion and the Plague." 19 (1826): 130-31.
       Classifies plague as contagious. See #2109.
243   [Wilson, John]. "Health and Longevity." 23 (1828): 96-111.
       Counts diet and exercise as significant for longevity.

244   [Wilson, John]. *"Anatomy of Drunkenness."* 23 (1828): 481-99.
Synopsizes, from a book by Robert Macnish, aspects of alcoholism.
245   [Robinson, David]. "The Poor Laws." 23 (1828): 923-36.
Validates a poor law for many reasons, among them relief of the ill and elderly.
246   [Alison, Archibald]. "Ireland." 33 (1833): 66-87, 223-42, 338-57, 561-82.
Narrative on Ireland touches on a poor law to sustain the sick and seniors.
247   [Wilson, John]. "The Factory System." 33 (1833): 419-50.
Exposes how detrimental the factory is for children and how machines endanger employees of all ages.
248   [Wilson, John]. "On Poor's [sic] Laws, and Their Introduction into Ireland." 33 (1833): 811-43.
Authorizes a poor law for Ireland to save, from starvation and disease, the large indigent population traditionally exploited by landlords.
249   [Alison, William P.]. "Evils of the State of Ireland." 40 (1836): 495-514.
Licenses an Irish poor law. Couples regularity of epidemics in Ireland and natives' inferior food and clothing.
250   [Eagles, John]. "Medical Attendance, and Other Parochials. By a Curate in a Letter to a Friend." 41 (1837): 629-42.
Remembers parishioners with illnesses, as cancer and fever, and their resort to charlatans and folk remedies.
251   [Murray, J.F.]. "The Lungs of London." 46 (1839): 212-27.
Chapter on London parks adds them to sufficient sewerage and purer water as priorities to combat persistent typhus and irregular cholera.
252   Tomkins [John Warner]. "Tea-Totalism [sic] and Total Abstinence." 48 (1840): 214-19.
Represents alcohol as medicinal and not more deleterious than polluted air and water.
253   [Alison, Archibald]. "Social and Moral Condition of the Manufacturing Districts in Scotland." 50 (1841): 659-73.
From census data, decides that typhus spreads quickly among the destitute and that their alcohol intake is substantial in Scotland.
254   [Sowler, Robert]. "Revolt of the Workers. The Employer and the Employed." 52 (1842): 642-53.
Study of recent workers' rioting has some words on unhealthy housing.

255   [Grove, William]. "Mesmerism." 57 (1845): 219-41.
        Perusal of instances of hypnosis reckons that evidence of its
        effects on the body is incomplete.
256   [Brady, J.D.]. "Ireland - Its Condition - The Life and Property Bill
        - The Debate, and the Famine." 59 (1846): 572-603.
        History of Irish peasantry denies that they are starving during the
        Famine.
257   [Aytoun, W.E.]. "Mesmeric Mountebanks." 60 (1846): 223-37.
        After watching a hypnotist perform, notes circumstances when
        hypnosis may be salutary.
258   [Gordon, J.T.]. "The Water-Cure." 60 (1846): 376-88.
        Disputes curative power of water but not its value as an
        alternative to liquor and for cleanliness.
259   Johnston, Professor [J.F.W.]. "On the Nutritive Qualities of the
        Bread Now in Use." 61 (1847): 768-72.
        Advertises whole meal bread as better for nutrition and digestion
        than white.
260   [Neaves, Charles]. "Highland Destitution." 62 (1847): 630-42.
        Paraphrases extensively *Observations on the Famine of 1846-7 in
        the Highlands of Scotland and in Ireland*, by W.P. Alison, M.D.,
        about the impact of the potato famine in Scotland.
261   [Alison, William P.]. "On the Miseries of Ireland, and Their
        Remedies." 64 (1848): 658-71.
        Tableau of Irish distress nods to lack of sanitation and
        overcrowded dwellings.
262   [Warren, Samuel]. "Modern State Trials." 68 (1850): 373-92, 545-
        72, 712-35; 69 (1851): 461-88, 733-47.
        Part II of an abstract of *Modern State Trials*, by William C.
        Townsend, Esq., is on insanity as a criminal defense.
263   [Eagles, John]. "What Is Mesmerism?" 70 (1851): 70-83.
        Attributes instances of hypnosis to the subject's physical or
        mental weakness.
264   [Johnston, J.F.W.]. "The Narcotics We Indulge In." 74 (1853):
        129-39, 605-28, 678-95.
        Warrants that tobacco, opium, cannabis, cocaine, thorn apple,
        lettuce, and peppergrass are not hazardous in small amounts. See
        #265 and #269.
265   [Johnston, J.F.W.]. "The Beverages We Infuse." 75 (1854): 86-
        112.
        Spells out the growth and properties of coffee, tea, and cocoa and
        their worth, coffee and tea as digestives and cocoa as a relaxant.
        See #264 and #269.

266   [Smith, William Henry]. *"The Epidemics of the Middle Ages."* 75 (1854): 352-66.
Excerpts, from a book by J.F.C. Harrison, M.D., episodes of plague and chorea.

267   [Smith, William Henry]. *"Psychological Inquiries."* 77 (1855): 402-20.
Text by Sir Benjamin Brodie inspires paragraphs on the brain, mainly in relation to memory and the nervous system.

268   [Johnston, J.F.W.]. "The Length of Human Life." 77 (1855): 499-508.
Plumbs the physiology and psychology of aging.

269   [Patterson, R.H.]. "Professor Johnston's Last Work." 78 (1855): 548-61.
Condenses concepts of J.F.W. Johnston as exhibited in #264 and #265.

270   [Burton, J.H.]. "Drinking and Smoking." 79 (1856): 103-14.
Countenances in moderation tobacco and alcohol but not earlier excessive drinking or contemporary teetotalism.

271   [Lewes, George Henry]. "Phrenology in France." 82 (1857): 665-74.
Brands phrenology inappropriate to understand psychology, physiology, or character, but theorizes that exceptions to its principal theorems might lead to penetration of brain functions and diseases.

272   [Lewes, George Henry]. "Hunger and Thirst." 83 (1858): 1-17.
Itemizes physical effects, as apparent coma and emaciation, of rationing the intake of water and food.

273   [Lewes, George Henry]. "Food and Drink." 83 (1858): 325-43, 402-15, 515-25.
Series on the physiology of eating articulates the nutritive value of many foods, notably milk. See #281.

274   [Lewes, George Henry]. "Blood." 83 (1858): 687-702.
Looks at the composition, functions, and transfusion of blood. See #275.

275   [Lewes, George Henry]. "Circulation of the Blood: Its Course and History." 84 (1858): 148-64.
Records past research on blood circulation and the tie between its process and rate and wellness. See #274.

276   [Lewes, George Henry]. "Respiration and Suffocation." 84 (1858): 296-312.
Describes respiration in several species and incidents of human suffocation.

277   [Lewes, George Henry]. "Animal Heat." 84 (1858): 414-30.
       Analysis of body temperature factors in age, sex, food intake, and
       respiration and circulation rates.

278   [Burton, J.H.]. "Mephitis and the Antidote." 85 (1859): 222-39.
       Overview on sanitation spans London sewers, housing of the poor,
       and the impact of Edwin Chadwick.

279   [Lewes, George Henry]. "Voluntary and Involuntary Actions." 86
       (1859): 295-306.
       Piece on muscles speculates that all involuntary activity can be
       mastered.

280   [Lewes, George Henry]. "Great Wits, Mad Wits?" 88 (1860): 302-
       11.
       Rejects the hypothesis of Dr. J. Moreau that genius and insanity
       are correlatives.

281   Lewes, George Henry. "Theories of Food." 88 (1860): 676-87.
       Responds to critics of ideas about food and drink. See #273.

282   [Lewes, George Henry]. "Mad Dogs." 90 (1861): 222-40.
       Focuses on symptoms and cases of rabies.

283   [Aytoun, W.E.]. "Meditations on Dyspepsia." 90 (1861): 302-22,
       406-19.
       Ascribes dyspepsia to irregular hours of sleep, lack of exercise,
       and improper fare. Glances at conventional neutralizers, as bathing
       and drinking mineral water.

284   [Collins, W. Lucas]. "Burton's *Anatomy of Melancholy*." 90
       (1861): 323-42.
       Captures Robert Burton's thoughts on the causes of and cures for
       melancholia.

285   [Lewes, George Henry]. "Physicians and Quacks." 91 (1862): 165-
       78.
       Avows that medical knowledge is still imperfect because of the
       complex origins of many diseases. Presumes physicians, because
       of their education and experience, to be more helpful to the ailing
       than are frauds with their certitude about recovery but not more
       than those offering atypical treatments, as homeopathy or
       hydropathy.

286   [Chambers, T.K.]. "The Renewal of Life." 91 (1862): 596-604.
       Cites coronary problems, colds, and anemia to validate how illness
       weakens the body.

287   [Aytoun, W.E.]. "Watering-Places." 92 (1862): 261-85.
       Glimpse of spas, primarily German, paints them as restorative.

288   [Boys, Thomas]. "Constitutional Tendencies." 93 (1863): 684-90.
       Parades people who deem themselves ill though apparently well.

289 [Aytoun, W.E.]. "Banting on Corpulence." 96 (1864): 607-17.
Challenges William Banting's diet as neither universally suitable
nor nutritionally sound.

290 [Mackay, Charles]. "Intemperance and Intolerance." 102 (1867):
208-20.
Vetoes Maine Liquor Law and similar temperance legislation.
Agrees that alcohol in excess is bad for health.

291 [Oliphant, Margaret]. "A City of the Plague." 102 (1867): 452-61.
Memorializes recent cholera epidemic in Albano, Italy.

292 [Mozley, Anne]. "Vapours, Fears, and Tremors." 105 (1869): 228-
37.
Epitomizes how stress, preeminently in women, is pernicious and
results in fainting.

293 [Skelton, John]. "Scotland in Parliament: The Poor-Law Inquiry."
106 (1869): 631-46.
Essay on Scottish poor relief prices care of the sick.

294 [Moncreiff, Henry J.]. "Dangerous Shots." 124 (1878): 572-75.
Delves into shooting accidents.

295 [Marshall, Frederic]. "Suicide." 127 (1880): 719-35.
Logs reasons for and methods of suicide.

296 [Pringle, R.O.]. "Irish Distress and Its Origin." 128 (1880): 244-
55.
Testifies that the Irish are susceptible to illness because of
improper diet.

297 [Hardy, H. Nelson]. "Proposed Medical Legislation." 135 (1884):
356-63.
Resists government interference in the medical profession as
dangerous to patient health and demeaning to doctors. See #298.

298 [Hardy, H. Nelson]. "The Government Medical Bill: A Radical
Cure." 135 (1884): 665-72.
Prolongs the message of #297.

299 [Oliphant, Margaret]. "A Scotch Physician." 138 (1885): 669-90.
Samples the autobiography of a Scot, Sir Robert Christison, M.D.

300 [Lewes, C.L.]. "The Need of Open Spaces." 141 (1887): 446-50.
Pairs more parks in London and good health.

301 Shand, Alex[ander] Innes. "The Pleasures of Sickness." 145
(1889): 546-56.
Conveys patients' enjoyment of being pampered.

302 [White, T. Pilkington]. "Modern Mannish Maidens." 147 (1890):
252-64.
Endorses some sports, as riding, rowing, skating, tennis,
badminton, and golf, as beneficial to women's health and grace.

303   DeFerro, A[nne]. "The Worishofen Water-Cure and Pfarrer
        Kneipp." 148 (1890): 816-28.
        Vaunts water cure of German pastor, Sebastian Kneipp.
304   Farquharson, Robert. "The Case for Moderate Drinking." 151
        (1892): 788-801.
        Controverts that the consumption of liquor is always baneful.
305   Shand, Alex[ander] Innes. "Aberdeen and Aberdeen Doctors." 153
        (1893): 425-40.
        Draws from words of Ella Hill Burton Roger on Aberdeen doctors.
306   Stewart, T. Grainger. "Notes on Scottish Medicine in the Days of
        Queen Mary." 153 (1893): 885-92.
        Recalls sixteenth-century afflictions and correctives of the Scots.
307   Robinson, Louis. "On Acquired Facial Expressions." 155 (1894):
        536-42.
        Scans muscles and nerves of the face.
308   Rawnsley, H.D. "The Village of Perfect Health: Leysin-sur-
        Aigle." 158 (1895): 680-84.
        Boasts that a sojourn in this Swiss village would heal diverse
        disorders.
309   [Collins, W.E.W.]. "My Friends Who Cycle." 159 (1896): 883-91.
        Notifies audience of injuries from bicycling.
310   Stewart, T. Grainger. "Our Duty in Regard to Vaccination." 160
        (1896): 703-14.
        Would compel smallpox vaccination.
311   [Steevens, George Warrington]. "The New Humanitarianism." 163
        (1898): 98-106.
        Meditates on the influence of humanitarians with respect to
        hospitals and smallpox vaccination.
312   [Burgess, R.J.]. "Physical Education in Schools." 165 (1899): 573-
        80.
        Discourses about rewards of exercise to youthful scholars.

THE BRITISH AND FOREIGN REVIEW, 1835-1844

Exhibiting bias only for betterment, the *British and Foreign* scattered
few but substantial items on wellness throughout its pages.

313   [French, Fitzjames]. "A Poor-Law for Ireland." 6 (1838): 338-71.
        Broadcasts that the Irish, without a poor law, have more fevers
        lately because of less food.

314 "Medical Reform." 11 (1840): 210-24.
Would abolish alternative ways for doctors' accreditation.
315 [?Harris, George]. "Phrenology: Combe's *Constitution of Man.*"
12 (1841): 142-80.
Acknowledges the validity of phrenology but not of George Combe's concepts.
316 [Banfield, Thomas Charles]. "State of the Nation: *Handloom Weavers' Report.*" 13 (1842): 111-62.
Points out perils of weaving and advantages of including exercise in any school program.
317 "Oriental Plague - Quarantine Laws." 13 (1842): 442-58.
Guesses that the plague is not contagious so quarantines are futile and oppressive.
318 [Harris, George]. "The Plea of Insanity in Criminal Cases: The Criminality of the Insane." 15 (1843): 152-69.
Story on insanity as a criminal defense apprehends some difficulties of diagnosis.

THE BRITISH QUARTERLY REVIEW, 1845-1886

Aimed at a nonconformist audience of middling rank, the *British Quarterly* concentrated on the plethora of pains of the municipal poor.

319 [Baines, Edward]. "The Factory System and Factory Legislation." 1 (1845): 117-57.
Foe of factory legislation would not standardize hours since there is no proof that long days are detrimental to employees.
320 [Skae, David]. "Animal Magnetism and Ghost-Seeing." 2 (1845): 402-27.
Divulges physical symptoms of those with visions of ghosts.
321 [Skae, David]. "Phrenology." 4 (1846): 397-419.
Queries the value of phrenology in the study of insanity.
322 [Smith, Robert A.]. "Supplies of Water." 4 (1846): 427-43.
Brackets insufficient or contaminated water and illness.
323 *"Moral Aspects of Medical Life."* 5 (1847): 186-206.
Abridges opinions of Professor K.F.H. Marx on medical training and practice.
324 [Godkin, James]. "Ireland and Its Famine." 5 (1847): 504-40.
Text on the "condition-of-Ireland" yokes unhealthiness and starvation during the potato famine.

325   "Sanitary Reform." 9 (1849): 41-70.
        Imputes maladies, notably fevers, to little sewerage, inadequate
        water, and improper ventilation.

326   [Beard, J.R.]. "Factory Life - *Mary Barton*." 9 (1849): 117-36.
        Contradicts novel's theme that factories are debilitating.

327   [Dauglish, John]. "Thoughts on the Labour Question." 14 (1851):
        67-87.
        Disquisition on workers assigns their alcoholism to poverty.

328   "The Smoke Nuisance - Its Cause and Cure." 25 (1857): 47-62.
        Labels air polluted by smoke unsalutary.

329   [Leifchild, J.R.]. "Coal Mines and Their Accidents." 25 (1857):
        86-110.
        Exhibits hazards of mining.

330   "Physical and Moral Heritage." 29 (1859): 3-56.
        Article on heredity sees it as a prerequisite for some physical and
        mental ailments.

331   [Spencer, Herbert]. "Physical Training." 29 (1859): 362-97.
        Marks diet, clothing, exercise, and education as crucial for
        juvenile vigor.

332   "Phases of London Life." 35 (1862): 341-66.
        Entry on crime marginalizes the venereal diseases of prostitutes
        and their patrons.

333   "Mind and Brain." 40 (1864): 440-63.
        Compendium on functions and malfunctions of the brain and
        nervous system impugns merits of phrenology.

334   [Anstie, Francis E.]. "British Epidemics." 43 (1866): 29-60.
        Singles out a multitude of communicable diseases allegedly
        accelerated by lack of sanitation.

335   "Our Poor Law Administration." 47 (1868): 297-326.
        Tract on the poor law bemoans treatment of the destitute sick.

336   [Torrens, W.T.M.]. "Artizans' Dwellings." 51 (1870): 343-61.
        Forwards better housing to improve workers' well-being.

337   [Conder, Francis R.]. "Report of the Commissioners on Coal." 56
        (1872): 66-98.
        Dissertation on the coal industry discerns how detrimental mining
        is for miners.

338   [Conder, Francis R.]. "The Public Health." 58 (1873): 29-60.
        Designates difficulties in developing an efficient national
        sewerage system and dangers of communicable diseases without
        one.

339   [Browne, J.H. Balfour]. "*Sin and Madness*." 62 (1875): 114-26.
        Reviews Henry Maudsley's book on causes of insanity.

340   Sandwith, Humphrey. "The London Water Question." 72 (1880): 144-71.
       Allies impure water and the proliferation of disease.
341   Crofts, H. Baptist, B.A. "The Relation of Drugs to Medicine." 78 (1883): 1-29.
       Prefers health maintenance, by clean air and water, proper diet and exercise, and sanitation, to illness necessitating drugs.
342   Rawlings, B. Burford. "Lay and Medical Functions in Hospital Administration." 79 (1884): 84-100.
       Expounds on medical and administrative duties in hospitals.

THE CONTEMPORARY REVIEW, 1866-1900

Manifesting an interest in social improvement, the *Contemporary*, established by Alexander Strahan of *Good Words* and the *Sunday Magazine*, spoke significantly about health. Preoccupations were the deleteriousness of poverty, the debate about vivisection, the situation of hospitals, and the safeguard of food.

343   Drew, G.S. "On the Social and Sanitary Laws of Moses." 2 (1866): 514-34.
       Treatise on Mosaic law accords with its sections on communicable diseases.
344   Markby, Thomas. "Athletics." 3 (1866): 374-91.
       Doubts that athletic training ameliorates salubrity.
345   Ludlow, J.M. "The Social Legislation of 1867, and Its New Year's Gifts for 1868." 7 (1868): 86-97.
       Skims several statutes of 1867, among them those on occupational health and safety.
346   Shaw, Benjamin. "The Food of the People." 7 (1868): 174-84.
       Directs readers' attention to foods vital for wellness.
347   Routledge, James. "The Food Supply of London." 9 (1868): 261-81, 502-18.
       Speaks about the amount and quality of food available in London.
348   Markby, Thomas. "Cholera." 10 (1869): 114-21.
       Assays treatments for cholera.
349   Merivale, Charles. "Remarks on the Physique of the Rural Population." 10 (1869): 255-62.
       Surmises that the rural poor, even with better medical care, are still disease-prone because of inadequate sanitation and food.

350   Hill, Florence. "The Family System for Workhouse Children." 15 (1870): 240-73.
Elects boarding out, as in Scotland, rather than workhouses for juvenile shelter and feeding. See #2497.

351   Potter, George. "The First Point of the New Charter: Improved Dwellings for the People." 18 (1871): 547-58.
Deems residences of laborers unhealthy.

352   [Winkworth, Susanna]. "The Alice Ladies' Society of Darmstadt." 21 (1872-73): 138-58.
Illuminates nursing in Germany.

353   Carpenter, W[illiam] B[enjamin]. "On the Hereditary Transmission of Acquired Psychical Habits." 21 (1872-73): 295-314, 779-95, 867-85.
Weighs the evidence for titled transmission and the sway of the mind on the salubrity of the body.

354   Darwin, George [H.]. "On Beneficial Restrictions to Liberty of Marriage." 22 (1873): 412-26.
Upholds marital laws on consanguinity as deterrents to inheritance of certain diseases.

355   Thompson, Henry. "The Treatment of the Body after Death." 23 (1873-74): 319-28.
Sanctions cremation for salubrity, among other reasons. See #356 and #357.

356   Holland, P.H. "Burial or Cremation." 23 (1873-74): 477-84.
Answers #355 that burial of the dead does not harm the living. See #357.

357   Thompson, Henry. "Cremation: A Reply to Critics and an Exposition of the Process." 23 (1873-74): 553-71.
Refutes #356 with the thesis in #355. See #1785.

358   Fairfax-Taylor, E. "Longevity in a New Light." 24 (1874): 606-26.
Searches for bases of longevity.

359   Tyndall, John. "On the Atmosphere in Relation to Fog-Signalling." 24 (1874): 819-41; 25 (1874-75): 148-68.
Would install sound and light signals along coasts to slow shipwrecks.

360   Synnot, Henrietta L. "Little Paupers." 24 (1874): 954-72.
Tale on workhouse waifs pronounces junior rural boarders more robust.

361   Greg, W.R. "Life at High Pressure." 25 (1874-75): 623-38.
Would offset the heart attacks, job anxiety, and nervous breakdowns catalyzed by a stressful lifestyle with ample exercise, food, and sleep.

362   Watson, Thomas. "Vivisection." 25 (1874-75): 867-70.
Would permit vivisection if animals are anesthetized or decapitated immediately after, but not random, unskilled, or unnecessary procedures, the last from curiosity or for fame.

363   [Edwards, W. Walter]. "The Poor Law: A Proposal for Its Abolition." 26 (1875): 639-49.
Considers the poor law less effective than private charity to protect the ill and aged.

364   Galton, Francis. "A Theory of Heredity." 27 (1875-76): 80-95.
Elaborates on heredity, briefly in the context of disease.

365   Lowe, Robert. "The Vivisection Act." 28 (1876): 713-24.
Assails the Act for Amending the Law Relating to Cruelty to Animals as superfluous and libelous to researchers.

366   Bucknill, John Charles. "Habitual Drunkenness." 29 (1876-77): 431-47.
Grounds many disorders in alcoholism.

367   Pettenkofer, Max von. "Liebig's Scientific Achievements." 29 (1876-77): 865-87.
Retrospective of the chemist, Justus von Liebig, has some paragraphs on his research on nutrition, particularly fats.

368   Gray, A.M. "Neglected Aspects of the Drink Question." 30 (1877): 454-65.
Wonders whether the government could police alcohol consumption, however toxic it was. See #568.

369   Tuke, D. Hack. "Legislation for the Insane." 30 (1877): 743-68.
Addresses legal issues in care of the insane.

370   Pettenkofer, Max von. "On the Hygienic Value of Plants in Rooms and the Open Air." 31 (1877-78): 68-81.
Enthuses about merits of plants indoors and shade outdoors.

371   Cobbe, Frances Power. "The Little Health of Ladies." 31 (1877-78): 276-96.
Sermonizes about the myriad roots of gentlewomen's unhealthiness and the want of female doctors.

372   Acland, Henry W. "Dog-Poison in Man." 31 (1877-78): 378-90.
Submits cases of rabies.

373   Gilbert, William. "The Abuse of Charity in London." 31 (1877-78): 770-89.
Watches Royal Hospitals, London. See #381 and #786.

374   Child, Gilbert W. "Sanitary Legislation and the Homes of the Poor." 32 (1878): 297-320.
Frets that current laws do not beget the clean dwellings fundamental to hinder contagions among the impoverished.

375   Paget, James, T. Lauder Brunton, and Albert J. Bernays. "The Alcohol Question." 33 (1878): 683-706.
      Multiple scribes debate whether alcohol is good or bad for health. See #376, # 377, and #567.

376   Gull, William [W.] [ed. by John Charles Bucknill], Charles Murchison, Walter Moxon, and Samuel Wilks. "The Alcohol Question." 34 (1878-79): 131-62.
      Augments #375. See #377 and #567.

377   Bennett, James Risdon, C.B. Radcliffe, Joseph Kidd, R. Brudenell Carter, and A.B. Garrod. "The Alcohol Question." 34 (1878-79): 341-72.
      Extends #375 and #376. See #567.

378   Haward, Warrington. "Ladies and Hospital Nursing." 34 (1878-79): 490-503.
      Capsulizes traits and duties of female hospital nurses.

379   Carter, R. Brudenell. "The London Medical Schools." 34 (1878-79): 582-93.
      Refutes criticisms of London medical students and their training. See #786.

380   Cowell, George. "Confession: Its Scientific and Medical Aspects." 34 (1878-79): 717-40.
      Desires same confidentiality between doctor and patient as between confessor and penitent.

381   Clarke, W. Fairlie. "How to Make Our Hospitals More Useful." 35 (1879): 91-106.
      Amends #373 on Royal Hospitals. Cheers the new medical schools and outpatient departments for former clients but not as clinics for the impoverished.

382   Blackley, W[illiam] Lewery. "Compulsory Providence as a Cure for Pauperism." 35 (1879): 608-29.
      Wants national dues to finance care of the ailing and aged.

383   Yeo, I. Burney. "Why Is Pain a Mystery?" 35 (1879): 630-47.
      Intellectualizes the physiology and psychology of pain.

384   Richardson, Benjamin Ward. "Chloral and Other Narcotics." 35 (1879): 719-39.
      Informs about uses of chloral hydrate and other narcotics in medicines and by addicts.

385   Miller, Henry J. "Lazarus Appeals to Dives." 36 (1879): 290-312.
      Prays for improvements for the indigent, such as cleaner residences conducive to wellness.

386   Pole, William. "Daltonism." 37 (1880): 821-36.
      Tutors on color blindness.

387   Moxon, W[alter]. "Miss Lonsdale on Guy's Hospital." 37 (1880): 872-92.
       Rebuts Margaret Lonsdale's ideas, in the *Nineteenth Century*, #1714, about nurses. Solicits quality nursing in workhouse infirmaries and as doctors' aides.
388   Knighton, William. "Suicidal Mania." 39 (1881): 81-90.
       Authenticates instances of and motives, as insanity, for suicide.
389   Jevons, W. Stanley. "Married Women in Factories." 41 (1882): 37-43.
       Charges infant mortality to mothers' factory labor. See #391.
390   Cobbe, Frances Power. "Vivisection and Its Two-Faced Advocates." 41 (1882): 610-26; with a response by Gerald F. Yeo: 897-98.
       Detests vivisection as unproductive medically, quite cruel, and yet widespread, although the press purportedly prints otherwise. For articles cited in this one relevant to health, see #1729 and #1730.
391   Cooke-Taylor, [Richard] Whately. "Married Women in Factories: A Reply." 42 (1882): 428-41.
       Contests thesis of #389.
392   DeCyon, E[lie]. "The Anti-Vivisectionist Agitation." 43 (1883): 498-510.
       Exonerates vivisectionists.
393   Hutton, Richard Holt. "The Anti-Vivisectionist Agitation." 43 (1883): 510-16.
       Parallels vivisection and torture of humans.
394   Mulhall, M.G. "Insanity, Suicide, and Civilization." 43 (1883): 901-08.
       Organizes insanity by rates, roots, as stress, and repercussions, chiefly suicide.
395   Lambert, Brooke and Andrew Mearns. "The Outcast Poor." 44 (1883): 916-33.
       Entries on the poor advert to their unsanitary and hence unsalutary domiciles.
396   Peek, Francis. "Lazarus at the Gate." 45 (1884): 81-96.
       Tarries at unsanitary dwellings, some of whose dwellers have smallpox. Laments that starving slum urchins are candidates for sickness.
397   Lidgett, George. "Shipowners, Seamen, and the Board of Trade." 45 (1884): 577-86.
       Swears that overloading and improper equipment kills merchant seamen. Concedes that some accidents have resulted from sailors' negligence when intoxicated.

398   Fothergill, J. Milner. "The Logic of Pain." 45 (1884): 680-86.
        Persuades that pain was utilitarian.
399   Chadwick, Edwin. "London Centralized." 45 (1884): 794-810.
        Would centralize London's government in order to have
        satisfactory house drainage and sewers, fire services, parks with
        unpolluted air, road cleaning (as accidents came from slippery
        streets), removal of the dead from lodgings, school health officers
        empowered to dismiss students with communicable diseases, and
        nuisance controls. Pictures London's environment as so noxious
        that it is an incentive to commuting from the suburbs.
400   Brassey, Thomas. "Tyrants of the Sea: Showing Some Tales of
        Suffering in the Merchant Service." 46 (1884): 403-12.
        Unmasks officers who have battered their men.
401   White, Arnold. "The Nomad Poor of London." 47 (1885): 714-26.
        Feature on the homeless has some words on adulterated food in
        London.
402   Burdon-Sanderson, J. [S.]. "Cholera: Its Cause and Prevention."
        48 (1885): 171-87.
        Speculates about causes of cholera.
403   Fuller, S.D. "Penny Dinners." 48 (1885): 424-32.
        Petitions for cheap meals for destitute youth debilitated by
        malnutrition.
404   Moxon, Walter. "Faith Healing." 48 (1885): 707-22.
        Dramatizes patients who have apparently been healed by the
        power of suggestion.
405   [Manning], Henry Edward, Cardinal Archbishop, and Benjamin
        Waugh. "The Child of the English Savage." 49 (1886): 687-700.
        Thanks the Society for the Prevention of Cruelty to Children for
        its efforts.
406   Wills, Freeman. "Meat for the People." 50 (1886): 80-87.
        Derives wellness from a diet high in meat.
407   Fawcett, Millicent Garrett. "Holes in the Education Net." 51
        (1887): 639-53.
        Broods about the health of minors on the stage.
408   Cobbe, Frances Power. "Faith Healing and Fear Killing." 51
        (1887): 794-813.
        Remonstrates against vivisectionists pursuing a remedy for rabies.
409   Hyndman, H.M. "The English Workers as They Are." 52 (1887):
        122-36.
        Personifies workers as pressured, women laborers by long hours
        and elderly ones by machinery, and all enervated by unsalutary
        housing, substandard food, noxious air, and little recreation.

410 Waugh, Benjamin. "Street Children." 53 (1888): 825-35.
Thunders that too many paupers abuse their offspring.

411 Tabor, Mary C. "The Rights of Children." 54 (1888): 408-17.
Ranks malnutrition as one form of juvenile victimization.

412 Picton, J. Allanson. "Compulsory Vaccination." 55 (1889): 114-31.
Would not compel vaccination for smallpox and syphilis.

413 Webb, Sidney. "The Limitation of the Hours of Labour." 56 (1889): 859-83.
Appeals for a multitude of labor reforms, such as an eight-hour day and the elimination of "sweating." See #414.

414 Haldane, R.B. "The Eight Hours Question." 57 (1890): 240-55.
Would substitute, for a statutory eight-hour day, each trade setting hours for its participants. See #413.

415 Rawnsley, H.D. "Sunlight or Smoke?" 57 (1890): 512-24.
Praises those who cut air pollution in mines and factories.

416 Waugh, Benjamin. "Baby-Farming." 57 (1890): 700-14.
Blames laxity in placements of infants for many of their maladies.

417 Waugh, Benjamin. "Child-Life Insurance." 58 (1890): 40-63.
Indicts those who abuse children and then murder them for their insurance.

418 Dolan, Thomas, M.D. "M. Pasteur and Hydrophobia." 58 (1890): 83-94.
Stamps Louis Pasteur's vaccine for rabies ineffective.

419 Webb, Sidney. "The Reform of the Poor Law." 58 (1890): 95-120.
Among other changes, would better the treatment of the needy ill and elderly under the law.

420 Mackenzie, Morell. "The Use and Abuse of Hospitals." 58 (1890): 501-19.
Typifies general hospitals as worthless to most patients and many doctors. Recommends strict criteria for free medical care.

421 Innes, A. Taylor. "Hypnotism in Relation to Crime and the Medical Faculty." 58 (1890): 555-66.
Underwrites more research on the consequences of hypnosis for health. See #1814.

422 Pike, Francis. "In Darkest England and the Way Out." 58 (1890): 796-807.
Dismisses the Salvation Army's suit for state action on salubrious housing.

423 Mackenzie, Morell. "Koch's Treatment of Tuberculosis." 59 (1891): 118-27.
Disseminates Robert Koch's study of tuberculosis.

424   Tolstoi, Leo. "The Ethics of Wine-Drinking and Tobacco-Smoking." 59 (1891): 170-87.
       Denominates alcohol and tobacco detrimental.

425   Schofield, Alfred T. "A Home for the Dying." 59 (1891): 423-27.
       Would dedicate some hospitals to comfort incurables who might otherwise die alone.

426   Romanes, George John. "Hydrophobia and the Muzzling Order." 59 (1891): 441-54.
       Depends on universal muzzling of dogs and quarantine law to stop rabies.

427   Ede, W. Moore. "National Pensions: One Way out of Darkest England." 59 (1891): 581-96.
       Predicts that pensions will be vital for the older poor.

428   Black, Clementina. "The Coming Factory Act." 59 (1891): 710-17.
       Decrees stringent standards of sanitation, safety, and working age in factories and stiff penalties for violaters.

429   Wager, Harold and Auberon Herbert. "Bad Air and Bad Health." 59 (1891): 852-72; with comments: 872-74.
       Yokes impure air and infirmity.

430   Mackenzie, W. Douglas. "The Ethics of Gambling." 60 (1891): 220-33.
       Prefaces suicide with gambling.

431   Rae, John. "The Balance Sheet of Short Hours." 60 (1891): 499-520.
       Heralds shorter hours for employees' wellness and owners' profits.

432   Tuckey, C. Lloyd, M.D. "The Applications of Hypnotism." 60 (1891): 672-86.
       Deliberates about the nexus between hypnosis and health.

433   Dobbs, Archibald E. "The London Water Companies: A Review and an Impeachment." 61 (1892): 26-38.
       Arraigns London water companies for overcharging and running contaminated water until government intervened.

434   Peek, Francis and Edwin T. Hall. "The Unhealthiness of the Cities: Its Cause and Cure." 61 (1892): 221-37.
       Stipulates that foul air and dangerous and unsanitary residences are major impediments to the vigor of urbanites.

435   Faithfull, Edith. "The Electrical Cure of Cancer." 61 (1892): 408-21.
       Picks electricity over surgery as a treatment for cancer.

436   Althaus, Julius, M.D. "Influenza: Its Origin and Mode of Spreading." 62 (1892): 225-39.
       Asserts that influenza is common and its origin still hidden.

437 Sellers, Edith. "The Story of a Colony for Epileptics." 62 (1892): 683-91.
Bruits German success in assisting epileptics.

438 Barnett, Samuel A. "Poor Law Reform." 63 (1893): 322-34.
Story on the poor law sympathizes with the sick and seniors.

439 Tuckey, C. Lloyd. "The New Hypnotism: A Reply." 63 (1893): 416-22.
Retorts to Ernest Hart, writing in the *Nineteenth Century* #1836, that hypnosis is a valid medical procedure. See #1792.

440 [Pringle-Pattison], Andrew Seth. "The 'New' Psychology and Automatism." 63 (1893): 555-74.
Decodes physiological psychology.

441 Spence, Frank. "How to Stop River Pollution." 64 (1893): 427-33.
Forecasts that ongoing disposal of sewage in rivers will expedite the onset of diseases, mainly cholera.

442 Farrar, F[rederic] W. "Mistakes about Abstainers." 65 (1894): 545-53.
Mirrors experts on the deleteriousness of alcohol.

443 Provand, A.D. "Employers' Liability." 66 (1894): 137-52.
From statistics, infers perils of several jobs for which employer liability is appropriate. See #1842.

444 Barnett, Henrietta O. "The Home or the Barrack for Children of the State." 66 (1894): 243-58.
Scorns children's barrack schools as debilitating.

445 Alexander, Joseph G. "Lotus Eating and Opium Eating." 66 (1894): 337-50.
Narrative on Indian and Chinese opium habits rejoices that few in Britain are addicted because Parliament, lobbied by the "medical profession," chartered only a "responsible and cautious class" of "licensed pharmaceutical chemists" to dispense the drug and thus opium is rarely prescribed.

446 Bainbridge, Emerson. "The Eight-Hours Bill for Miners." 66 (1894): 457-74.
Linchpin is the expense of the bill, with a gloss on the risks to colliers from improper ventilation and mishaps.

447 Wolff, Henry W. "Accident Insurance." 67 (1895): 68-80.
Would copy German legislation on insurance for job-related accidents.

448 Allbutt, T. Clifford. "Nervous Diseases and Modern Life." 67 (1895): 210-31.
Contravenes inflation in rates of insanity and nervous disorders. See #1108.

449   Roberts, Charles. "The Physiology of Recreation." 68 (1895): 103-13.
Grades recreational exercise high for fitness.

450   Geddes, Patrick and J. Arthur Thomson. "Louis Pasteur." 68 (1895): 632-44.
Pays tribute to Louis Pasteur for his research.

451   Boulger, Demetrius C. "Antitoxin, from a Patient's Point of View." 69 (1896): 177-89.
After use, disdains an antitoxin for diphtheria.

452   Browne, [Isaac] Lennox. "The Antitoxin Treatment of Diphtheria." 70 (1896): 119-35.
Induces, from statistics on diphtheria, that a serum was not therapeutic.

453   Picton, J. Allanson. "The Vaccination Commission." 70 (1896): 485-503.
Would not enforce compulsory vaccination because assumes that it does not arrest smallpox.

454   Nuttall, G. Clarke. "Bacteria and Butter." 71 (1897): 123-29.
Illustrates how bacteria are beneficial in some dairy products.

455   Lidgett, Elizabeth S. "Poor Law Children and the Departmental Committee." 71 (1897): 205-20.
Treatise on official action on behalf of the young poor spots the prevalence of disease among them, whether they live in institutions or homes.

456   Verney, Edmund. "The Inhabitants of Milk." 72 (1897): 709-21.
Theme is bacteria in milk.

457   Ellis, Havelock. "Mescal: A New Artificial Paradise." 73 (1898): 130-41.
Shares sensations after ingestion of mescaline. Without much evidence, declares persistent use as baneful, so would confine the alleged rapture of mescal visions to the robust.

458   Nutall, G. Clarke. "The Secret of Baldness." 73 (1898): 356-61.
Repudiates the theory of bacteria as the source of baldness.

459   Cullingworth, Charles J. "The Registration of Midwives." 73 (1898): 394-402.
Hopes that midwives with both formal training and experience will curtail puerperal fever.

460   Turner, E.B. "Health on the Bicycle." 73 (1898): 640-48.
Trumpets how invigorating bicycling is.

461   Harrison, Frederic. "Ideal London." 74 (1898): 139-52.
Would supplement improvements in air and water quality with more sanitary reform in London.

462   Barnett, Samuel A. "Twenty-Five Years of East London." 74 (1898): 280-89.
       Retrospective has some paragraphs on improvements in housing and water, yet construes East London as unhealthy.

463   Nash, Vaughan. "The East London Water Company." 74 (1898): 474-79.
       Castigates London company for pumping impure water.

464   Ensor, Ernest. "The Football Madness." 74 (1898): 751-60.
       Teams brutality of football spectators and subsequent enfeeblment.

465   Fawcett, Millicent Garrett. "The Vaccination Act of 1898." 75 (1899): 328-42.
       History of smallpox vaccination would not command it for infants.

466   Hutchinson, Woods. "The Republic of the Body." 75 (1899): 568-77.
       Text summarizes how the body reacts to illness.

467   Hutchinson, Woods. "The Cancer Problem: Treason in the Republic of the Body." 76 (1899): 105-17.
       Trails the inroads of cancer.

468   Shaw, Edith M. "The Workhouse from the Inside." 76 (1899): 564-72.
       Unveils the difficulties of tending sick and elderly paupers.

469   Holmes, Thomas. "Obscure Causes of Crime." 76 (1899): 577-88.
       Dubs insanity and epilepsy possible stimuli of crime.

470   Donald, Robert. "Housing the Poor." 77 (1900): 323-33.
       Generalizes that many abodes of the poor are dirty and crowded.

471   Coleridge, Stephen. "Some London Hospitals and Their Audited Accounts." 77 (1900): 343-50.
       Frowns on the transfer of hospital budgets to research laboratories or medical schools. See #472.

472   Thompson, Ralph. "Mr. Coleridge and the Middlesex Hospital." 77 (1900): 606-08.
       Would channel hospital money to cancer investigators. See #471.

473   Shadwell, Arthur. "The True Aim of Preventive Medicine." 78 (1900): 579-89.
       Backs sanitation, bacteriology, and immunity, natural and artificial, for health maintenance.

THE CORNHILL MAGAZINE, 1860-1900

Planned principally for relaxation, the *Cornhill* carried numerous notices on fitness. Emphasized were intoxicants, insanity, and, increasingly, exercise.

474   [Ansted, D.T.]. "Colour Blindness." 1 (1860): 403-11.
        Demystifies color blindness.
475   [Thompson, Henry]. "Under Chloroform." 1 (1860): 499-504.
        Would administer chloroform to patients undergoing surgery.
476   [Dallas, E.S.]. "The Poor Man's Kitchen." 1 (1860): 745-54.
        Mutters that the fare of prisoners is better than that of the honest
        but needy. Would make affordable, nourishing food available to
        trade unionists.
477   [Hinton, James]. "Physiological Riddles." 2 (1860): 21-32, 167-74,
        313-25, 421-31.
        Abridges functions of nerves and muscles, processes of growth,
        structure of the brain, and cell differentiation.
478   [Hassall, Arthur H.]. "Adulteration, and Its Remedy." 2 (1860):
        86-96.
        Because adulteration could physically harm buyers, rejects
        Parliamentary bill that does not subsume all ingestible goods.
479   [Hinton, James]. "Health." 3 (1861): 332-41.
        Tags clean air, exercise, food, sleep, temperance, hygiene, and less
        stress as necessary for wellness.
480   [Hinton, James]. "Food - What Is It?" 3 (1861): 460-72.
        Highlights the salubrity of food and minerals.
481   [Hinton, James]. "Food - What It Does." 4 (1861): 75-93.
        Dissects human digestion.
482   [Hinton, James]. "Food - How to Take It." 4 (1861): 281-94.
        Spells out when, what, and how to eat for health, with sentences
        on adulteration, alcohol, sleep, and stress.
483   [Hinton, James]. "What Are the Nerves?" 5 (1862): 153-66.
        Abstract on the nerves suggests how to maintain their
        effectiveness.
484   [Stephen, James Fitzjames]. "Commissions of Lunacy." 5 (1862):
        220-32.
        Gauges the impact of titled commissions.
485   [Hinton, James]. "The Brain and Its Use." 5 (1862): 409-25.
        Anatomizes the brain.
486   [Leifchild, J.R.]. "Fire-Damp and Its Victims." 5 (1862): 426-37.
        Campaigns for ventilation in coal mines, typically filled with
        dangerous gasses.
487   [Wood, J.G.]. "Inner Life of a Hospital." 5 (1862): 462-77.
        Traverses thoroughly all aspects of a hospital.

488   [Wynter, Andrew]. "First Beginnings." 5 (1862): 481-94.
Posts early symptoms of insanity, such as inattention, unusual behavior, and fixation, sometimes appearing years after a heavy blow to the head.

489   [Kaye, J.W.]. "On Growing Old." 5 (1862): 495-507.
Comprehends psychological benefits of aging.

490   [Anstie, Francis E.]. "Is It Food, Medicine, or Poison?" 5 (1862): 707-16.
Discusses how alcohol affects the body. See #492.

491   [Brady, J.D.]. "French System of Relieving the Poor." 6 (1862): 44-51.
Posits that French plan for support of the destitute is better and cheaper than is England's poor law.

492   [Anstie, Francis E.]. "Does Alcohol Act as Food?" 6 (1862): 319-29.
Broadens the assessment in #490. Appends a few words on chloroform.

493   [Lewes, George Henry]. "Effect of Railways on Health." 6 (1862): 480-89.
Balances boons and burdens, for vigor, of railroad commuting.

494   [Anstie, Francis E.]. "Tobacco: Its Use and Abuse." 6 (1862): 605-15.
Estimates values of smoking, chewing, and sniffing tobacco, in themselves and as against drinking liquor.

495   [McCroskey, H.]. "The Working Man's Restaurant." 7 (1863): 252-58.
Guest in working class cafeteria in Glasgow that serves inexpensive nutritious meals in scrubbed surroundings would replicate it elsewhere. See #1595.

496   [Lewes, George Henry]. "Aids to Beauty, Real and Artificial." 7 (1863): 391-400.
Growls that uncleanliness, cosmetics, and some attire interfere with vitality.

497   [Anstie, Francis E.]. "Corpulence." 7 (1863): 457-68.
Pertains to onset of and treatment for obesity.

498   [Hinton, James]. "A Meditation; On Skeletons - and Some Other Things." 7 (1863): 622-28.
Essay on skeletons, human and other, has a few lines on illness.

499   [Lewes, George Henry]. "The Mental Condition of Babies." 7 (1863): 649-56.
Synopsizes recent experiments in which healthy babies reacted to sensation and expressed emotion.

500   [Anstie, Francis E.]. "Over-Eating and Under-Eating." 8 (1863): 35-47.
        Monitors consequences of malnutrition, primarily in infants, and overindulgence.

501   [Anstie, Francis E.]. "Medical Etiquette." 8 (1863): 154-63.
        Pierces doctor-doctor and doctor-patient relationships.

502   [Stratton, J.Y.]. "The Life of a Farm Labourer." 9 (1864): 178-86.
        Biography of an agricultural laborer parenthesizes the high price of illness without insurance.

503   [Lewes, George Henry]. "Training in Relation to Health." 9 (1864): 219-31.
        Depends on exercise and prudent eating, not special training, for health maintenance.

504   [Richardson, Coke]. "Sentence of Death Recorded." 9 (1864): 304-08.
        Imparts the mood of someone diagnosed with a fatal malady.

505   [Gilbert, William]. "Club-House Sobriety." 9 (1863): 480-86.
        Would spur workers to emulate current sobriety of the upper and middle classes.

506   [Martin, Frances]. "Blind Workers and Blind Helpers." 9 (1864): 603-17.
        Has a program to stabilize psychologically the vision impaired.

507   [Gilbert, William]. "A Visit to the Convict Lunatic Asylum." 10 (1864): 448-60.
        Lingers on facilities and inmate management of an asylum for insane criminals.

508   [Martineau, Harriet]. "Nurses Wanted." 11 (1865): 409-25.
        Steers women to nursing as an excellent job opportunity as skilled stewards of the sick.

509   [Morris, Miss]. "The Devils of Morzine." 11 (1865): 468-81.
        Tells of French village where residents had severe seizures, which doctors christened epilepsy, hysteria, insanity, or gastritis, but not demonic possession, contrary to peasants' belief.

510   [Strange, William]. "Plague and Pestilence." 11 (1865): 591-603.
        Overview of epidemics has paragraphs on plague, typhus, cholera, and scarlet fever.

511   [Blandford, G. Fielding]. " 'Acquitted on the Ground of Insanity'." 12 (1865): 426-40.
        Tract on insanity as a criminal defense demarcates it as a species.

512   [Carter, R. Brudenell]. "Provincial Medical Charities." 12 (1865): 555-67.
        Enumerates financial and staffing problems of provincial hospitals.

513   [Hannay, James]. "Greenwich Hospital." 12 (1865): 631-40.
Shifts from early days to modern budget and status of institution
for old and ailing seamen.

514   [Stillman, W.J.]. "My Experiences in a Greek Quarantine." 13
(1866): 173-83.
Recalls cholera episode.

515   [Blandford, G. Fielding]. "Sleep." 14 (1866): 226-37.
Disquisition on sleep mates it with fettle.

516   [Blandford, G. Fielding]. "Training." 15 (1867): 92-103.
Supervises training regimen for rowing and other sports.

517   [Clayden, P.W.]. " 'Off for the Holidays'." 16 (1867): 315-22.
Sells vacations as physically and mentally energizing.

518   [Armfield, H.T.]. "Dumb Men's Speech: A Belgian Experiment."
16 (1867): 693-703.
Primes the hearing impaired on how to speak.

519   [Ritchie, Anne]. "A City of Refuge." 17 (1868): 735-44.
Tarries at a sanctuary for incurables.

520   [Ritchie, Anne]. "Chirping Crickets." 19 (1869): 235-42.
Peeks at juvenile hospitals and shelters.

521   [Wolfe-Barry, J.W.]. "Railway Signalling." 19 (1869): 280-93.
Drills readers on procedures for safety on railroads.

522   [Pole, William]. "Fog-Signals." 21 (1870): 470-82.
Would install foghorns along coasts in order to avert shipwrecks.

523   An Optimist [J.W. Kaye]. "Rest." 22 (1870): 223-38.
Article on the value of rest times it ideally during convalescence.

524   [Hinton, James]. "On Nursing as a Profession." 22 (1870): 451-56.
Expounds on the education and salary of nurses, assumed to be
females.

525   [Burgess, R.B.]. "Rocket and Mortar Apparatus for Saving Life
from Shipwreck, and Volunteer Life Brigades." 28 (1873): 72-87.
Sketches brigades involved in rescuing the shipwrecked.

526   [Mew, James]. "Physical Education." 28 (1873): 345-55.
Noises how salutary exercise was.

527   [Proctor, R.A.]. "Growth and Decay of Mind." 28 (1873): 541-55.
Pores over effects of aging on the mind.

528   [Lathbury, D.C.]. "Houses of the Poor in Towns." 30 (1874): 74-
83.
Affiliates illness among the urban poor and their dirty, dank
domiciles.

529   [Proctor, R.A.]. "Have We Two Brains?" 31 (1875): 149-66.
Familiarizes readers with malfunctions of left and right brain. See
#533.

530   [Cobbe, Frances Power]. "Sacrificial Medicine." 32 (1875): 427-38.
Disparages prescriptions that are either painful or overly expensive.

531   [Ritchie, Anne]. "Mr. Campbell's Pupils." 33 (1876): 349-57.
Chats about student musicians at the Normal College for the Blind.

532   [Sully, James]. "The Laws of Dream-Fancy." 34 (1876): 536-55.
Widens knowledge of the physiology and psychology of dreams.

533   [Proctor, R.A.]. "Dual Consciousness." 35 (1877): 86-105.
Extends, through examples, #529 on brain malfunctions.

534   [Proctor, R.A.]. "Hereditary Traits." 37 (1878): 411-31.
Slates insanity, alcoholism, and mental underdevelopment as inherited.

535   [Proctor, R.A.]. "Bodily Illness as a Mental Stimulant." 39 (1879): 412-26.
Thesis is that sickness sires a host of mental reactions. See #536.

536   [Proctor, R.A.]. "Influence of the Mind on the Body." 40 (1879): 148-70.
Reverses #535 with instances wherein the mind had caused or cured illness.

537   S[ully], J[ames]. "Babies and Science." 43 (1881): 539-54.
Describes the progress of a healthy infant, with evidence allegedly from both scientific and parental studies.

538   P[roctor], R.A. "Living Death-Germs." 45 (1882): 303-18.
Paen to Louis Pasteur licenses smallpox vaccination.

539   [Patterson, R.H.]. "Longer Life." n.s., 3, o.s., 50 (1884): 175-84.
Keys longevity to more recreation and better health care, both possible because of prosperity and legislation on sanitation and occupational safety.

540   "Dynamite." n.s., 3, o.s., 50 (1884): 273-91.
Markets dynamite to reduce risks to miners.

541   "Leeches." n.s., 4, o.s., 51 (1885): 326-36.
Notices that leeches are still applied as a medical remedy.

542   [Mawer, Mrs. E.B.]. "Hachisch [sic] Eating." n.s., 22, o.s., 69 (1894): 500-05.
Records sensations while under the influence of cannabis.

543   "The Humours of Hospital Life." 3d ser., 5, o.s., 78 (1898): 549-52.
Shadows hospital patients' interactions with doctors and chaplains.

544   Thomas, W. Beach. "Athletics and Health." 3d ser., 8, o.s., 81 (1900): 537-48.
Proclaims how important exercise is for salubrity.

THE DARK BLUE, 1871-1873

Organized by Oxonians, the *Dark Blue* did not much deliberate issues of illness.

545   [Freund, Amelia Lewis]. "Recreation a Religious Duty." 1 (1871): 346-50.
       Points out how recreation improves mental and physical health.
546   [Redgrave, Alexander]. "The London Needlewoman." 2 (1871-72): 66-75.
       Looks at laws that lessen the job hazards of needlewomen.
547   Wilson, Edward D.J. "Preservation of the National Health." 2 (1871-72): 327-35.
       Indicts local officials for nonfeasance with respect to statutes on sanitation and water, expediting typhus, cholera, and smallpox.
548   Barraclough, George, M.A., M.R.C.S. "On Physical Education: The Turn-Verein in England." 2 (1871-72): 450-65.
       Would imitate German gymnastics for fitness.

THE DUBLIN REVIEW, 1836-1900

Conceived for an English congregation, the *Dublin Review* nonetheless made prominent the plight of the Irish, in Ireland and in other precincts.

549   [Palmer, J.F.]. "Medical Statistics." 2 (1836-37): 95-111.
       Hinges improved physical and mental health to diet, doctors, smallpox vaccination, and sanitation.
550   [Palmer, J.F.]. "Mesmerism, or Animal Magnetism." 4 (1838): 202-32.
       Chapter on hypnosis tabs it therapy for hysteria.
551   [Palmer, J.F.]. "Medical Notices." 7 (1839): 301-33.
       Story on doctors acquaints the subscriber with their practices.
552   [Palmer, J.F.]. "Statistics of Population." 7 (1839): 454-83.
       Translates data into a discourse on decline in mortality rates.
553   [Quin, M.J.]. "Mental Epidemics." 10 (1841): 348-82.
       Earmarks roots and genres of insanity.
554   [Symons, Jelinger C.]. "Education of the Working Classes." 14 (1843): 141-77.
       Proponent of education wakens to how workplaces impair juvenile health.

555   [Campbell, John Shaw]. "A Bill for the Better Regulation of Medical Practice Throughout the United Kingdom." 18 (1845): 174-205.
        Predicts that captioned bill would propagate quackery and divisiveness between surgeons and general practitioners.

556   [Russell, C.W.]. "The Deaf and Dumb in Ireland: Dr. Kitto's *Lost Senses*." 20 (1846): 291-319.
        Rephrases a book by John Kitto, D.D., on the hearing impaired, notably Irish Catholic children who also do not speak.

557   [Kemp, T.L.]. "Liebig's Philosophy." 25 (1848): 179-204.
        Abbreviates notions of Justus von Liebig on food chemistry.

558   [Hawkins, Charles]. "Ether and Chloroform." 29 (1850): 226-47.
        Recommends ether and chloroform only for major surgery because they are dangerous for all patients, not merely those with weak hearts.

559   [?Brooks, Charles W.S.]. "The Age of Honesty." 31 (1851): 589-611.
        Reviles those who adulterate food or pump foul water.

560   [Kemp, T.L.]. "Food and Its Adulteration." 39 (1855): 60-75.
        Rages about the adulteration of food.

561   [Abraham, G.W.]. "Epidemic Disease in Ireland." 42 (1857): 76-95.
        Surveys outcomes of pestilence generally in Ireland.

562   [Crolly, George]. "Obstetric Morality." 44 (1858): 100-30.
        Lectures on various procedures for child delivery, all in a Catholic context.

563   [Ryan, William Burke]. "Child-Murder - Obstetric Morality." 45 (1858): 54-106.
        Damns those who perform abortion and craniotomy.

564   [Finalson, W.F.]. "The Plea of Insanity in Trials for Murder." 46 (1859): 58-92.
        Topic is whether doctors can determine insanity in criminal circumstances.

565   "London Poor and London Work." n.s., 23, o.s., 75 (1874): 29-53.
        Observer of the poor despairs about their unwholesome domiciles.

566   M[ivart, St. George]. "An Examination of Mr. Herbert Spencer's Psychology." n.s., 23, o.s., 75 (1874): 476-508; n.s., 25, o.s., 77 (1875): 143-72; n.s., 28, o.s., 80 (1877): 192-219; n.s., 30, o.s., 82 (1878): 154-94; n.s., 31, o.s., 83 (1878): 412-39; 3d ser., 1, o.s., 84 (1879): 141-63, 368-96.
        Exegesis on Herbert Spencer's psychology does not neglect the nervous system.

567 Gasquet, J.R. "Alcohol: Its Action and Use." 3d ser., 1, o.s., 84 (1879): 447-54.
Announces a few boons to health from alcohol. See #375, #376, and #377.

568 Whittaker, Thomas P. "The Liquor Traffic; Should It Be Prohibited?" 3d ser., 2, o.s., 85 (1879): 1-32.
Would ban liquor sales on the ground that alcohol is damaging to health. See #368.

569 Gasquet, J.R. "Recent Research on the Nerves and Brain." 3d ser., 3, o.s., 86 (1880): 372-81.
Subject is research on the brain and the nervous system in relation to consciousness.

570 "The Distress in Ireland." 3d ser., 3, o.s., 86 (1880): 464-91.
Rumors that starvation and then dysentery are rampant in Ireland. *Edinburgh Review* article noted does not address health.

571 Mackey, E., M.D. "Miracles and Medical Science." 3d ser., 4, o.s., 87 (1880): 386-98.
Disbelieves that sudden recoveries, particularly from hysteria, are miracles.

572 [Gasquet, J.R.]. "The Brain and the Mind." 3d ser., 5, o.s., 88 (1881): 25-56.
Simplifies theses of H. Charlton Bastian, M.D., mainly on maladies affected by the nerves.

573 Harrod, Henry D. "The Dwellings of the Poor." 3d ser., 11, o.s., 94 (1884): 414-37.
Sermonizes that the housing of the poor is unsalutary because sanitary laws are not always enforced. See #575, #807, and #1747, but *National Review* citation is not pertinent.

574 Sibbald, Andrew T. "The Brain and the Mind." 3d ser., 13, o.s., 96 (1885): 381-92.
Comments on how the brain and nerves interact with the body.

575 Harrod, Henry D. "The Royal Commission and the Homes of the Poor." 3d ser., 14, o.s., 97 (1885): 102-19.
Returns to the topic of #573.

576 Sibbald, Andrew T. "The Nerves and Over-Pressure." 3d ser., 15, o.s., 98 (1886): 40-57.
Anchors disorders of the nerves in educational methods.

577 Gasquet, J.R. "Hypnotism." 3d ser., 25, o.s., 108 (1891): 241-54.
Entry on hypnosis has some lines on it as a medical treatment.

578 Waugh, Benjamin. "Prevention of Cruelty to Children." 4th ser., 1, o.s., 110 (1892): 140-51.
Accentuates detrimental effects of child abuse.

579   Griffith, T.B. "An Aspect of the Temperance Question." 4th ser., 1, o.s., 110 (1892): 363-71.
Points out how deleterious alcohol is for the undernourished.

580   Bruce, Eric Stuart, M.A. Oxon., F.R. Met. Soc. "Town Fogs: Their Amelioration and Prevention." 4th ser., 5, o.s., 114 (1894): 132-44.
Core is the harm of urban air pollution, worse during fogs.

581   Clarke, Robert F. "The Vivisection Controversy." 4th ser., 6, o.s., 115 (1894): 96-121.
Referees the debate on vivisection.

582   Snow, T.B., Abbot. "Hallucinations." 4th ser., 8, o.s., 117 (1895): 245-64.
Inventories types of and reasons for hallucinations.

THE DUBLIN UNIVERSITY MAGAZINE, 1833-1880

Reflecting initially Anglo-Irish ideas, the *Dublin University*, and its successor, the *University Magazine*, 1878-1880, studied sickness in Gaellic and other venues. Hypnosis and the brain, hydropathy and bathing, and how to train doctors were typical topics.

583   "The Scottish System of Poor Laws." 3 (1834): 508-22.
Would cap, akin to Scottish law, aid to ailing and aged paupers.

584   "Phrenology and Its Opponents." 3 (1834): 570-78.
Transcribes phrenologists' views on the brain.

585   [Butt, Isaac]. "Medical Education." 3 (1834): 592-96.
Ordains higher standards for medical education in order to achieve skilled and fewer doctors.

586   "Some Effects of Unnoticed Insanity." 6 (1835): 666-75.
Describes symptoms of paranoia.

587   [Butt, Isaac]. "The Surgeon-General's Introductory Lecture." 7 (1836): 163-76.
Based on recent talk by Philip Crampton, M.D., would integrate clinical training in medical education, principally for aspiring surgeons.

588   "The Royal Hospital, Kilmainham." 7 (1836): 222-26.
Reproves managers of this Irish hospital.

589   "The State of the Irish Poor." 7 (1836): 349-64.
From evidence given before Royal Commissioners, 1835, briefs on illnesses of and treatments available to the Irish poor.

590 [Lever, Charles]. "Post-Mortem Recollections of a Medical Lecturer." 7 (1836): 623-28.
Relives near-death experience caused by nervous disorder.
591 "Ellis' Treatise on Insanity." 12 (1838): 459-71.
Borrows from W.C. Ellis, M.D., sources of insanity, namely heredity, physical trauma, and stress.
592 [Lever, Charles]. *"Physic and Physicians."* 14 (1839): 653-64.
Reviews a book by F.B. Winslow on lifestyles of physicians.
593 Walsh, R[obert], LL.D., M.D. "Our Fellow Lodgers." 15 (1840): 617-24.
Describes cases of insect infestation of humans.
594 [Lever, Charles]. "The Water Cure - Mr. Claridge." 19 (1842): 729-35.
Confutes opinions of R.T. Claridge, Esq., on the worth of hydropathy.
595 [Marsh, Henry]. "The Medical Charities of Ireland." 20 (1842): 88-101.
Objects to legislative alteration of care of indigents in Irish hospitals and dispensaries.
596 [Lever, Charles]. "Dr. Graves on *Clinical Medicine*." 21 (1843): 307-17.
Promulgates theories of R.J. Graves, M.D., on medical education. See #2138.
597 A[nster, John]. "Criminal Responsibility of the Insane." 21 (1843): 626-46.
Ignores medical aspects of insanity.
598 "The Factory System of England." 22 (1843): 435-41.
Flags the unwholesomeness of workers' housing.
599 Herfner, Irys [Henry Ferris]. "Mesmerism." 23 (1844): 37-53, 286-301.
Series on F.A. Mesmer's concepts has some sentences on the curative value of hypnosis. See #601.
600 [Hayman, Samuel]. *"Essays by an Invalid*: Harriet Martineau's *Life in the Sick Room*." 23 (1844): 573-82.
Focus is Martineau's book on being a patient.
601 Herfner, Irys [Henry Ferris]. "A Few More Words about Mesmerism - The State of Sleep-Waking." 24 (1844): 78-90.
Deepens #599.
602 [Ferris, Henry]. "Of the Nightmare." 25 (1845): 32-44.
Offers examples of psychosomatic illness.
603 A[nster, John]. *"The Claims of Labour*." 25 (1845): 45-57.
Listens to Arthur Helps about perils in factories.

604   J[errold], W.B. "Warm Water *versus* Cold; or, a Visit to Warmbrunn in Prussian and Graefenberg in Austrian Silesia." 38 (1851): 223-33, 283-97.
        Encounters invalids at contintental spas.

605   "Animal Magnetism." 38 (1851): 383-406.
        Muses about hypnosis as a medical treatment.

606   F[erguson], S[amuel]. "Divination, Witchcraft, and Mesmerism." 38 (1851): 687-707.
        Presages that hypnosis would relieve some physical symptoms heretofore mistaken as supernatural.

607   "The Epidemics of the Famine Years." 40 (1852): 653-63.
        Attaches Irish susceptibility to diseases, such as typhus and cholera, to the potato blight.

608   [Wilde, W.R.]. "The Food of the Irish." 43 (1854): 127-46, 317-33.
        Item on Irish diet recollects the Great Famine and its aftermath, disease.

609   "Food - Drink - Drugs." 47 (1856): 78-90.
        Complains about adulterated food, drink, and drugs.

610   [Dunlop, Durham]. "The Doctor in the Witness-Box." 47 (1856): 178-95.
        Reports on doctors as experts in criminal trials.

611   [Dunlop, Durham]. "What Shall We Do with the Poison Trade?" 49 (1857): 160-76.
        Rants about the toxicity of adulterated drugs.

612   S[coffern], J[ohn]. "The Fire-Damp's Family Circle." 50 (1857): 185-91, 345-52.
        Spotlights firedamp explosions in mines.

613   [Spender, Edward]. "Charity at Home." 55 (1860): 617-27.
        Would transform housing in order to boost inhabitants' health.

614   "Thermal Antiquae Redivivae: or the Thermal and Vapour Baths of the Ancients, Revived." 57 (1861): 29-39.
        Fancies thermal and vapor bathing as therapy for sundry ailments.

615   [Scott, J.A.]. "Emigration as an Agency of Lancashire Relief." 61 (1863): 595-99.
        Perceives that typhus flourishes as unemployment mandates sharing rooms.

616   [Irwin, T.C.]. "Phrenology." 64 (1864): 158-60.
        Paragraphs on phrenology do not overlook brain functions.

617   [Cole, J.W.]. "Are the Pygmies to be Revived?" 65 (1865): 506-17.
        Assent to own query has instances of dwarfism. See #618.

618 [Cole, J.W.]. "Of Giants." 66 (1865): 193-205.
Reverses #617 with examples of gigantism.
619 [Hennessy, W.M.]. "Mad Men of Letters." 66 (1865): 276-86.
Profile of individuals sketches alleged peculiarities of the insane.
620 [Merrifield, Mary P.]. "The Need of Sanitary Knowledge to Women." 76 (1870): 343-48.
Reprint from *St. James's Magazine* binds nutrition, exercise, and knowledge of hygienic precepts to the salubrity of women and their progeny.
621 "Chemistry in the Kitchen." 77 (1871): 461-65.
Piece on foods of many lands links diet to wellness.
622 M., S.D. "Visiting in London Hospitals." 77 (1871): 584-89.
Fan of salaried nurses in hospitals also spends time on patients' vulnerability to visitors.
623 [Axon, W.E.A.]. "The Tobacco Question." 78 (1871): 279-89.
Underlines health hazards of smoking. See #627.
624 P[icciotto], J[ames]. "Fevers." 79 (1872): 184-94.
Incorporates sources and signs of fevers, chiefly typhoid fever and typhus.
625 Beard, George M., M.D. "The Extent of Insanity." 79 (1872): 688-702.
Discusses roots, signs, and rampancy of insanity.
626 [Adams, Charles F.]. "German Wines." 80 (1872): 168-76.
Tickets German wines invigorating.
627 [Axon, W.E.A.]. "Juvenile Smoking." 80 (1872): 289-99.
With medical evidence, asseverates how risky tobacco smoking is for the young. See #623.
628 Spencer, H.B., M.D. "Cheap Wines." 80 (1872): 357-59.
Dictates drinking light wines to speed recuperation.
629 P[icciotto], J[ames]. "Beautiful for Ever [sic]." 81 (1873): 301-11.
Hitches hygiene and habits to well-being.
630 P[icciotto], J[ames]. "Our Hair." 81 (1873): 394-404.
Considers the nexus between health and hair, especially its loss.
631 [Dunlop, Durham]. "Public Bathing - The Hot-Air Bath." 82 (1873): 1-13.
Disquisition on steam and hot and cold water baths concludes that steam is best for fitness and good skin.
632 Pennefather, J.P., Esq. "Cremation." 83 (1874): 592-93.
Would cremate the dead to decontaminate air and water.
633 "Alcohol as a Medicine." 85 (1875): 230-47, 324-35, 467-79.
With medical evidence of alcohol's harm, depreciates it as a nostrum. See #2483.

634 Pennefather, J.P. "The Sense of Hearing." 85 (1875): 733-38.
Explains the structure and function of the ear.
635 The London Hermit [Walter Parke]. "On Spectacles and Weak
Nerves." 89 (1877): 780-86.
Beseeches individuals with stress from the clamor of civilization
to empathize with those with impaired vision.
636 Huxley, Prof. [T.H.], F.R.S. "On Elementary Instruction in
Physiology." 90 (1877): 129-32.
Entreats readers to learn some physiology in order to safeguard
their health.
637 Blake, Edward T., M.D., M.R.C.S.E., F.B.H.S. "The Medical
Basis of Charms." 90 (1877): 159-73.
Tale of numerous charms confesses the curative power of some.

The University Magazine

638 Shore, Thomas. "Human Harriers." n.s., 1, o.s., 91 (1878): 488-92.
Teams cross-country running and wellness.
639 [Whittaker, Thomas]. "The Philosophy of Stimulants, with Special
Reference to Opium and Hashish." n.s., 5, o.s., 95 (1880): 493-
503.
Illustrates effects of alcohol, opium, and cannabis on the body.

THE EDINBURGH REVIEW, 1802-1900

Rooted in Whig theory and reveling in new science, the *Edinburgh*
examined health extensively. Observations ranged from drink to diseases
of the mind, from surgery to statistics on job mortality.

640 [Thomson, John]. "Morveau on the Means of Purifying Infected
Air." 1 (1802-03): 237-52.
Records how L.B. Guyton Morveau would halt contagious
diseases by air purification.
641 [Thomson, John]. "Dr. Haygarth on *Infectious Fevers*." 1 (1802-
03): 245-52.
Annotates a text on fevers by John Haygarth, M.D.
642 [Thomson, John]. "Heberden on the *History and Cure of
Diseases*." 1 (1802-03): 466-74.
Broadcasts William Heberden's treatments for gout, fever, and
hernia.

643 [Brown, Thomas]. "Villiers, *Sur une Nouvelle Theorie du Cerveau.* " 2 (1803): 147-60.
Quotes ideas of Dr. F.J. Gall about mental illness.

644 [Reeve, Henry]. "Pinel, *Traite sur l'Alienation Mentale.*" 2 (1803): 160-72.
Previews Philip Pinel's work on origins and kinds of insanity and care of its victims.

645 [Brougham, Henry]. *"Memoirs of the Philosophical Society of Manchester."* 2 (1803): 192-96.
Presents notions of John Gough on hearing.

646 [Thomson, John]. "Hey's *Practical Observations in Surgery.*" 2 (1803): 261-68.
Memorializes William Hey's treatments for cataract and hernia.

647 [Thomson, John]. "Nicholas and Gueudeville, *Sur la Diabete Sucre.*" 3 (1803-04): 410-22.
Citing C.C. Nicholas and Victor Gueudeville, discusses French cases of diabetes with their causes and symptoms.

648 [Thomson, John]. "Abernethy's Surgical Observations." 5 (1804-05): 168-79.
Comments on John Abernethy's procedures for tumor surgery.

649 [Thomson, John]. "Spallanzani, *Memoirs sur la Respiration.*" 5 (1804-05): 362-71.
Summarizes thoughts of Lazarus Spallanzani on respiration.

650 "Currie's *Medical Reports.*" 7 (1805-06): 42-63.
Gleans from a book by James Currie, M.D., that heat, cold, and water are remedies for typhus, influenza, and insanity.

651 [Duncan, Andrew and Francis Jeffrey]. "Willan and Others on Vaccination." 9 (1806-07): 32-66.
Collects views on smallpox vaccination of Robert Willan, M.D., Benjamin Moseley, M.D., James Moore, F.R.C.S., and Robert Squirrel.

652 [Jeffrey, Francis]. "Sir John Sinclair on Health and Longevity." 11 (1807-08): 195-214.
Recounts John Sinclair's reasons for longevity, such as heredity, diet, and occupation.

653 [Jeffrey, Francis]. "Pamphlets on Vaccination." 15 (1809-10): 322-51.
Confronts foes of smallpox vaccination.

654 [Brougham, Henry]. "Papers on the Stone." 17 (1810-11): 155-67.
Pens therapy for stones in the gall bladder or kidneys.

655 "Experiments on Vegetable Poisons." 18 (1811): 370-79.
Remarks on experiments showing perils of alcohol and tobacco.

656　　[Gordon, John]. "Ellis on Respiration." 19 (1811-12): 41-63.
　　　　Theme is a study of respiration by Daniel Ellis.

657　　[Mackintosh, James]. *"Account of a Boy Born Blind and Deaf."* 20
　　　　(1812): 462-71.
　　　　Synopsizes a story by Dugald Stewart, Esq., F.R.S., of Scottish
　　　　child who is vision and hearing impaired.

658　　[Brougham, Henry]. "Brande on the Blood." 22 (1813-14): 178-
　　　　84.
　　　　Centers on the research of W.T. Brande on blood.

659　　"Appert on the Preservation of Food." 23 (1814): 104-31.
　　　　Offers techniques of food preservation from Charles Appert.

660　　[Smith, Sydney]. "Tuke's Account of the Retreat near York." 23
　　　　(1814): 189-98.
　　　　Following Samuel Tuke's tour of Quaker establishment for the
　　　　insane, speculates about roots of insanity and treatments for mania,
　　　　melancholia, and dementia.

661　　[Gordon, John]. "Functions of the Nervous System." 24 (1814-15):
　　　　439-52.
　　　　Highlights instances of brain injury and disease.

662　　"Lunatic Asylums." 28 (1817): 432-71.
　　　　Scrutinizer of several asylums would improve care of the insane.

663　　"On the Causes, Cure, and Prevention of Contagious Fever." 31
　　　　(1818-19): 413-40.
　　　　Would slow typhus, whose origin was purportedly murky, by
　　　　hygiene and isolation of the afflicted.

664　　[Gordon, John, Leonard Horner, and John Macculloch]. "Marcet
　　　　on Calculous Disorders." 32 (1819): 418-30.
　　　　Topic is the research of A.J.G. Marcet, M.D., on urinary stones.

665　　"Adulterated Provisions." 33 (1820): 131-44.
　　　　Chapter on the illegality of adulterating comestibles mentions their
　　　　deleteriousness.

666　　[Marcet, A.J.G.]. "Malaria." 36 (1821-22): 536-52.
　　　　Catalogs signs and spread of malaria in Italy.

667　　[Smith, Sydney]. "Vaccination and Small-Pox." 38 (1822): 325-
　　　　37.
　　　　Endorses smallpox vaccination.

668　　[Smith, Sydney]. "Licensing of Alehouses." 45 (1826): 441-57.
　　　　Anti-licenser nods to the adulteration of ale.

669　　[McCulloch, J.R.]. "Rise, Progress, Present State, and Prospects
　　　　of the British Cotton Manufacture." 46 (1827): 1-39.
　　　　Minimizes the unhealthiness of mills and child labor, but ratifies
　　　　protective legislation for the immature.

670   "Dietetics." 47 (1828): 37-59.
        Talks about the relationship of food to wellness.
671   [Conolly, John]. "Nervous System." 47 (1828): 441-81.
        Describes functions and malfunctions of nerves.
672   [Sandford, D.K.]. "New Systems of Cure - Hahnemann's
        Homeopathie." 50 (1829-30): 504-27.
        Appraises ideas of Dr. Samuel Hahnemann on homeopathy.
673   [Spring-Rice, Thomas]. "Proposed Introduction of Poor Laws into
        Ireland." 59 (1834): 227-61.
        Seeks Irish poor law for the sick, the old, and the young.
674   "Monypenny on the Scottish Poor Laws." 59 (1834): 425-38.
        Concurs with David Monypenny, Esq. that there must be a poor
        law for the Scottish ill and aged.
675   [Brewster, David]. "Dr. Roget's *Bridgewater Treatise - Animal
        and Vegetable Physiology.*" 60 (1834-35): 142-79.
        Based on a book by Peter Mark Roget, M.D., concentrates on
        plants and animals with an aside on human digestion.
676   [McCulloch, J.R.]. "On the Frequency of Shipwreck." 60 (1834-
        35): 338-53.
        Attributes deaths of seamen to official classification of vessels and
        ignorance of officers.
677   [Hamilton, William]. "Dalgarno's *Works.*" 61 (1835): 407-17.
        Refers to George Dalgarno on the education of the hearing
        impaired who do not speak.
678   [Chadwick, Edwin]. "The New Poor Law." 63 (1836): 487-537.
        Pages on former and current poor laws distinguish the elderly and
        ailing.
679   [Wrightson, W.B.]. "The Workhouse System -The Irish Poor Bill."
        66 (1837-38): 186-208.
        Essay on potential Irish legislation features care of the indigent ill.
680   [Senior, N.W.]. "Poor Law Reform." 74 (1841-42): 1-44.
        History of poor relief glances at the unwell.
681   [Spring-Rice, Thomas]. "Distress in the Manufacturing Districts -
        Causes and Remedies." 77 (1843): 190-227.
        Treks to regions of great poverty with sentences on the sick.
682   [Merivale, Herman]. "*Life of a Travelling Physician.*" 78 (1843):
        47-67.
        Profiles Sir George Lefevre, a physician who practiced mainly in
        Russia.
683   [Greg, W.R.]. "Juvenile and Female Labour." 79 (1844): 130-56.
        Ascribes many ailments of women and children to work, primarily
        in mills and mining.

684   [Phipps, Edmund]. "The Late Census." 80 (1844): 67-104.
        Tract on the Census of 1841 offers some data on causes of deaths.

685   [Christison, Robert]. "Medical Reform." 81 (1845): 235-72.
        Article on medical education, licensing, and practice votes for Sir
        James Graham's regulatory bill.

686   [Mill, J.S.]. *The Claims of Labour.* 81 (1845): 498-525.
        Overview on concepts of Arthur Helps on workers whispers about
        lack of sanitation as a source of their indispositions.

687   [Trevelyan, Charles E.]. "The Irish Crisis." 87 (1848): 229-320.
        Treatise on potato blight identifies it as a forerunner of disease
        among the Irish.

688   [Senior, N.W.]. "Relief of Irish Distress." 89 (1849): 221-68.
        Dissertation on Irish Famine downplays its relation to unwellness.

689   [O'Brien, W.]. "Transportation as It Now Is." 90 (1849): 1-39.
        Narrative on secondary punishments couples convicts' fare and
        fitness.

690   [Greg, W.R.]. "Unsound Social Philosophy." 90 (1849): 496-524.
        Explores the rationale for poor relief with a nod to the ill.

691   [Bainbridge, William]. "The British Mines: Mining Records." 91
        (1850): 62-87.
        Reveals mining perils that can be reducted by state intervention.

692   [Burton, J.H.]. "Sanitary Reform." 91 (1850): 210-28.
        Argues that absent sanitation, epidemic diseases, as cholera,
        proliferate.

693   [O'Brien, W.]. "Supply of Water to the Metropolis." 91 (1850):
        377-408.
        Asserts that, because London water is impure and insufficient,
        disorders from drinking and uncleanliness are likely.

694   [Greg, W.R.]. *England as It Is.* 93 (1851): 305-39.
        Disagrees with William Johnstone, author of captioned book.
        Believes that sanitation, railroads to the country, more food, less
        alcohol, shorter hours, and better job conditions will promote
        workers' health.

695   [Burton, J.H.]. "Fatal Accidents: How Far Preventible." 94 (1851):
        98-127.
        Finds most fatalities came from structural fires and the operation
        of railroads and machines. Projects that such mishaps will
        diminish with official inspection.

696   [Greg, W.R.]. "Investments for the Working Classes." 95 (1852):
        405-53.
        Lists a variety of laborers' investments, such as bank savings,
        cooperative business ventures, and health insurance.

697 [Howell, T. James]. "Cholera and Quarantine." 96 (1852): 403-35.
Spotlights an episode of and societal answers to cholera.

698 [Howell, T. James]. "Quarantine, Small Pox, and Yellow Fever." 98 (1853): 191-215.
Details symptoms and outbreak of yellow fever, not smallpox.

699 [Johns, B.G.]. "The Blind, Their Works and Ways." 99 (1854): 61-93.
Emphasizes education of the vision impaired.

700 [Conybeare, W.J.]. "Teatotalism [sic], and Laws Against the Liquor Trade." 100 (1854): 43-79.
Opponent of teetotalism weighs alcohol's effects on health.

701 [Laycock, Thomas]. "Body and Mind." 103 (1856): 423-52.
Probes the physiology of the brain in relation to dreams, memory, use of narcotics, and sleep.

702 [Holland, Henry]. "Human Longevity." 105 (1857): 46-77.
Moors longevity to heredity, environment, and freedom from sickness.

703 [Carpenter, William Benjamin]. "Binocular Vision." 108 (1858): 437-73.
Explicates how eyes function.

704 [Leifchild, J.R]. "Life Assurance." 109 (1859): 37-65.
Chapter on insurance business has information on mortality rates and policies for illness.

705 [Martineau, Harriet]. "Female Industry." 109 (1859): 293-336.
Text on women's work interweaves circumstances affecting the wellness of farm workers and governesses. Promises that women doctors will safeguard their sisters' salubrity.

706 [Mill, J.S.]. "Bain's *Psychology*." 110 (1859): 287-321.
Considers opinions of Alexander Bain on association as a technique of psychology.

707 [Wynter, Andrew]. "Mortality in Trades and Professions." 111 (1860): 1-31.
Connects occupations with myriad maladies, notably of lungs and skin.

708 [Wynter, Andrew]. "Brain Difficulties." 112 (1860): 526-45.
Concerns some manifestations of insanity and consequences to the brain of fever, concussion, and lesion.

709 [Leifchild, J.R.]. "Wrecks, Life-Boats, and Lighthouses." 115 (1862): 153-84.
Worries about potential deaths in ship collisions, notwithstanding the National Lifeboat Institution, so seeks more coastal lighting.

710   [Cheney, R.H.]. "The Black Country." 117 (1863): 406-43.
       Labels miners' jobs and drinking pernicious.
711   [Sidney, Edwin]. "Idiot Asylums." 122 (1865): 37-74.
       Covers characteristics, care, and education of those mentally
       challenged since birth.
712   [Leifchild, J.R.]. "Water Supply." 123 (1866): 384-422.
       Brands London's water scarce and polluted.
713   [Leifchild, J.R.]. "Fatal Accidents in Coal Mines." 125 (1867):
       549-77.
       Indicates reasons for and deterrents to deaths in collieries.
714   [Rickards, G.K.]. "The Agricultural Labourers of England." 128
       (1868): 489-523.
       Notices unsanitary abodes and inadequate diet of rural toilers.
715   [Wynter, Andrew]. "Non-Restraint in the Treatment of the
       Insane." 131 (1870): 418-49.
       Evaluates theories and practices of therapy for the insane.
716   [Mann, R.J.]. "Researches on Life and Disease." 136 (1872): 216-
       44.
       Theme is blood circulation in relation to wellness and illness,
       specifically tuberculosis.
717   [Wynter, Andrew]. "The Progress of Medicine and Surgery." 136
       (1872): 488-515.
       Logs advancements in surgery, namely anesthetics, instruments,
       techniques, and hospital cleanliness, and in the treatment of
       insanity.
718   [Holland, Henry]. "Maury on Sleep and Dreams." 137 (1873):
       330-63.
       Condenses views of Alfred Maury on sleep, with sentences on its
       value for vitality.
719   [Croskerry, Thomas]. "Drunkenness, Abstinence, and Restraint."
       137 (1873): 398-421.
       Story on alcohol recognizes how baneful it is.
720   [Stanhope, Edward]. "The Agricultural Labourers of England."
       141 (1875): 126-49.
       Feature on agricultural union assigns members' wellness to their
       steady meals.
721   [Mann, R.J.]. "The Physiological Influence of Alcohol." 142
       (1875): 145-73.
       Documents the aftermath of drinking on the body.
722   [Clarke, W. Fairlie]. "Metropolitan Medical Relief." 146 (1877):
       146-65.
       Registers hospitals and dispensaries for London's sick poor.

723   [Mann, R.J.]. "Mental Physiology." 149 (1879): 58-83.
       Examines the nervous system.
724   [Mann, R.J.]. "Helmholtz and Carter on Eyesight." 154 (1881):
       516-46.
       Borrows from Hermann von Helmholtz and R. Brudenell Carter
       ideas about eye functions and diseases.
725   [Mann, R.J.]. "The Present State of Medical Science." 157 (1883):
       481-508.
       Ties recent cures to greater medical knowledge.
726   [Crespi, Alfred J.H.]. "Recent Advances in Surgery and
       Medicine." 168 (1888): 491-515.
       Headlines Victorian progress in pharmacy, medical discovery, and
       surgery.
727   [Phelps, L.R.]. "The Relief of the Destitute." 169 (1889): 398-415.
       Estimate of the poor law incorporates care of the sick, especially
       in hospitals.
728   [Tait, P.M.]. "Life Assurance." 172 (1890): 491-520.
       Script on life insurance has mortality tables.
729   [Phelps, L.R.]. "Sanitary Progress." 173 (1891): 65-92.
       Contends that clean air, job sites, and residences enhance life.
730   [Johns, B.G.]. "The Care and Education of the Blind." 173 (1891):
       123-44.
       Publicizes methods, notably braille, and price of teaching the
       vision impaired. See #1476.
731   [Johns, B.G.]. "Colour-Blindness." 177 (1893): 129-44.
       Primer on tests for color blindness mandates them for railroad
       signalers.
732   [Galton, Douglas]. "The Purification of Sewage and Water." 188
       (1898): 151-74.
       Clarifies how to detoxify sewage that pollutes water.
733   [Anderson, Elizabeth Garrett]. "The History and Effects of
       Vaccination." 189 (1899): 335-68.
       Piece on remedies for smallpox before vaccination hails it.
734   [Anderson, Elizabeth Garrett]. "The Ethics of Vivisection." 190
       (1899): 147-69.
       Pairs vivisection and medical headway.

THE FOREIGN QUARTERLY REVIEW, 1827-1846

Pledged to an international perspective, the *Foreign Quarterly*, which eventually merged with the *Westminster Review*, logged infirmity largely in figures.

735   [Ferguson, Robert]. "Berard - *Influence of Civilization on Public Health.*" 1 (1827): 178-88.
       Paraphrases F. Berard on downturn in mortality rates.
736   [Conolly, John]. "Andral, on Consumption." 7 (1831): 52-68.
       Transmits notions of G. Andral on symptoms of and treatments for tuberculosis.
737   [Copland, James]. "Pestilential Cholera." 8 (1831): 461-96.
       Abridges roots and signs of cholera and ways to check it.
738   [Conolly, John]. "Philosophical History of Hypochondriasis and Hysteria." 12 (1833): 110-30.
       Delineates causes and symptoms of hypochondria and hysteria.
739   [Lord, Percival B.]. "Animal Magnetism." 12 (1833): 413-44.
       Measures modes of hypnosis and its utility to medicine.
740   [Nichol, J.P.]. "Comparative Mortality of Different Populations." 13 (1834): 272-82.
       From birth/death statistics of England, France, Switzerland, and Russia, postulates why some populations are healthier.
741   [Taylor, William Cooke]. "Objects and Advantages of Statistical Science." 16 (1835-36): 205-29.
       Contains data on mortality and on the weight and height of youths in and out of factories.
742   [?Williams, Edmund Sydney]. "Ideler's System of Psychology." 18 (1836-37): 203-18.
       Ponders the thinking of K.W. Ideler on the interaction between mind and body.
743   [Conolly, John]. "French and English Schools of Medicine." 18 (1836-37): 304-16.
       Avers that medical research in France is superior to that in England.
744   [Conolly, John]. "Statistics of Insanity in Europe." 20 (1837-38): 39-54.
       Focuses on the etiology of insanity.

THE FORTNIGHTLY REVIEW, 1865-1900

Committed to no cause or sect, the *Fortnightly* circulated thoughtful and telling material on vitality. Entries on the hazards of labor and the housing of the impoverished ran regularly. Fascination with medicine and its practioners was both customary and comprehensive.

745   Editor [George Henry Lewes]. "The Heart and the Brain." 1 (1865): 66-74.
        Sketches the interrelationship between heart and brain.
746   Dennis, John. "Our Rural Poor." 1 (1865): 257-77.
        Discloses noxious living and working situations of rural dwellers.
747   Sayer, Frederic. "The Dangers of Madeira." 1 (1865): 612-22.
        Warns that Madeira's climate is inappropriate for those with tuberculosis.
748   Adam, William. "Consanguinity in Marriage." 2 (1865): 710-30; 3 (1865-66): 74-88.
        Prose on the historical, legal, and biological aspects of intrafamily marriages conjectures that their offspring are unhealthy.
749   Hart, Ernest. "The Condition of Our State Hospitals." 3 (1865-66): 217-26.
        Declares that many workhouse infirmaries do not have the prerequisites of good hospitals.
750   Bain, Alexander. "The Feelings and the Will, Viewed Physiologically." 3 (1865-66): 575-88.
        Pinpoints the nervous system. See #753.
751   Arnold, R. Arthur. "Sanitary Reform - Water Supply." 3 (1865-66): 607-16.
        Submits plans to improve the quantity and quality of water.
752   Bevan, [George] Phillips. "Underground Perils." 3 (1865-66): 617-25.
        Catalogs hazards of coal mining.
753   Bain, Alexander. "The Intellect, Viewed Physiologically." 3 (1865-66): 735-48.
        Elaborates on brain functions. See #750.
754   Parkinson, J[oseph] C[harles]. "On a Uniform Poor-Rate for London." 4 (1866): 184-92.
        Would revise the poor law for efficiency and clients' health.
755   Hart, Ernest. "Metropolitan Infirmaries for the Pauper Sick." 4 (1866): 459-63.
        Solicits better hospitals in London for the needy.
756   Foster, M[ichael], Jun. "The Elements of Muscular Strength." 6 (1866): 189-99.
        Ruminates about muscle physiology.
757   Cheadle, W.B. "The Progress of Medicine." 6 (1866): 567-78.
        Follows the evolution of medical knowledge.

758   Abram, W.A. "Social Conditions and Political Prospects of the Lancashire Workmen." n.s., 4, o.s., 10 (1868): 426-41.
        Tale of Lancashire credits the law for fewer job-related illnesses.

759   Fawcett, Millicent Garrett. "The Medical and General Education of Women." n.s., 4, o.s., 10 (1868): 554-17.
        Pleads for excellence in female education, for doctors and others.

760   Tollemache, Lionel A. "Sir G.C. Lewis and Longevity." n.s., 5, o.s., 11 (1869): 454-72.
        From cases of longevity, hypothesizes reasons for it.

761   Blandford, G. Fielding. "On the Nature of Emotion." n.s., 6, o.s., 12 (1869): 103-15.
        Attaches emotions to brain-nerve functions.

762   Bridges, John Henry. "Influence of Civilisation on Health." n.s., 6, o.s., 12 (1869): 140-61.
        Lesson on social and physical well-being reminds readers of the dirt and infant mortality in industrial towns.

763   Huxley, T.H. "Administrative Nihilism." n.s., 10, o.s., 16 (1871): 525-43.
        Supports some government action to stall smallpox and venereal diseases. See #764.

764   Spencer, Herbert. "Specialized Administration." n.s., 10, o.s., 16 (1871): 627-54.
        Amends #763. Chooses insurance and benefit societies for security against illness and accidents because government interference has usually been improper and ineffective.

765   Tollemache, Lionel A. "The New Cure for Incurables." n.s., 13, o.s., 19 (1873): 218-30.
        Judges merits of euthanasia.

766   Storr, John S. "The Anarchy of London." n.s., 13, o.s., 19 (1873): 754-68.
        Blames London's administration for the city's unsanitary milieu and unwholesome residences.

767   Phillips, Edwin. "The Internal Working of Railways." n.s., 15, o.s., 21 (1874): 372-84.
        Enumerates risks to employees of railroads.

768   [Maudsley, Henry]. "Sex in Mind and Education." n.s., 15, o.s., 21 (1874): 466-83.
        Insists that females' fitness will evaporate if they are educated as were males. See #769 and #2506.

769   Anderson, Elizabeth Garrett. "Sex in Mind and Education: A Reply." n.s., 15, o.s., 21 (1874): 582-97.
        Challenges thesis of #768.

770   Freeman, Edward A. "Field Sports and Vivisection." n.s., 15, o.s.,
      21 (1874): 618-29.
      Condemns cruelty to animals in all circumstances, medical and
      otherwise. See #2507.
771   Clifford, W.K. "Body and Mind." n.s., 16, o.s., 22 (1874): 714-36.
      Depicts brain activities.
772   Sandwith, Humphrey. "Public Health." n.s., 17, o.s., 23 (1875):
      254-70.
      Thunders that impure air and water and styles of sewage disposal
      abet disease.
773   Jex-Blake, Sophia. "The Practice of Medicine by Women." n.s.,
      17, o.s, 23 (1875): 392-407.
      Bruits legal and professional bars to women doctors.
774   Congreve, Richard, M.R.C.P., and J[ohn] H[enry] Bridges,
      M.R.C.P. "Vivisection." n.s., 17, o.s., 23 (1875): 435-37.
      Deems vivisection generally unwarranted for medical knowledge.
775   Roberts, W.H. "The Poor Laws and the Peasantry." n.s., 17, o.s.,
      23 (1875): 508-21.
      Illuminates sections on sickness in the poor law.
776   Cooke-Taylor, [Richard] Whately. "The Employment of Mothers
      in Factories." n.s., 17, o.s., 23 (1875): 664-79.
      Imagines that mills are not particularly deleterious for mothers.
777   Carroll, Lewis [Charles Lutwidge Dodgson]. "Some Popular
      Fallacies about Vivisection." n.s., 17, o.s., 23 (1875): 847-55.
      Rejects vivisection as valid research technique.
778   Darwin, George H. "Marriages Between First Cousins in England
      and Their Effects." n.s., 18, o.s., 24 (1875): 22-41.
      Concludes from statistics that consanguineous marriages do not
      breed insane or infertile descendants. See #2484, #2510, and
      #2513.
779   Bridges, J[ohn] H[enry]. "Harvey and Vivisection." n.s., 20, o.s.,
      26 (1876): 1-17.
      Salute to William Harvey contends that a distant immunity from
      rabies or cancer is not enough to excuse the brutality of animal
      handlers, with its consequences for popular morality.
780   Sully, James. "Hartmann's Philosophy of the Unconscious." n.s.,
      20, o.s., 26 (1876): 242-62.
      Reveals notions of Edward von Hartmann on the nature and
      manifestations of the unconscious.
781   Tyndall, J[ohn]. "Fermentation and Its Bearings on the Phenomena
      of Disease." n.s., 20, o.s., 26 (1876): 547-72.
      Thanks Louis Pasteur and Justus von Liebig for studying bacteria.

782   Yeo, J. [I.] Burney, M.D. "On Stimulants." n.s., 21, o.s., 27 (1877): 538-58.
       Reflects on how alcoholic and non-alcoholic beverages affect wellness.

783   Yeo, J. [I.] Burney, M.D. "Sea or Mountain?" n.s., 22, o.s., 28 (1877): 195-218.
       Gauges how sea and mountain locales moderate illness.

784   Bridges, J[ohn] H[enry]. "The Moral and Social Aspects of Health." n.s., 22, o.s., 28 (1877): 562-80.
       Associates physical vigor with mindset and milieu.

785   Maudsley, Henry. "Hallucinations of the Senses." n.s., 24, o.s., 30 (1878): 370-86.
       Propounds causes of hallucinations.

786   Gilbert, William. "The London Medical Schools." n.s., 25, o.s., 31 (1879): 47-61.
       Objects to the funding and faculty of London medical schools and to hospital care that they tender because students are ignorant, charity funds are redirected, and the poor, the pregnant, and outpatients suffer. See #373 and #379.

787   Scott, Francis. "English County Asylums." n.s., 26, o.s., 32 (1879): 114-43.
       Ruminates about many asylums for the insane.

788   Maudsley, Henry. "Materialism and Its Lessons." n.s., 26, o.s., 32 (1879): 244-60.
       Brackets brain damage with physical injury and disease, insanity with lack of morality.

789   Simcox, Edith. "Ideals of Feminine Usefulness." n.s., 27, o.s., 33 (1880): 656-71.
       Praises Dorothy Pattison, "Sister Dora," a nurse in the Black Country.

790   Yeo, J. [I.] Burney. "Health Resorts in the Pyrenees." n.s., 28, o.s., 34 (1880): 164-75.
       Lists assets and liabilities for British invalids of spas in the Pyrenees. See #795.

791   Brand, Henry R. "The Dwellings of the Poor." n.s., 29, o.s., 35 (1881): 218-28.
       Grumbles that habitations of the poor are still unsanitary and overcrowded, so the salubrity of inhabitants is in jeopardy.

792   Cameron, Charles. "Has Our Vaccination Degenerated?" n.s., 29, o.s., 35 (1881): 592-605.
       From statistics on deaths of those inoculated with smallpox vaccine, deems it less potent.

793   Gurney, Edmund. "A Chapter in the Ethics of Pain." n.s., 30, o.s.,
       36 (1881): 778-96.
       Orders a board to oversee vivisection. See #794 and #796.

794   Cobbe, Frances Power. "Vivisection: Four Replies." n.s., 31, o.s.,
       37 (1882): 88-104.
       Opposes, contrary to #793 and #1726, medical research using
       animals. See #796.

795   Yeo, J. [I.] Burney, M.D. "The Health Resorts of the Western
       Riviera." n.s., 31, o.s., 37 (1882): 198-224.
       Appraises resorts of southern France for British invalids. See
       #790.

796   Coleridge, [John Duke]. "The Nineteenth Century Defenders of
       Vivisection." n.s., 31, o.s., 37 (1882): 225-36.
       Denounces vivisection and its proponents. See #793, #794, and
       #1726.

797   Carpenter, William B[enjamin]. "The Ethics of Vivisection." n.s.,
       31, o.s., 37 (1882): 237-46.
       Endorses vivisection.

798   Galton, Francis. "The Anthropometric Laboratory." n.s., 31, o.s.,
       37 (1882): 332-38.
       Realizes the importance of records on physical history for health
       maintenance and medical treatment. See #805.

799   Yeo, Gerald F. "The Practice of Vivisection in England." n.s., 31,
       o.s., 37 (1882): 352-68.
       Backs vivisection to increase medical knowledge.

800   Carpenter, William B[enjamin]. "Sir Charles Bell and
       Physiological Experiments." n.s., 31, o.s., 37 (1882): 468-75.
       Declares that although Charles Bell's research on nerves was
       inaccurate, not all experiments with animals are flawed.

801   Lubbock, Montagu. "On the Development of the Colour-Sense."
       n.s., 31, o.s., 37 (1882): 518-29.
       Deals with color blindness.

802   Rossiter, Elizabeth. "Unnatural Children." n.s., 31, o.s., 37 (1882):
       612-19.
       Calculates that ill indigent children cost more than will the food
       and exercise opportunities to keep them well.

803   Broderick, W. St. John, [1st Earl Midleton]. "The Homes of the
       Poor." n.s., 32, o.s., 38 (1882): 420-31.
       Tags lodgings of the London poor unsanitary.

804   Creighton, C[harles]. "Importation of Disease." n.s., 34, o.s., 40
       (1883): 175-88.
       Treatise on communicable diseases alludes to cholera.

805   Galton, Francis. "Medical Family Registers." n.s., 34, o.s., 40
        (1883): 244-50.
        Reiterates motif of #798.

806   [Harris, Frank]. "The Radical Programme - The Housing of the
        Poor in Towns." n.s., 34, o.s., 40 (1883): 587-600.
        Allies dirty abodes to disease among townspeople.

807   Chamberlain, J. "Labourers' and Artisans' Dwellings." n.s., 34,
        o.s., 40 (1883): 761-76.
        Repeats that urban domiciles are dirty and comrades of disease.
        See #573 and #2189.

808   Corbet, W.J. "Is Insanity on the Increase?" n.s., 35, o.s., 41
        (1884): 482-94.
        From data on all of Great Britain, confirms that insanity is
        escalating, and expresses reasons for this surge. See #2574.

809   Blackley, William Lewery. "The Juggernaut of Poor Men's
        Providence." n.s., 35, o.s., 41 (1884): 537-48.
        Focuses on sick benefit societies.

810   Bazalgette, C. Norman. "London Water Supply." n.s., 36, o.s., 42
        (1884): 378-84.
        Proclaims that London water is not a carrier of cholera or other
        diseases.

811   Sharpe, Sutton. "Moderation and Total Abstinence." n.s., 36, o.s.,
        42 (1884): 675-87.
        Suggests that drinking alcohol in moderation is not detrimental.

812   Robertson, Eric S. "Education for the Hungry." n.s., 37, o.s., 43
        (1885): 95-104.
        Divulges that school meals are the only substantial fare that
        sustains some impoverished youths.

813   Mackenzie, Morell. "Specialism in Medicine." n.s., 37, o.s., 43
        (1885): 772-87.
        Approves of a trend among doctors toward specialization. See
        #814 and #815.

814   Donkin, H.B. "The Dangers of Medical Specialism." n.s., 38, o.s.,
        44 (1885): 67-78.
        Opposes specialization by doctors. See #813 and #815.

815   Mackenzie, Morell. "Medical Specialism: A Rejoinder." n.s., 38,
        o.s., 44 (1885): 267-76.
        Replies to #814, and restates the theme of #813.

816   Jeune, Mary. "Saving the Innocents." n.s., 38, o.s., 44 (1885): 345-
        56.
        Frets about society's inattention to the lack of vigor of illegitimate
        children.

817 Roose, Robson. "Health-Resorts and Their Uses." n.s., 38, o.s., 44 (1885): 382-94.
Categorizes resorts according to their restorative effects on various maladies.

818 Myers, Frederic W.H. "Human Personality." n.s., 38, o.s., 44 (1885): 637-55.
Entry on hypnosis has some lines on it as a therapy.

819 Edis, Robert W. "Health and Taste in English Homes." n.s., 38, o.s., 44 (1885): 711-21.
Supposes that mansions of the rich are unsalutary because of the means of ventilation and drainage.

820 Wilson, Robert. "Aesculapia Victrix." n.s., 39, o.s., 45 (1886): 18-33.
History of female medical education claims that women in the kingdom and the empire want doctors of their own sex.

821 Roose, Robson. "Wear and Tear of London Life." n.s., 39, o.s., 45 (1886): 200-08.
Announces job-related health problems of doctors, barristers, and members of Parliament. See #823.

822 Fenn, W.W. "The Welfare of the Blind." n.s., 39, o.s., 45 (1886): 472-79.
Proposes alternative training of the vision impaired.

823 Roose, Robson. "Rest and Repair in London Life." n.s., 39, o.s., 45 (1886): 500-08.
Cites ways to maintain the robustness of those in #821.

824 Maudsley, Henry. "Heredity in Health and Disease." n.s., 39, o.s., 45 (1886): 648-59.
Posits that heredity is significant for both sickness and wellness.

825 Heather-Bigg, Ada. "Female Labour in the Nail Trade." n.s., 39, o.s., 45 (1886): 829-38.
Assures readers that nail making is not dangerous for women.

826 Mackenzie, Morell. "Is Medicine a Progressive Science?" n.s., 39, o.s., 45 (1886): 845-54.
Extols developments in medical knowledge.

827 Crawford, G.M. "Pasteur." n.s., 40, o.s., 46 (1886): 9-22.
Mulls over Louis Pasteur's vaccine for rabies.

828 Jones, Alfred S. "Pollution of the Thames." n.s., 40, o.s., 46 (1886): 79-90.
Ranks sewage in the Thames as a serious risk to health.

829 [Manning], Henry Edward, Cardinal Archbishop. "Our National Vice." n.s., 40, o.s., 46 (1886): 388-94.
Singles out alcohol as antithetical to fitness.

830   Allen, Grant. "Falling in Love." n.s., 40, o.s., 46 (1886): 452-62.
       Disquisition on mating habits hints about eugenics.
831   Roose, Robson. "Infection and Disinfection." n.s., 41, o.s., 47
       (1887): 249-61.
       Includes causes of and curbs for communicable diseases.
832   DeWatteville, A., M.D. "Sleep and Its Counterfeits." n.s., 41, o.s.,
       47 (1887): 732-42.
       Pictures those illnesses accompanied by coma or trance.
833   Sargant, George Herbert. "Free Dinners at National Schools." n.s.,
       42, o.s., 48 (1887): 372-78.
       Prizes free school meals for juvenile robustness.
834   Roberts, Charles. "The Physical Condition of the Masses." n.s.,
       42, o.s., 48 (1887): 482-90.
       Assays statistics on diseases of the poor and sanitation and diet as
       factors for health.
835   Schloss, David F. "The Sweating System." n.s., 42, o.s., 48
       (1887): 835-56.
       Accents perils of sweated trades.
836   Schloss, David F. "Healthy Homes for the Working Classes." n.s.,
       43, o.s., 49 (1888): 526-37.
       Demands more sanitary housing for workers.
837   Savage, George H. "Homicidal Mania." n.s., 44, o.s., 50 (1888):
       448-63.
       Links insanity and the commission of murder.
838   Tyndall, John. "A Story of the Lighthouses." n.s., 44, o.s., 50
       (1888): 805-28; n.s., 45, o.s., 51 (1889): 198-219.
       Would electrify fog lamps to slow shipwrecks.
839   Roose, Robson. "The London Water Supply." n.s., 45, o.s., 51
       (1889): 325-38.
       Tracks purification of London water. Advocates two supplies, one
       for drinking and one for sewage disposal.
840   Thornton, Thomas Henry. "Two Centuries of Magistrates' Work
       in Surrey." n.s., 45, o.s., 51 (1889): 693-710.
       Overview on Surrey magistrates detects belated care of the insane.
841   Roose, Robson. "The Art of Prolonging Life." n.s., 45, o.s., 51
       (1889): 857-70.
       Attributes longevity to moderate meals and exercise, sufficient
       sleep, hygiene, heredity, and keeping busy. See #1471.
842   Abraham, Phineas S. "Leprosy and Its Causes." n.s., 46, o.s., 52
       (1889): 150-52.
       Dismisses heredity and contagiousness of the afflicted as sources
       of leprosy.

843 Jeune, Mary. "The Homes of the Poor." n.s., 47, o.s., 53 (1890): 67-80.
Denigrates tenements as filthy and overflowing with people.

844 Bradlaugh, Charles. "Regulation by Statute of the Hours of Adult Labour." n.s., 47, o.s., 53 (1890): 440-54; with letters: 454-60.
Denies that an eight-hour day is essential for laborers' health.

845 Mackenzie, Morell. "The Reform of the College of Surgeons." n.s., 47, o.s., 53 (1890): 601-20.
Applauds legislation to end patronage by and monopoly of the governing board of the College of Surgeons.

846 Luys, J. "The Latest Discoveries in Hypnotism." n.s., 47, o.s., 53 (1890): 896-921; n.s., 48, o.s., 54 (1890): 168-93.
Tells of methods and uses of hypnosis, principally as therapy.

847 Eccles, A. Symons. "The Tenth International Medical Congress." n.s., 48, o.s., 54 (1890): 581-88.
Quotes medical congress on recent improvements and ongoing difficulties in surgery.

848 Berdoe, Edward. "Dr. Koch's Consumption-Cure." n.s., 48, o.s., 54 (1890): 914-24.
Doubts the efficacy of tuberculosis vaccine of Berlin doctor, Robert Koch.

849 Mackenzie, Morell. "Influenza." n.s., 49, o.s., 55 (1891): 877-86.
Banners signs of influenza and its effect on the nerves.

850 Mecredy, R.J. "Cycling." n.s., 50, o.s., 56 (1891): 75-88.
Tale of bicycling understands its value for vitality.

851 Tyndall, John. "On the Origin, Propagation, and Prevention of Phthisis." n.s., 50, o.s., 56 (1891): 293-309.
Abbreviates the research of Dr. George Cornet on tuberculosis.

852 Mecredy, R.J. "Winter Cycling." n.s., 50, o.s., 56 (1891): 822-32.
Sponsors winter cycling with a caution against chills.

853 Lombroso, C. "The Physical Insensibility of Woman." n.s., 51, o.s., 57 (1892): 354-57.
Surmises that women feel less pain than men from the same maladies.

854 Corbet, W.J. "The Increase of Insanity." n.s., 53, o.s., 59 (1893): 7-19.
Holds that insanity is increasing throughout Great Britain. See #867, #869, #2558, #2574, and #2576.

855 Jones, A. Coppen. "The Benefits of Vivisection." n.s., 53, o.s., 59 (1893): 112-15.
Validates vivisection because of its role in the isolation of the cause of tetanus.

856   Nash, Vaughan. "The Home Office and the Deadly Trades." n.s., 53, o.s., 59 (1893): 169-83.
        Inventories dangers of numerous occupations.

857   Haffkine, Waldemar-Mardochee. "Vaccination Against Asiatic Cholera." n.s., 53, o.s., 59 (1893): 316-29.
        Confesses own efforts to concoct a cholera vaccine. See #2551.

858   Anderson, E[lizabeth] Garrett. "The History of a Movement." n.s., 53, o.s., 59 (1893): 404-17.
        Commemorates the success of women in becoming doctors.

859   Bevan-Lewis, W. "The Origins of Crime." n.s., 54, o.s., 60 (1893): 329-44.
        Judges alcoholism, insanity, and epilepsy common in criminals.

860   Nash, Vaughan. "The Employers' Liability Bill." n.s., 55, o.s., 61 (1894): 244-54.
        Lobbies for a bill to compensate for employment-related injuries.

861   Pearson, Karl. "Woman and Labour." n.s., 55, o.s., 61 (1894): 561-77.
        Agrees that women have a stake in state action on the health of workers because of the effect of female work on pregnancy.

862   Phillipps, Evelyn March. "The New Factory Bill: As It Affects Women." n.s., 55, o.s., 61 (1894): 738-48.
        Parades hazards of female occupations in factories.

863   Oliver, Thomas. "Our Workmen's Diet and Wages." n.s., 56, o.s., 62 (1894): 513-26.
        Yokes toilers' disorders to their food and jobs.

864   Roose, Robson, M.D. "The Spread of Diphtheria." n.s., 56, o.s., 62 (1894): 873-81.
        Instructs on symptoms and scope of diphtheria.

865   Phillipps, Evelyn March. "Factory Legislation for Women." n.s., 57, o.s., 63 (1895): 733-44.
        Certifies a host of threats to health for females in factories.

866   Smith, T.P., M.B. "Vegetarianism." n.s., 58, o.s., 64 (1895): 753-64.
        Controverts any bond between vegetarianism and salubrity. See #868 and #2566.

867   Corbet, W.J. "The Increase of Insanity." n.s., 59, o.s., 65 (1896): 431-42.
        Assumes that insanity is burgeoning throughout the kingdom. See #854, #869, and #2574.

868   Salt, Henry S. "The Humanities of Diet." n.s., 60, o.s., 66 (1896): 426-35.
        Rebuts anti-vegetarianism of #866.

869   Drapes, Thomas, M.B. "Is Insanity Increasing?" n.s., 60, o.s., 66
        (1896): 483-93.
        Disputes that there are more insane, speculating instead that there
        are merely more confinements. Puts alcoholism and heredity at the
        center of insanity. See #854, #867, and #2574.
870   Morris, Malcolm. "The Prevention of Consumption." n.s., 64, o.s.,
        70 (1898): 307-16.
        Parallels the decline of tuberculosis and inauguration of sanitation.
871   Tennant, H.J. "Dangerous Trades: A Case for Legislation." n.s.,
        65, o.s., 71 (1899): 316-25.
        Would legally protect persons in unsafe trades.
872   Tuckwell, Gertrude M. "A Seventeen Hours' Working Day." n.s.,
        65, o.s., 71 (1899): 783-88.
        Stipulates that exceptions to a reasonable working day adversely
        affect employee health.
873   Tuckwell, Gertrude M. "The Government Factory Bill of 1900."
        n.s., 67, o.s., 73 (1900): 972-79.
        Swears that new factory law weakens safeguards for laborers'
        wellness.
874   Parry, Edward Abbott. "The Workmen's Compensation Act; What
        It Was to Be and What It Is." n.s., 68, o.s., 74 (1900), 67-73.
        Alerts that universal compensation for job injuries is not available
        in law, either statutory or common.

FRASER'S MAGAZINE, 1830-1882

Opening and closing with a conservative overview, *Fraser's*, captioned
for Hugh, not publisher James, investigated the communal impact of
illness. Hence, hospitals, sanitation, and safe occupations were standard
subjects.

875   [Carlyle, J.A.]. "On Medical Quackery and Mr. St. John Long."
        1 (1830): 451-56; 2 (1830-31): 264-65.
        Accuses John St. John Long of puffing panaceas.
876   [Carlyle, J.A.]. "Animal Magnetism." 1 (1830): 673-84.
        Ponders hypnosis as therapy.
877   [?Moir, D.M.]. "The Asiatic Cholera." 4 (1831-32): 613-25.
        Covers cholera's symptoms and contagiousness.
878   [Macnish, Robert]. "The Philosophy of Burking." 5 (1832): 52-65.
        Satirizes murderers whose victims' bodies go to anatomists.

879   [Moir, D.M.]. "The Contagious Character of Cholera: England and
        America." 6 (1832): 119-23.
        From its rapid expansion, deduces that cholera is contagious.
880   [Maginn, William]. "National Economy: Surplus Labour and the
        Remedies Proposed - Poor Law for Ireland." 7 (1833): 282-91.
        Comprehends that Irish peasants starve without a poor law.
881   [Maginn, William]. "National Economy: The Factory System -
        The Ten Hours Bill." 7 (1833): 377-92.
        Vividly portrays the deleteriousness of factories for young
        workers.
882   "The Commission for Perpetuating Factory Infanticide." 7 (1833):
        707-15.
        Deplores laws that permit parents to expose their children to
        excessive and hence debilitating factory labor.
883   The Author of 'Old Bailey Experience' [Charles Wall].
        "Metropolis Water Supply." 10 (1834): 561-72.
        Hinges health in London to clean water.
884   "Oneiromancy." 19 (1839): 513-28.
        Has instances of people purportedly simulating death.
885   [Moir, D.M.]. "Occult Science." 22 (1840): 1-16.
        Reckons that medical progress will eliminate reputedly magical
        cures.
886   "Winslow's *Physic and Physicians*." 23 (1841): 149-53.
        Assails, as unflattering to physicians, the prose of F.B. Winslow.
887   "*The Spas of England, and Principal Sea-Bathing Places*." 25
        (1842): 182-91.
        Quotes A.B. Granville, M.D., F.R.S., on the roles of spas and sea
        bathing in salubrity.
888   "Trial of Daniel M'Naughten, the Bar of the Criminal Court, and
        the Plea of Insanity." 27 (1843): 444-54.
        Contemplates insanity in the context of a trial for murder.
889   "The Factory Bill." 29 (1844): 617-28.
        Associates ten-hour day for factory workers with better health.
890   S., R.S. "Animal Magnetism and Neurhypnotism." 29 (1844): 681-
        99; 32 (1845): 1-19.
        Text on hypnosis glances at its medical applications.
891   "Hints on the Modern Governess System." 30 (1844): 571-83.
        Bewails that too many governesses finish their careers insane or
        destitute.
892   [Guy, W.A.]. "The Sanitary Question." 36 (1847): 366-78.
        Rebukes local governments for tardiness in implementing salutary
        sanitary projects.

893   [Guy, W.A.]. "The Sanitary Commission and the Health of the Metropolis." 36 (1847): 505-17.
       Marks London's environment as less baneful than that of other cities but tainted by slum lodgings.

894   [Guy, W.A.]. "1774 and 1844; or, the Prisoner and the Labourer." 37 (1848): 40-54.
       Sees similarities in sanitation between prisons in 1774 and laborers' residences in 1844.

895   [Guy, W.A.]. "Church Lane, St. Giles." 37 (1848): 257-60.
       Thunders that the titled area of London is rampant with disease because of impure air and water.

896   "A Plea for Physicians." 37 (1848): 286-94.
       Core is the schooling and practice of physicians.

897   "Hospital Nurses, as They Are and as They Ought to Be." 37 (1848): 539-42.
       Recommends better training for hospital nurses.

898   "Quackery and the Quacked." 37 (1848): 645-57.
       Censures advertising about homeopathy, hydropathy, and hypnosis that is aimed at the uneducated.

899   [Guy, W.A.]. "The Public Health Bill: Its Letter and Its Spirit." 38 (1848): 444-46.
       Fixes on sewerage clauses of public health bill.

900   "The Thames: Its Uses and Abuses." 38 (1848): 685-88.
       Decries ongoing pollution of the Thames.

901   "The Lord Chief Baron's Law of Lunacy." 40 (1849): 363-73.
       Meditates on the reliability of procedures for certifying the insane for commitment.

902   [Guy, W.A.]. "Work and Wages." 40 (1849): 522-30.
       Paper on employment has a gloss on cholera outbreak.

903   [Guy, W.A.]. "Cholera Gossip." 40 (1849): 702-11.
       Enlightens audience about the incidence and prevention of cholera.

904   "The Drainage of the Metropolis." 41 (1850): 190-99.
       Spells out the perniciousness of having the same water supply for drinking and sewage in London.

905   "The Mineral Waters of Germany." 44 (1851): 149-55.
       Enthuses about the salubriousness of German spas.

906   [Wynter, Andrew]. "Preserved Meats." 45 (1852): 410-17.
       Demonstrates how tinned meat may be contaminated.

907   "Quarantine." 47 (1853): 74-83.
       Pens reasons for and against quarantine for cholera and typhus.

908   "A Visit to the Hospital for Sick Children." 49 (1854): 62-67.
       Vignette of a London hospital for children justifies the genre.

909   [Guy, W.A.]. "Neglected Health." 50 (1854): 238-44.
        Solicits government action to foster wellness.

910   "*Psychological Inquiries.*" 50 (1854): 371-87.
        Borrowing from Benajmin Brodie, seeks ties between mind and
        body, insanity and disorders of the brain and nervous system.

911   "Moral Insanity - Dr. Mayo's Croonian Lectures." 51 (1855): 245-
        59.
        Interprets Thomas Mayo's lectures in 1853 on insanity as a
        criminal defense.

912   "The Adulteration of Food." 52 (1855): 191-202.
        Explores prevalent, deliberate adulteration of food and fouling
        of water.

913   L[ewes], G[eorge] H[enry]. "The Story of a Great Discovery." 52
        (1855): 352-56.
        Remembers William Harvey's research on blood circulation.

914   L[ewes], G[eorge] H[enry]. "Dwarfs and Giants." 54 (1856): 140-
        53, 286-93.
        Exhibits cases of dwarfism and gigantism.

915   [Boyd, A.K.H.]. "Life at the Water Cure." 54 (1856): 197-207.
        Acclaims hydropathy.

916   H[umphreys], E[dward] R[upert]. "Some Talk about Food." 55
        (1857): 474-84.
        History of food has some sentences on nutrition.

917   [Lewes, George Henry]. "The Physician's Art: Dr. Watson." 57
        (1858): 94-104.
        Honors Thomas Watson, a physician.

918   A Sanitary Reformer [Charles Kingsley]. " 'A Mad World, My
        Masters'." 57 (1858): 133-42.
        Scolds government for indifference to sanitary reform.

919   "*Phantasmata.*" 57 (1858): 376-85.
        Introduces a study by R.R. Madden on insanity due to possession
        by devils.

920   H[elps], A[rthur]. "The Thames and Its Difficulties." 58 (1858):
        167-72.
        Pleads for decontamination of the Thames.

921   P[arker, John W.]. "The Expensive Luxury of Waste." 58 (1858):
        614-17.
        Learns, from a bluebook on sanitation, about official apathy to
        sewerage and water pollution.

922   G. "Hallucinations." 60 (1859): 625-31.
        Compresses notions of A. Brierre de Boismont, M.D., on
        hallucination.

923 Bain, Alexander. "Phrenology and Psychology." 61 (1860): 692-708.
Accentuates the power of mind over body.

924 Mayo, Thomas, President of the Royal College of Physicians. "On the Relations of the Public to the Science and Practice of Medicine." 62 (1860): 179-90.
Articulates how doctors diagnose maladies generally and insanity particularly.

925 Brodie, Sir Benjamin C., Bart. "Homeopathy." 64 (1861): 337-40.
Grades homeopathy as therapy.

926 "Mental Epidemics." 65 (1862): 490-505.
Silhouettes people who simultaneously display similar physical symptoms that are apparently both mental in origin and group-induced.

927 A Man on the Shady Side of Fifty [A.V. Kirwan]. "Physicians and Surgeons of a Bygone Generation." 66 (1862): 566-78.
Commends several physicians and surgeons.

928 B[eaton], P[atrick] C. "A Chapter on Innocents." 67 (1863): 333-48.
Recites activities of "innocents," that is, persons reputedly with signs of insanity.

929 W[hyte]-M[elville], G. "A Week in Bed." 69 (1864): 327-35.
Rhapsodizes about pleasures of recuperation from a minor disturbance.

930 [Cobbe, Frances Power]. "The Philosophy of the Poor Laws and the Report of the Commission on Poor Relief." 70 (1864): 373-94.
Borrowing from an official report, a survey on workhouse infirmaries, asylums for the insane and the vision and hearing impaired, maternity wards, and the treatment of the mentally challenged and epileptics, wants more establishments, and more inspections therein, for the sick poor.

931 "The Embankment of the Thames." 70 (1864): 466-77.
Enumerates major engineering obstacles to sound sewerage in London.

932 "Late Operations on the Serpentine." 72 (1865): 125-34.
Motif is sewerage in London.

933 A[ustin], S[arah]. "The Cholera in Malta." 73 (1866): 93-103.
Reminisces about an 1837 cholera episode.

934 Cobbe, Frances Power. "The Indigent Class - Their Schools and Dwellings." 73 (1866): 143-60.
Bemoans risks to personal and public health of schools and teeming tenements.

935   Chadwick, Edwin, Esq., C.B. "Administration of Medical Relief to the Destitute Sick of the Metropolis." 74 (1866): 353-65.
        Bewails the failure of London officials to implement, with respect to the indigent ill, the poor law so that problems prevalent in 1834 survived. Would consolidate care, thereby expanding supplies and contracting costs, prohibit staff doctors from private practice, and appoint inspectors to monitor both personnel and sites. Would supplement such care with sewerage, clean water, and health officers to audit dwellings and deaths, both causes and interments.

936   [Cobbe, Frances Power]. "The American Sanitary Commission." 75 (1867): 401-14.
        Petitions for the reform of hospital nursing and for Parliament and volunteers to extirpate slums, hubs of communicable diseases.

937   "The Alcoholic Controversy." 78 (1868): 277-99.
        Article on the temperance movement acknowledges the menace of alcohol to wellness.

938   [Greg, W.R.]. "On the Failure of 'Natural Selection' in the Case of Man." 78 (1868): 353-62.
        Mutters that only those debilitated by indulgence or privation reproduce rapidly.

939   Tyndall, John, LL.D., F.R.S. "On Dust and Disease." n.s., 1, o.s., 81 (1870): 302-10.
        Preaches about the harm of air pollution.

940   "The Agricultural Labourer." n.s., 1, o.s., 81 (1870): 427-43.
        Narrative on farm employment avows that it is unhealthy, notably for juveniles.

941   "The Adulteration of Food and Drugs." n.s., 1, o.s., 81 (1870): 718-30.
        Reveals frauds in food and drug manufacture that threaten salubrity.

942   Higgins, W.M. "The Water We Should Not Drink." n.s., 2, o.s., 82 (1870): 66-72.
        Rages about water pollution, chiefly from sewage.

943   Stephen, Leslie. "Athletic Sports and University Studies." n.s., 2, o.s., 82 (1870): 691-704.
        Warns that some sports at university are perilous.

944   Wright, Thomas, the 'Journeyman Engineer'. "On the Condition of the Working Classes." n.s., 4, o.s., 84 (1871): 426-40.
        Tract on the lifestyle of workers says that their congested abodes contribute to disease.

945   Owen, Richard. "On Longevity." n.s., 5, o.s., 85 (1872): 218-33.
        Draws from physiological probes of longevity.

946 "The Agricultural Strike." n.s., 5, o.s., 85 (1872): 651-66.
Professes that farm workers are often sick because they cannot afford proper food and lodging.

947 [Stack, J. Herbert]. "The Duties of the State." n.s., 5, o.s., 85 (1872): 737-50.
Ratifies the regulation of communicable diseases and sewerage.

948 Rawlinson, Robert, C.E., C.B. "Domestic Sanitary Arrangements." n.s., 6, o.s., 86 (1872): 775-81.
Parrots dangers of inadequate sewerage and dirty air and water.

949 Galton, Francis. "Hereditary Improvement." n.s., 7, o.s., 87 (1873): 116-30.
Sanctions eugenics to improve physical and mental health.

950 Jefferies, Richard. "A Railway-Accidents Bill." n.s., 9, o.s., 89 (1874): 658-70.
Attests to the likelihood of injury in railroad travel. See #954.

951 H[ardy], H. N[elson]. "Our Great London Hospitals." n.s., 10, o.s., 90 (1874): 179-85, 670-78.
Tracks the administration of and medical care, mainly of outpatients, in London hospitals.

952 "Training-Schools for Nurses." n.s., 10, o.s., 90 (1874): 706-13.
Encompasses not only the preparation of nurses for private and hospital duty but also assets and liabilities of their career.

953 Newman, Francis William. "Vegetarianism." n.s., 11, o.s., 91 (1875): 156-72.
Favors vegetarian menus for vigor.

954 Jefferies, Richard. "The Shipton Accident." n.s., 11, o.s., 91 (1875): 234-42.
Echoes #950.

955 Hoggan, George, M.B., C.M. "Vivisection." n.s., 11, o.s., 91 (1875): 521-28.
Stamps vivisection cruel and its practioners insensitive to animals.

956 H[ardy], H. N[elson]. "The First London Dispensaries." n.s., 11, o.s., 91 (1875): 598-607.
Retrospective of London dispensaries moves to Irish ones as examples of effective curbs to contagions.

957 Jefferies, Richard. "Field-Faring Women." n.s., 12, o.s., 92 (1875): 382-95.
Text on female farm laborers tells of their unhealthy pregnancies.

958 Galton, Francis, F.R.S. "The History of Twins, as a Criterion of the Relative Powers of Nature and Nurture." n.s., 12, o.s., 92 (1875): 566-76.
Expects twins to have parallel pains and illnesses.

959   E., S. "The Ventilation of Hospitals." n.s., 12, o.s., 92 (1875): 577-91.
        Would change the air quality in hospitals.

960   Baker, George Sherston, Barrister-at-Law. "A Few Words on Interment." n.s., 13, o.s., 93 (1876): 81-85.
        Prefers cremation as more sanitary than burial of the dead.

961   C[onder], F[rancis] R. "Waste of Power in Sanitary Improvement." n.s., 13, o.s., 93 (1876): 506-13.
        Protests that government reports on sanitation are invisible, so studies are unnecessarily duplicated.

962   Newman, Francis W[illiam]. "On Cruelty." n.s., 13, o.s., 93 (1876): 523-36.
        Dissertation on cruelty disputes merits of vivisection, and designates it retrogressive for society.

963   E., S. "The Poor and the Hospitals." n.s., 13, o.s., 93 (1876): 715-27.
        Would alter hospital care of the sick poor in numerous ways.

964   C[onder], F[rancis] R. "The Future Sources of the Illumination and Water Supply of London." n.s., 14, o.s., 94 (1876): 45-52.
        Supports unpolluted water for London.

965   Horne, Richard Hengist. "Eyes and Eye-Glasses: A Friendly Treatise." n.s., 14, o.s., 94 (1876): 698-722.
        Item on malfunctions of the eye separates oculists and opticians.

966   Hopkins, Ellice. "The Moral Treatment of Insanity: A Sketch of Its Rise and Progress." n.s., 15, o.s., 95 (1877): 444-59.
        Praises current treatments for insanity.

967   Conder, F[rancis] R., C.E. "The Battles of Peace." n.s., 15, o.s., 95 (1877): 797-806.
        Pinpoints mineral traffic as a key to casualties among railroaders.

968   Bell, Horace. "The Functions of Government Regarding Public Works." n.s., 17, o.s., 97 (1878): 309-14.
        Countenances state-run railroads for safety.

969   Conder, F[rancis] R., C.E. "The Limit of the Habitability of London." n.s., 17, o.s., 97 (1878): 482-92.
        Tags mishandled sewage and impure water bad for Londoners.

970   Conder, F[rancis] R., C.E. "The Question of the Thames." n.s., 18, o.s., 98 (1878): 726-36.
        Thesis is the befouling of the Thames.

971   Cooke-Taylor, [Richard] Whately. "The New Factory Act." n.s., 19, o.s., 99 (1879): 55-62.
        Cheers clauses in factory law on occupational health. Rues that there are not similar statutes for other workers.

972 Barraclough, George, M.R.C.S. Eng. "On Nursing as a Career for Ladies." n.s., 19, o.s., 99 (1879): 468-79.
Familiarizes readers with the training, duties, and salaries of nurses.

973 Conder, Francis R., C.E. "Are Explosions in Coal Mines Preventible?" n.s., 19, o.s., 99 (1879): 557-68.
Shares ideas about how to decrease accidents in coal mines.

974 Burdett, Henry C. "Hospital Nursing." n.s., 22, o.s., 102 (1880): 112-25.
Monitors the education and tasks of hospital nurses. See #1713.

975 Richardson, Benjamin Ward, M.D., LL.D., F.R.S. "Woman as a Sanitary Reformer." n.s., 22, o.s., 102 (1880): 667-83.
Would enlighten women about physiology, food and drink, and disease in order to secure family health.

976 Conder, F[rancis] R. "The Problem of Railway Safety." n.s., 22, o.s., 102 (1880): 798-805.
Would not mix freight and human traffic on railroads because to do so is dangerous and expensive.

977 Burdett, Henry C. "Hospital Reform." n.s., 23, o.s., 103 (1881): 501-14.
Laments that many wealthy patients in hospitals and their clinics pay nothing.

978 Chadwick, Edwin. "Employer Liability for Accidents to Workpeople." n.s., 23, o.s., 103 (1881): 680-92.
Predicts that employers' liability for employee mishaps will speed owners' adoption of safer techniques.

979 Rawlings, B. Burford. "The Honorary Element in Hospital Administration." n.s., 24, o.s., 104 (1881): 57-67.
Befriends hospital administrators trained in medicine.

980 Rawlings, B. Burford. "The Finance of Unendowed Hospitals." n.s., 24, o.s., 104 (1881): 212-23.
Would channel monetary donations only to hospitals accredited by government.

981 Richardson, Benjamin Ward, M.D., LL.D., F.R.S., President of the Brighton Health Congress. "The Seed-Time of Health." n.s., 25, o.s., 105 (1882): 28-45.
Categorizes unwellness as inherited, accidental, inflicted, and acquired.

982 Rawlings, B. Burford. "The Case of the Special Hospitals." n.s., 25, o.s., 105 (1882): 720-33.
Demystifies the medical and fiscal management of special hospitals.

GOOD WORDS, 1860-1900

Seeking to span the gap between godly and earthly affairs, *Good Words* surveyed sickness. The paper, with ties to the *Contemporary Review* and the *Sunday Magazine*, sermonized most about the needy, notably children. Consequently, hospitals and nursing also captured headlines.

983   Brown, John. "The Doctor: A Lay Sermon for Working People, by the Author of 'Rab and His Friends'." 2 (1861): 30-32.
        Advises workers to trust, obey, and reward doctors and to disdain quacks. See #986.

984   The Author of 'John Halifax, Gentleman' [Dinah Maria Mulock]. "Give Us Air!" 2 (1861): 38-42.
        Suspects that without fresh air, people are susceptible to illness.

985   Hollingshead, John. "Huddled Together in London." 2 (1861): 110-13.
        Blares that London's congested and filthy houses are unsalutary.

986   Brown, J[ohn]. "The Doctor: His Duties to You." 2 (1861): 168-70.
        Counsels doctors not only to heal but also to be trustworthy, compassionate, and grateful for patients. See #983.

987   Hollingshead, John. "London Model Lodging-Houses." 2 (1861): 170-74.
        Cautions that even model interiors in titled domiciles have some hazards, such as steps too winding for the young.

988   Smith, Angus. "Light and Scenery as Affecting Health." 2 (1861): 236-40.
        Presumes that light and color contribute to robustness.

989   Brown, John. "Children and How to Guide Them." 2 (1861): 309-13.
        Story on juvenile fitness promotes nutrition and smallpox vaccination but not laudanum.

990   Fyfe, J.H. "The Ways and Works of the Blind." 2 (1861): 313-18.
        Extols achievements of the vision impaired.

991   Jones, Thomas Herbert. "Patent Medicines: What They Are, and How They Are Sold - A Candid Confession." 2 (1861): 371-75.
        Purveyor of patent medicines recalls his career.

992   Brown, John. "Health." 2 (1861): 493-96.
        Prefaces vigor with sleep, diet, and hygiene.

993   Brown, John. "Medical Odds and Ends." 2 (1861): 651-56.
        Chats about teeth, beards, and shoes as elements of wellness.

994   Leifchild, J.R. "Causes and Remedies of Colliery Calamities." 3 (1862): 137-43.
Would modify mining methods and milieu to cut job fatalities.

995   Brewster, David. "The Eye - Its Structure and Powers." 3 (1862): 170-76.
Has illustrations of the eye and prose on its functions. See #998.

996   Leifchild, J.R. "Colliers in Their Homes and at Their Work." 3 (1862): 213-20.
Piece on miners roots many of their maladies in their occupation.

997   Gairdner, W.T. "Houses and Homes." 3 (1862): 411-16.
Taps clean air and water and nutritious fare as fundamental for vitality.

998   Brewster, David. "The Human Eye: Its Phenomena and Illusions." 3 (1862): 498-503.
Has cases of optical illusions and color blindness. See #995.

999   Crosswaithe, John. "Needlewomen." 4 (1863): 684-88.
Posts dangers to women's health from sewing for pay.

1000   Brewster, David. "The Life-Boat and Its Work." 4 (1863): 688-97.
Credits Lifeboat Institution for services to the shipwrecked.

1001   Almond, James. "A Fireside Wrong." 4 (1863): 873-78.
Swears that, notwithstanding 1840 Act for the Regulation of Chimney Sweepers, climbing boys are still in jeopardy.

1002   By the Author of 'John Halifax, Gentleman' [Dinah Maria Mulock]. "Meadowside House." 5 (1864): 19-23.
Tarries at the Hospital for Sick Children, Edinburgh, which caters to the poor.

1003   Stevenson, David, F.R.S.E. "Our Lighthouses." 5 (1864): 105-15, 233-42.
Salutes lighthouses for curtailing shipwrecks.

1004   Wilson, F.E. "Keeping Up the Fire." 5 (1864): 567-69.
Blesses hospital night nurses.

1005   Taylor, Isaac. "Country Life - Routine of the Seasons - Family Health." 5 (1864): 625-31.
Guesses that rural air is much more conducive to health than is urban.

1006   Wynter, Andrew. "The Water Supply of London." 5 (1864): 769-76.
Admits that London's water is not always pure.

1007   Playfair, Lyon, C.B., LL.D. "On the Nature and Composition of Food." 6 (1865): 24-31, 156-64.
Expounds on nutritional value of some foods. Would tailor diet to lifestyle.

1008   Hollingshead, John. "Tiny Needleworkers." 6 (1865): 124-25.
         Repines because needlework is so deleterious for very young
         sewers.

1009   Wynter, Andrew. "Longevity." 6 (1865): 492-94.
         Names digestion, state-of-mind, and heredity as important for
         longevity.

1010   Rogers, Henry. "Railway Accidents and Securities Against Them."
         6 (1865): 578-86.
         Grounds railroad accidents in passenger overcrowding and
         luggage handling.

1011   Wilkinson, W.F. "Health of Body and Mind." 7 (1866): 48-54,
         116-23, 181-88.
         Tabs menu, air, exercise, hygiene, and clothing as factors in well-
         being of mind and body.

1012   Fox, Tilbury. "A Day with the Out-Patients of a Hospital." 7
         (1866): 232-37.
         Witnesses a diversity of cases in a hospital clinic.

1013   Gilmore, John. "A Night with the Ramsgate Life-Boat: One
         Hundred Twenty Lives Saved." 7 (1866): 244-52.
         Reports on the rescue of shipwrecked passengers.

1014   Wynter, Andrew. "Village Hospitals." 7 (1866): 348-55.
         Subsumes administration and activities, notably of nurses and
         surgeons, in country hospitals.

1015   A Medical Man. "Some Effects of Intemperance on the Brain." 7
         (1866): 395-401.
         Gathers instances of the harm of alcohol on the brain.

1016   Wynter, Andrew. "London Street Traffic." 7 (1866): 401-06.
         Regrets the plethora of serious accidents due to congestion in
         London lanes.

1017   The Author of 'Quaker Philanthropy.' "Johanna Chandler." 7
         (1866): 537-42.
         Eulogizes woman behind the Northern Hospital for the Paralysed
         and Epileptic. See #1019.

1018   Browne, Matthew [William Brighty Rands]. "The Deformed and
         the Stricken." 7 (1866): 737-40.
         Pertains to the physically challenged, from birth or after.

1019   The Author of 'Quaker Philanthropy.' "Mary Merryweather." 7
         (1866): 748-52.
         Bows to the founder of Liverpool Nurses' Home and Training
         School. See #1017.

1020   Wynter, Andrew. "Meat at Starvation Prices." 7 (1866): 839-42.
         Concentrates on how to add more meat to diets of the poor.

1021 Hollingshead, John. "Unhealthy Humour." 8 (1867): 106-07.
Castigates comedies about illness.

1022 Gilbert, William. "The English Demoniac." 8 (1867): 116-24.
Demarcates as insane those alleging demonic possession.

1023 Murray, Andrew. "A Personal Experience of Fire-Damp." 8
(1867): 326-28.
Reputed onlooker relives mining explosion.

1024 Skirving, Robert Scot. "The Agricultural Labourer and His Food."
8 (1867): 387-92.
Ponders the size not the nutritiousness of the farm laborer's menu.

1025 "The Sewing Machine." 8 (1867): 417-20.
Boosts sewing machine to alleviate needlewomen's fatigue and to
employ the vision impaired.

1026 DeMorgan, S.E. "Playgrounds for Poor Children." 8 (1867): 727-
30.
Would supplement ragged schools with playgrounds for the
salubrity of city urchins.

1027 Nightingale, Florence. "Una and the Lion." 9 (1868): 360-66.
Entreats women to become nurses.

1028 Kingsley, Charles. "The Two Breaths." 10 (1869): 498-504.
Prioritizes fresh air and exercise for fitness.

1029 Betham-Edwards, M. "Cottage Homes for Workhouse Children;
or, 'The Boarding-Out System'." 11 (1870): 173-75.
Would send waifs in workhouses to rural homes for mental even
more than physical health.

1030 Lynn-Linton, E[liza]. "A Small Hospital with a Large Name." 12
(1871): 790-94.
Acquaints audience with the Great Northern Hospital, London, a
purportedly small but necessary institution for its neigborhood.

1031 Camden, Charles. " 'Pity the Poor Blind'." 13 (1872): 205-10,
284-88.
Concentrates on endeavors, such as working and begging, of the
vision impaired.

1032 Gilbert, William. "The Idiot Colony at Caterham." 13 (1872): 271-
77.
Profiles the mentally challenged in a care facility.

1033 Kingsley, C[harles]. "The Science of Health." 14 (1873): 44-50.
Forecasts that health education will elevate and prolong life and
perhaps phase out hereditary ailments.

1034 Thomson, Sir William, LL.D., F.R.S. "Lighthouses of the Future."
14 (1873): 217-24.
Topic is new ways for lighthouses to foil shipwrecks.

1035   Page, H.A. "Our Merchant Seamen." 14 (1873): 246-52.
        Conjectures that official guidelines on ship load and equipment
        and crew numbers and meals will arrest job-related deaths.

1036   Gilbert, William. "Deaf and Dumb Asylum." 14 (1873): 252-56.
        Grieves that the hearing impaired who do not speak are often
        mistaken as mentally challenged because they are not trained.

1037   A Riverside Visitor. "A Half-Yearly Overhaul." 14 (1873): 612-
        16.
        Oversees applications by the impoverished ill and elderly for
        outdoor relief.

1038   Author of 'John Halifax, Gentleman' [Dinah Maria Mulock].
        "Fighting in the Dark." 14 (1873): 634-39.
        Journeys to music school for the vision impaired.

1039   Kingsley, C[harles]. "Nausicaa in London: The Lower Education
        of Women." 15 (1874): 18-23.
        Earmarks incorrect eating and apparel and little exercise as sources
        of female debility. Would have the sex wholesome, as was
        Nausicaa, rather than learned.

1040   Page, H.A. "Sisters and Orphans." 15 (1874): 49-54.
        Compliments Tottenham Training Hospital and Orphan Home for
        its training of nurses and ministration to sick children.

1041   Kingsley, C[harles]. "Pure Water; or, a Substitute for Latin
        Verses." 15 (1874): 169-76.
        Allies epidemic disease and polluted water.

1042   Page, H.A. "A Day down at Ratcliffe." 15 (1874): 307-11.
        Chapter on East London children's hospital, directed by a doctor
        and a nurse, derives local infant mortality from impure air and
        water and overpopulated quarters.

1043   Esdaile, D., D.D. "Pneumatic Drainage." 15 (1874): 404-08; 17
        (1876): 773.
        Markets for public health a means to dispose, without water, of
        sewage.

1044   A Riverside Visitor. "The Dwellings Improvement Question." 15
        (1874): 515-19.
        Rules London housing, with its crowds, detrimental to wellness.

1045   Arnold, F. "Convalescent Homes and Hospitals." 15 (1874): 659-
        64.
        Esteems establishments for recuperation.

1046   Reid, P.Y. "A Successful Physician." 15 (1874): 738-43.
        Solemnizes the career of David Simpson (1810-67), a physician.

1047   A Riverside Visitor. " 'The House'." 15 (1874): 769-73.
        Vignette of a workhouse has some lines on care of the sick.

1048 Lees, Florence S. "District Nursing in a Large Town." 16 (1875): 318-20.
Scans cases of district nurses in Liverpool.

1049 Japp, Alex[ander] H. "In a Low Quarter." 16 (1875): 536-40.
Indicates improper sanitation as a major cause of illness among impoverished urbanites.

1050 Page, H.A. "Homes of the London Poor." 17 (1876): 140-44.
Lauds Octavia Hill for opening healthier homes for Londoners.

1051 Richardson, Benjamin W[ard]. "National Health." 17 (1876): 386-93, 498-504, 569-76, 642-48, 713-20, 785-92, 851-58.
Has paragraphs on health legislation, doctors, sanitation, food, lodging, and recreation.

1052 Scott, Adam. "Compulsory Registration of Infectious Diseases." 18 (1877): 410-414.
Guarantees greater public health if doctors have to register outbreaks of communicable diseases.

1053 Gilbert, William. "A Sawdust Pie." 19 (1878): 126-29.
Discusses the young vision impaired.

1054 Stanley, Arthur Penrhyn, D.D., Dean of Westminster. "Sick Children." 19 (1878): 140-43.
Sermonizes about juvenile patients.

1055 Williams, B.T., Q.C., M.P. "The Story of the Rhondda Valley." 19 (1878): 474-79.
Dramatizes the rescue of Welsh miners in a flood.

1056 Fletcher, J. Hamilton. "Feminine Athletics." 20 (1879): 533-36.
Would compel girls to exercise, walk, row, swim, and do gymnastics in order to be well women.

1057 Poore, G.V., M.D. "Hygiene and the 'Parkes' Museum." 20 (1879): 553-58.
Raves about *Practical Hygiene* by Edmund A. Parkes, M.D.

1058 Farrar, Joseph, L.R.C.P.ED. "Respiration and the Respirator." 20 (1879): 619-22.
Concern is nasal passages.

1059 Gilbert, William. "Savernake Cottage Hospital." 20 (1879): 841-44.
Penetrates the management and activities of rural hospital.

1060 The Riverside Visitor. "A Little Ireland." 20 (1879): 857-61.
Assumes that the Irish in England die because diseases speed through their supposedly teeming and dirty abodes.

1061 Fothergill, J. Milner, M.D. "Food for the Economical." 21 (1880): 18-21, 123-26.
Ranks foods according to nutritional value.

1062   McKendrick, Professor J.G., M.D. "The Ear and Its Mechanism."
        21 (1880): 55-60, 140-44.
        Describes the structure and functions of the ear.

1063   Richardson, B[enjamin] W[ard], M.D., F.R.S. "Health at Home."
        21 (1880): 64-70, 98-102, 282-87, 382-87, 569-74, 848-53.
        Sets forth salutary benefits of sunlight and sleep at home and
        instructions on how to secure and maintain cleanliness there. See
        #1066.

1064   Farrar, Joseph, L.R.C.P.ED. "Lung Capacity and Tight-Lacing."
        21 (1880): 202-05.
        Flags the peril to female lungs of tight corsets.

1065   Macquoid, Katharine S. "City Courts and Country Lanes." 21
        (1880): 429-32.
        Tickets country holidays to invigorate city children.

1066   Richardson, B[enjamin] W[ard], M.D., F.R.S. "Health at Home.-
        Second Series." 22 (1881): 50-55, 753-58, 817-22.
        Continues #1063.

1067   Hope, Lady [?E.W.], of Carriden. "Trained Nursing in Workhouse
        Infirmaries." 22 (1881): 351-54.
        Prays for qualified nurses for the ill in workhouses.

1068   Wagstaff, Frederic. "Children in the Black Country." 22 (1881):
        614-16.
        Indicts government for negligence whereby brickyard owners
        exploit junior employees without penalty.

1069   Granville, J. Mortimer, M.D. "Fish as Food and Physic." 22
        (1881): 676-77.
        Relies on fish for nutrition and for curing nervous disorders.

1070   Greville, Lady Violet. "The Sunshine of the Sick Poor in the East-
        End." 22 (1881): 693-97.
        Respects the service of district nurses to London's indigent ill.

1071   Granville, J. Mortimer, M.D. "The Wooing of Sleep." 23 (1882):
        70-72.
        Boosts ways to sleep without drugs.

1072   Fothergill, J. Milner, M.D. "Fashions and Physiology." 23 (1882):
        136-38.
        Damns most female apparel as unhealthy.

1073   Richardson, B[enjamin] W[ard], M.D., F.R.S. "Tricycling in
        Relation to Health." 23 (1882): 177-80, 679-83, 734-37.
        Views tricycling as salubrious for everyone.

1074   Fothergill, J. Milner, M.D. "Work and Overwork." 23 (1882): 571-
        76.
        Conveys the harm of mental and physical overwork.

1075 Simpson, Professor P.A., M.A., M.D. "Poison in Common Things." 23 (1882): 635-40, 807-12.
Brands polluted air, food, and water obstacles to wellness.

1076 Doyle, A. Conan. "Life and Death in the Blood." 24 (1883): 178-81.
Reveres researchers who demystify diseases.

1077 Strange-Butson, A.A. "Country Holidays for City Children." 24 (1883): 262-63.
Champions rural vacations to animate urban juveniles. See #1083.

1078 The Riverside Visitor. "London Haunts: A Rookery District." 24 (1883): 542-45.
Paints London paupers as chronically ill or genetically weak.

1079 Sharp, William. "Dust and Fog." 24 (1883): 721-23.
Headlines air pollution.

1080 Jones, Rev. Harry, M.A. "Life and Work among the East-London Poor." 25 (1884): 50-54, 107-11, 252-55.
Deplores foul air and insufficient food and sewerage in East London. Concedes that dispensaries assist victims of accidents and some maladies.

1081 Walford, L.B. "Our Vile Body." 25 (1884): 245-47.
Guides readers on diet, exercise, and recreation for health.

1082 Collier, J.F. "The Prevention of Cruelty to Children: Some Account of What Has Been Done in Liverpool." 25 (1884): 337-40.
Congratulates local branch of captioned society for guarding progeny from injury inflicted by parents.

1083 Rossiter, Mrs. Elizabeth. "Country Life for Poor Town Children." 25 (1884): 357-59.
Mirrors opinions of #1077.

1084 Granville, J. Mortimer, M.D. "How and When Stimulants Are Hurtful." 26 (1885): 46-47.
Discourages taking narcotics in excess or when exhausted or depressed.

1085 A Social Explorer. "London Opium Dens: Notes of a Visit to the Chinaman's East-End Haunts." 26 (1885): 188-92.
Peek at a London opium house has an aside on low salary and social indifference as elements of debility.

1086 Mitchell, William, Vice-Chairman of the Glasgow School Board. "Twelve Years' Dealing with Neglected Children." 26 (1885): 260-63, 391-94.
Would utilize volunteer societies and state schools to upgrade the health of neglected waifs in Scotland and the kingdom.

1087   Playfair, Right Hon. Sir Lyon, K.C.B., M.P., F.R.S. "The Disposal of the Dead." 26 (1885): 437-40.
Frowns on burial procedures that defile soil, air, and water.

1088   Mitchell, William, Vice-Chairman of the Glasgow School Board. "Pantomime Children." 26 (1885): 580-83.
Deprecates employment of juveniles in evening theatre because of risks to their physical and mental health.

1089   Twining, Louisa. "State Hospitals; or, Nursing in Workhouse Infirmaries." 26 (1885): 667-70.
Commends nurses in workhouses.

1090   McGregor-Robertson, J., Muirhead-Demonstrator of Physiology, Glasgow University. "The Relation of Living Organisms to Putrefaction and Disease." 27 (1886): 256-61, 611-16, 827-31.
Unmasks bacteria, chiefly in food preparation and preservation.

1091   Mitchell, William, Vice-Chairman of the Glasgow School Board. "The Infirm Children of Our Great Cities." 27 (1886): 478-82.
Wants facilities for ill and mentally or physically challenged waifs.

1092   Mitchell, William, Vice-Chairman of the Glasgow School Board. " 'Homes' of Poor Children." 27 (1886): 618-22.
Hitches unwellness of destitute young to unsanitary domiciles.

1093   Thorpe, Professor T.E., F.R.S. "A Colliery Explosion." 28 (1887): 96-102.
Pens reasons for explosions in coal mines.

1094   Ingelow, Jean. "On the Culture of the Senses: The Colour Blind." 29 (1888): 195-99, 247-51.
Inquires about the nature of color blindness and its impact on the job performance of doctors, nurses, pharmacists, and railroad signalers.

1095   Ingelow, Jean. "Taste." 29 (1888): 413-15.
Notifies that taste is not a barrier to swallowing poison. Also has words on nutritious fare.

1096   Rossiter, W. "The Originator of 'Country Life for Poor Town Children' - Mrs. Elizabeth Rossiter." 29 (1888): 702-03.
Extols Elizabeth Rossiter's plan to restore urban children by rural sojourns.

1097   Waugh, Rev. Benjamin. "Cruelty to Children." 29 (1888): 818-22.
Arraigns parents and guardians for endangering juvenile health by beating or dereliction.

1098   Japp, Alex[ander] H., LL.D. "A Railway Whistle." 29 (1888): 850-54.
Validates the whistle to halt railroad accidents at night, in bad weather, or because of signalers' weariness or distraction.

1099   Rae, John, M.A. "English Industrial Insurance." 30 (1889): 406-11, 466-70.
Rules on societies that insure workers' against sickness or disability.

1100   Jones, Rev. Harry. "The Amusements of the People." 32 (1891): 163-66.
Prompts recreation and exercise for robustness.

1101   Preston, William C. "The London City Mission." 32 (1891): 241-48.
Interweaves titled Mission's attention to the ailing poor.

1102   Bolton, Mary P. "A Noble Work." 34 (1893): 563-64.
Glorifies those who rescue children from parental abuse.

1103   Preston, William C. "The Deptford Medical Mission." 34 (1893): 821-27.
Scans a doctor's tending of the impoverished ill.

1104   Frankland, Mrs. Percy [G.C.]. "Half an Hour with the Microbes." 35 (1894): 266-70.
With drawings, elucidates bacterial contamination of food and causality of tetanus.

1105   Tait, E.C. "Wanted a House." 35 (1894): 475-79.
Teams residential cleanliness and ventilation with wellness.

1106   Jones, Rev. Prebendary Harry, M.A. "Nurses and Nursing." 35 (1894): 554-56.
Idealizes nurses as competent, calm, responsible, and vigilant.

1107   Fleming, W.J., M.D. "About the New Cure for Diphtheria." 36 (1895): 115-17.
Targets an antitoxin for diphtheria.

1108   Haweis, Mrs. [?M.E.]. "The Soft Sex." 37 (1896): 36-40.
Would not pamper female patients lest that catalyze nervous disorders. See #448.

1109   Aikman, C.M., D.Sc., F.R.S.E. "Milk." 37 (1896): 763-69.
Fan of milk as nutritious would pasteurize it.

1110   Sorrel, Lucian. "In a Hospital Receiving Room." 38 (1897): 188-94.
Travels to hospital outpatient department.

1111   Frankland, Mrs. Percy [G.C.]. "Microbes and Mineral Waters." 38 (1897): 243-47.
Pinpoints the unhealthiness of mineral waters allegedly filled with bacteria. See #1118.

1112   Ward, B.M. "Recalled to Life." 38 (1897): 272-75.
Comments on how Therese Exner, both vision and hearing impaired, learned to speak.

1113   "An Accident Ward in Sunshine." 38 (1897): 476-77.
        Touches on the behavior of accident victims.

1114   Frankland, Mrs. Percy [G.C.]. "Louis Pasteur: A Sketch." 38
        (1897): 490-94.
        Appreciates achievements of Louis Pasteur.

1115   Whitechurch, V.L. "Fog Signalling on Our Railways." 39 (1898):
        173-78.
        Verifies that railroad fogmen are not at risk and are crucial for
        passenger safety.

1116   Lillingston, Leonard W. "Frozen Food." 39 (1898): 237-44.
        Would import frozen food, particularly meat, to enrich popular
        menus.

1117   Somerset, Duchess of [?Rowena Wall]. "A Plea for Workhouse
        Inmates." 39 (1898): 396-400.
        Guest in a workhouse thereafter importunes for better treatment for
        the sick poor.

1118   Frankland, Mrs. Percy [G.C.]. "Natural Mineral Waters and
        Bacteria." 39 (1898): 843-46.
        Amplifies the motif of #1111.

1119   Nuttall, G. Clarke, B.Sc. "The Inhabitants of an Egg-Shell." 40
        (1899): 20-22.
        Interest is bacteria that befoul eggs.

1120   Nuttall, G. Clarke, B.Sc. "A New Light on Cheese." 40 (1899):
        554-56.
        Pursues effects of bacteria in cheese.

1121   Dron, Rev. J.A. "Infant Chimney Sweepers." 40 (1899): 668-90.
        Recollects the concern, in 1840 and again in 1870, for the health
        of junior chimney sweepers.

1122   Jones, Rev. Harry, M.A. "Sickness." 40 (1899): 739-42.
        Pontificates, from a religious perspective, on how to cope with
        illness.

1123   Mackenzie, W.C. "Seaweed: Its Uses and Possibilities." 41
        (1900): 315-19.
        Boasts of seaweed's value as a food and as therapy for anemia,
        chiefly chlorosis.

1124   Cameron, Professor Sir Herbert C., M.D. "Present-Day Leaders of
        Science: Lord Lister." 41 (1900): 516-22.
        Lionizes Joseph Lister for his contributions to safer surgery.

1125   Lillingston, Leonard W. "The Underworld of London." 41 (1900):
        679-85.
        Observes that digging sewers in London is no longer dangerous
        employment.

HOGG'S (WEEKLY) INSTRUCTOR, 1845-1856

Dedicated to the dissemination of knowledge and virtue, *Hogg's*, sire of *Titan*, was an inexpensive collection of concise comments. Its primary concerns were public health and proper nutrition.

1126 "Steam - Its Influence on Society." 1 (1845): 33-36.
      Tract on steam power expects it to reduce mishaps of rail travelers.
1127 *"Lectures on the Ordinary Agents of Life."* 1 (1845): 39-41.
      Conveys the wisdom of Alexander Kilgour, M.D., on how air, climate, clothing, housing, and alcohol affect workers' fitness.
1128 "The Language of the Deaf and Dumb." 1 (1845): 253-55.
      Forwards programs to teach the hearing impaired to speak. See #1129.
1129 "The Method of Teaching the Deaf and Dumb." 1 (1845): 266-68.
      Broadens #1128.
1130 "Vaccination - Its Nature and Advantages." 1 (1845): 393-96.
      Corroborates the success of smallpox vaccination.
1131 "Vegetables Forming the Food of Man." 2 (1845-46): 81-83, 153-55.
      Passes on nutritional worth of grains, vegetables, and sugar.
1132 Landless, W. "The Amusements of the People." 2 (1845-46): 85-87.
      Dubs exercise and recreation linchpins of vitality for the poor.
1133 "Influence of External Agents on the Welfare of the People." 2 (1845-46): 97-98, 131-33, 218-21, 326-28.
      Calculates the influence of food, water, hygiene, housing, sewerage, and climate on health.
1134 M'Michael, Rev. Prof. "Benefit Societies." 2 (1845-46): 337-39, 353-56.
      Details the scope of benefit societies.
1135 "Manufacture and Adulteration of Champagne." 3 (1846): 72-73.
      Pivot is the toxicity of contaminated champagne.
1136 "The Cold Water Cure." 3 (1846): 163-66.
      Voices theories of E.L. Bulwer on hydropathy. See #1647.
1137 "Italy Considered as a Place of Residence for Invalids." 3 (1846): 189-92.
      Objects to habitation in Italy for invalids.
1138 "Dangerous Bleeding." 3 (1846): 305-06.
      Commands compression for excessive bleeding after tooth extractions.

1139	"Hallucinations." 4 (1846-47): 4-6, 28-31.
Displays victims of hallucinations.

1140	"Function of Digestion." 4 (1846-47): 104-07.
Essay on digestion schedules food intake to facilitate processing.

1141	"Spontaneous Combustion of the Human Body." 4 (1846-47): 237-39.
Has cases of death ostensibly by spontaneous combustion.

1142	"Health of Towns." 4 (1846-47): 267-70.
Hinges debility of impoverished urbanites to air and water quality, inadequate sewerage and quarters.

1143	"Health of Towns' Association." 5 (1847): 15-16.
Encourages groups dedicated to the wellness of townspeople.

1144	"The Food of the Million." 5 (1847): 65-67.
Juxtaposes diet and salubrity, especially for workers.

1145	"Our Famishing Neighbours." 5 (1847): 197-99.
Appeals for aid to stop starvation during the Famine in Ireland.

1146	"Education of the People by the State." 5 (1847): 225-27.
Growls that schools had insufficient ventilation and sewerage.

1147	"Sulphuric Ether - Use in Operations." 5 (1847): 241-43.
Elects ether as a painkiller in surgery irrespective of past fatalities.

1148	"Interment in Towns." 5 (1847): 295-97.
Defines municipal burials as health hazards.

1149	"New Method of Bread-Making." 5 (1847): 305-07.
Relies on the addition of salt for more wholesome bread.

1150	"Impudence and Quackery." 5 (1847): 327-29.
Inculpates the press for publicizing many nostrums.

1151	"Bleaching Greens and Gymnasiums for the People." 5 (1847): 329-31.
Anticipates that sites for laundry and exercise will spur a clean and sturdy populace.

1152	"The Disinfecting Fluid." 6 (1847-48): 68-70.
Charges government with indifference to public health. Would require disinfectant for sewage handlers.

1153	"New Baths and Wash-Houses for the People, in Liverpool." 6 (1847-48): 108-09.
Affiliates cleanliness of the body and clothes with wellness.

1154	"Hints on Houses." 6 (1847-48): 284-86.
Anchors vigor in ventilated and spotless homes.

1155	"Chloroform." 6 (1847-48): 328-31.
Votes for chloroform in surgery and in childbirth.

1156	"Inquiry on the Sanitary State of London." 6 (1847-48): 380-82.
Decries London housing without enough water and drainage.

1157 "Notes on Diet." n.s., 1 (1848): 7-8.
Would eat grains, potatoes, and fish, and would correlate menu and climate for salubrity.

1158 "Sanitary Reform and Agricultural Improvement." n.s., 1 (1848): 67-69.
Would manufacture manure from sewage otherwise dumped into the Thames.

1159 "Human Physiology - Absorption and Circulation." n.s., 1 (1848): 343-45.
Plumbs the role of blood in nutrition.

1160 "Public Health Act." n.s., 2 (1848-49): 105-07.
Introduces captioned Act as important for disease prevention.

1161 "What Is Cholera?" n.s., 2 (1848-49): 273-75.
States society's ignorance about origins of cholera, hence its rapid diffusion.

1162 "Apparent and Real Death." n.s., 3 (1849): 307-08.
Promulgates ways to ascertain death in order to avoid premature interment.

1163 "Town and Country." n.s., 4 (1849-50): 126-27.
Promises that rural excursions will revivify most municipal inhabitants.

1164 "North Wales Lunatic Asylum, Denbigh." n.s., 5 (1850): 249-50.
Confides that the insane, if treated at first symptoms and with kindness, can be cured as in the titled establishment in Wales. Worries about relapses because the indigent have no support after release.

1165 "Filtration of Water." n.s., 5 (1850): 274-77.
Proposes techniques to purify water.

1166 "Sanitary Improvements - Cemeteries and Public Walks." n.s., 6 (1850-51): 78-80.
Announces that crowded urban cemeteries jeopardize public health.

1167 "Hydrophobia." n.s., 6 (1850-51): 96.
Rephrases the notion of a M. Buisson that vapor baths counter rabies.

1168 "Innovations and Novelties." n.s., 7 (1851): 196-98.
Queries why people frequently resist reputed progress, such as smallpox vaccination.

1169 "Dreaming and Somnambulism." n.s., 7 (1851): 215-16.
Labels somnambulism a sign of stress.

1170 "Provision for Aged Females." n.s., 7 (1851): 310-12.
Begs on behalf of older, ailing gentlewomen.

1171   Eothen. "Impressions and Recollections of Hanwell Asylum." n.s.,
         8 (1851-52): 129-32, 193-96, 232-36, 296-300, 328-33, 361-64;
         n.s., 9 (1852): 8-10, 72-76, 120-23, 237-40.
         Narrative on a shelter for the insane has some of their literary
         compositions.

1172   "The Theory, Practice, and Capabilities of Insurance." n.s., 8
         (1851-52): 161-64, 241-43; n.s., 9 (1852): 65-66, 145-46, 253-55,
         299-301.
         Essay on insurance has a few words on policies for accidents, fire
         and travel, principally on railroads.

1173   *"God in Disease."* n.s., 8 (1851-52): 219-21.
         Pirates opinions of James Duncan, M.D., on how nature, by pain,
         fainting, and vomiting, warns of and wards off illness and repairs
         the body.

1174   "Houses for the Working Classes." n.s., 9 (1852): 296-98.
         Treatise on laborers' abodes noises about their unsanitary
         environment.

1175   "Memory and Its Caprices." n.s., 9 (1852): 377-80.
         Cases of amnesia cue such causes as trauma and illness.

1176   "Geographical Distribution of Health and Disease." n.s., 9 (1852):
         415-16.
         Attributes sickness, with some variations because of climate, to
         poverty, improper ventilation, work on dangerous jobs by or
         overwork of children and adults, alcoholism, "dissolute habits,"
         and war.

1177   "The Vital Fluid." n.s., 10 (1852-53): 49-52, 257-60, 470-72.
         Explains the function of blood in humans and other species and the
         nexus between blood and illness or poison circulation.

1178   "The Early Closing Movement in Manchester." n.s., 10 (1852-53):
         281-84.
         Essay on shorter workday fulminates that long hours are ruining
         the health of needlewomen.

1179   "Scenes from the Life of a Sufferer." 3d ser., 1 (1853): 316-24; 3d
         ser., 2 (1854): 78-84, 323-32.
         Writes, from patient's perspective, about the causes of insanity and
         asylum life.

1180   "Old Age, and Institutions for Its Amelioration." 3d ser., 4 (1855):
         121-28.
         Requests more facilities for care of the aged poor.

1181   "Man and His Surroundings." 3d ser., 4 (1855): 337-48.
         Discusses the aftermath of food, tea, tobacco, and opium ingestion
         for the body.

1182 "Noxious Occupations *versus* Public Health." 3d ser., 5 (1855): 405-16.
Summarizes Parisian attempts to control nuisances, such as slaughterhouses, and to reduce dust and skin contacts in workplaces. Also notices the deleteriousness of tobacco.

1183 "The Adulteration of Food, Drink, and Drugs." 3d ser., 6 (1856): 57-66.
Testifies to universal adulteration of bread, beer, and drugs.

1184 "The Blind - How Do We Treat Them?" 3d ser., 6 (1856): 130-46.
Covers education of and institutions for the vision impaired.

THE HOME AND FOREIGN REVIEW, 1862-1864

Replacing the *Rambler*, the *Home and Foreign* hardly whispered about wellness.

1185 Block, Maurice. "Poor-Relief in England and France." 1 (1862): 312-34.
Contrasts French programs for indigent insane, young, and hospital cases with English neglect of the starving.

1186 [Block, Maurice]. "Foundlings." 3 (1863): 497-521.
Dissertation on French schemes for foundlings has some sentences on hospitals.

HOUSEHOLD WORDS, 1850-1859

Resolved to reach many without being crude, *Household Words* counseled chiefly the comfortable. Edited by Charles Dickens, this progenitor of *All the Year Round* arraigned the town as the source of myriad maladies. Likewise, the journal lingered on perilous trades and polluted fare.

1187 [Wills, W.H.]. "The Troubled Water Question." 1 (1850): 49-54.
Recognizes difficulties in delivering pure water to London.

1188 [Wills, W.H.]. "A Coroner's Inquest." 1 (1850): 109-13.
Would move dissection sites of coroners for public health.

1189 [Horne, Richard Hengist]. "The Fire Brigade of London." 1 (1850): 145-51.
Paen to London fire brigade has lines on job and house blazes.

1190   [Morley, Henry]. "Letter from a Highly Respected Old Lady." 1 (1850): 186-87.
        Deplores jaw disease that afflicts makers of matches.
1191   Hunt, Frederick Knight. "The Registrar-General on 'Life' in London." 1 (1850): 330-33.
        Validates salutary London districts from official statements.
1192   [Wills, W.H.]. "Lungs for London." 1 (1850): 451-52.
        Associates fresh air in parks and vitality of Londoners.
1193   [Wills, W.H. and ?John Joseph Shillinglaw]. "The Preservation of Life from Shipwreck." 1 (1850): 452-54.
        Pumps for government inspection of lifesaving equipment before sailing in order to preclude deaths from shipwreck.
1194   [Wills, W.H.]. "Health by Act of Parliament." 1 (1850): 460-63.
        Would spend taxes on sewers, nuisance removal, and water purification.
1195   [Morley, Henry]. "The Water-Drops." 1 (1850): 482-89.
        Ridicules London's polluted water.
1196   [Wills, W.H.]. "No Hospital for Incurables." 1 (1850): 517.
        Petitions for a hospital for the dying.
1197   [Hunt, Frederick Knight]. "London Pauper Children." 1 (1850): 549-52.
        Celebrates suburban institute that offers nutitious meals, exercise, and clean air to destitute London children.
1198   [Jerrold, W.B.]. "The Methuselah Pill." 2 (1850-51): 36-38.
        Derides catholic elixirs.
1199   [Wills, W.H. and Thomas Stone]. "Hints on Emergencies." 2 (1850-51): 47-48.
        Refers to a volume on handling medical emergencies at home.
1200   [Hunt, Frederick Knight]. "A Great Day for the Doctors." 2 (1850-51): 137-39.
        Captions 1 October 1850 when some medical classes began.
1201   [Hunt, Frederick Knight]. "A Visit to the Registrar-General." 2 (1850-51): 235-40.
        Questions the accuracy of official birth and death statistics.
1202   [Horne, Richard Hengist]. "A Coal Miner's Evidence." 2 (1850-51): 245-50; with letters: 323-25, 427.
        Highlights risks to miners of explosions and other catastrophes.
1203   [Dickens, Charles]. "A December Vision." 2 (1850-51): 265-67.
        Broods about dirt as an ally of disease.
1204   [Strange, Charles and W.H. Wills]. "Death in the Teapot." 2 (1850-51): 277.
        Broadcasts evils of adulterated tea.

1205 [Hunt, Frederick Knight]. "Christmas among the London Poor and Sick." 2 (1850-51): 304-05.
Follows festivities on Christmas with injuries on Boxing Day.

1206 [Strange, Charles and W.H. Wills]. "Death in the Bread-Basket." 2 (1850-51): 323.
Protests the adulteration of bread.

1207 [Dickens, Charles]. "The Last Words of the Old Year." 2 (1850-51): 337-39.
Seeks safety devices for passenger ships.

1208 [Stone, Thomas]. "Physiology of Intemperance." 2 (1850-51): 413-17.
Publicizes the harm of substantial liquor drinking.

1209 [Wills, W.H.]. "Death in the Sugar Plum." 2 (1850-51): 426-27.
Claims that cheap sweets contain lead or poison.

1210 [Horne, Richard Hengist]. "Father Thames." 2 (1850-51): 445-50.
Bemoans the pollution of the Thames.

1211 [Hunt, Frederick Knight]. "Twenty-Four Hours in a London Hospital." 2 (1850-51): 457-65.
Details furnishings, organization, and patient care of a London hospital.

1212 [Stone, Thomas]. "Sleep." 2 (1850-51): 470-75.
Teams sleep and wellness.

1213 By an Eye-Witness and Sufferer [Richard Hengist Horne]. "The Builder's House and the Bricklayer's Garden." 2 (1850-51): 513-16.
Criticizes the construction of and sanitation in current residences.

1214 [Thomas, T.M.]. "A Suburban Connemara." 2 (1850-51): 562-65.
Ascribes the debility of inhabitants in Irish section of London to inadequate housing and sewers.

1215 [Horne, Richard Hengist]. "Lives and Cargoes." 3 (1851): 18-19.
Laments that rescuers of persons after shipwreck are less compensated than are those who salvage cargoes.

1216 [Stone, Thomas]. "Somnambulism." 3 (1851): 132-38.
Describes symptoms of and treatments for somnambulism.

1217 [Leigh, Percival]. "Some Account of Chloroform." 3 (1851): 151-55.
Illuminates chloroform's origin and its utility in surgery and in childbirth.

1218 [Horne, Richard Hengist]. "The Pen and the Pickaxe." 3 (1851): 193-96.
Blames administrative confusion for lack of sewers in many towns.

1219   [Morley, Henry]. "Fish Dinners." 3 (1851): 421-25.
        Would develop fish farms as an alternative to seafood from
        befouled waters.

1220   [Morley, Henry]. "Foreign Airs and Native Places." 3 (1851): 446-
        50.
        Prefers British sanitariums, with controlled environments, for
        those with lung disorders.

1221   [Jerrold, W.B.]. "Science at Sea." 3 (1851): 468-71.
        Verbalizes seasickness.

1222   [Hannay, James]. "The 'Dreadnought'." 3 (1851): 516-19.
        Subject is the Seamen's Hospital.

1223   [Oliver, Richard]. "The Treatment of the Insane." 3 (1851): 572-
        76.
        Considers causes of and remedies for insanity of the poor. Frets
        about the absence of government standards for private patients.

1224   [Martineau, Harriet]. "Malvern Water." 4 (1851-52): 67-71.
        Treasures water, drinking and cleaning, as salutary but not tight
        corsets that obstruct respiration and blood circulation.

1225   [Horne, Richard Hengist]. "Life and Luggage." 4 (1851-52): 152-
        56.
        Applauds saviors of the shipwrecked.

1226   [Morley, Henry]. "Need Railway Travelers Be Smashed?" 4
        (1851-52): 217-21.
        Beseeches railroads not to dismiss potential anti-accident devices.

1227   [Dickens, Charles and W.H. Wills]. "A Curious Dance Round a
        Curious Tree." 4 (1851-52): 385-89.
        Journeys to an institution for the insane.

1228   [Martineau, Harriet]. "Needles." 4 (1851-52): 540-46.
        After a visit to a needleworks, concludes that the occupation does
        not damage health.

1229   [Dickens, Charles and Henry Morley]. "Drooping Buds." 5 (1852):
        45-48.
        Welcomes the Hospital for Sick Children, London. See #37.

1230   [Wynter, Andrew]. "Saint George and the Dragon." 5 (1852): 77-
        80.
        Chats about the routine of metropolitan hospital.

1231   [Morley, Henry]. "One of the Evils of Match-Making." 5 (1852):
        152-55.
        Bruits perils, chiefly jaw disease, to match workers.

1232   [Morley, Henry and ?Richard Oliver]. "The Treatment of the
        Insane." 5 (1852): 270-73.
        Sketches a variety of facilities for the insane.

1233 [Morley, Henry]. "Constitutional Trials." 5 (1852): 423-26.
Condemns those who adulterate food.
1234 [Morley, Henry]. "A Wholesome Policy." 5 (1852): 577-80.
Would notify life insurers when policyholders move to unhealthy homes.
1235 [Morley, Henry]. "Our Own Temperature." 6 (1852-53): 11-12.
Divulges circumstances and activities that change body temperature.
1236 [Martineau, Harriet]. "The Irish Union." 6 (1852-53): 169-75.
Tale of Irish workhouses mentions the frequency of ophthalmia among paupers.
1237 [Owen, Richard]. "Poisonous Serpents." 6 (1852-53): 186-88.
Chronicles the death from snakebite of a guest and a keeper at London zoo.
1238 [Morley, Henry]. "Justice to Chicory." 6 (1852-53): 208-10.
Assesses chicory as an adulterant of coffee.
1239 [Murray, Grenville]. "The Roving Englishman - His Philosophy of Dining." 6 (1852-53): 231-33.
Opponent of vegetarianism suggests when and how to dine.
1240 [Morley, Henry]. "A Foe under Foot." 6 (1852-53): 289-92.
Links the spread of diseases, as typhus, to insufficient or improper sewers. See #1275.
1241 [Capper, John]. "Really a Temperance Question." 6 (1852-53): 296-300.
Tabs uncontaminated wine medicinal.
1242 [Morley, Henry]. "Information Against a Poisoner." 6 (1852-53): 427-30.
Mutters about the occurrence of malaria.
1243 [Morley, Henry]. "The Club Surgeon." 6 (1852-53): 433-37.
Theme is the difficulty of prospering in medicine.
1244 [Wills, W.H.]. "Clean Water and Dirty Water." 6 (1852-53): 496-97.
Salutes sewers and water in Barnard Castle.
1245 [Dickens, Charles and W.H. Wills]. "Received, A Blank Child." 7 (1853): 49-53.
Sketches the past and present of the Foundling Hospital, London.
1246 [Morley, Henry]. "How to Kill Labourers." 7 (1853): 97-102.
Believes that the great distance many rural toilers walk from hovels to jobs is detrimental.
1247 [Morley, Henry]. "Fresh Air in Finsbury." 7 (1853): 107-08.
Anticipates that new titled park, with fresh air, will animate Londoners.

1248   [Morley, Henry]. "Chloroform." 7 (1853): 179-81.
        Assures that, notwithstanding a recent fatality, chloroform reduces the risks of surgery.
1249   [Morley, Henry]. "Our Last Parochial War." 7 (1853): 265-70.
        Satirizes those who resist sewers and other projects for public health.
1250   [Dickens, Charles and W.H. Wills]. "Idiots." 7 (1853): 313-17.
        Profiles the mentally challenged, their training and talents. See #1264.
1251   [Morley, Henry]. "Magazines of Meat." 7 (1853): 356-57.
        Demonstrates how to preserve meat and vegetables.
1252   [Dodd, George]. "Books for the Blind." 7 (1853): 421-25.
        Outlines tactile methods by which the vision impaired "read."
1253   [Morley, Henry and W.H. Wills]. "Lilliput in London." 7 (1853): 573-76.
        Objects to the exhibition of children with dwarfism.
1254   [Morley, Henry]. "The Modern Practice of Physic." 8 (1853-54): 169-73.
        Urges readers to select doctors for skill, not charm or appearance.
1255   [Knox, James and W.H. Wills]. "Colour-Blindness." 8 (1853-54): 255-57.
        Headlines types of color blindness. See #1290.
1256   [Dodd, George]. "The House That Jack Built." 8 (1853-54): 286-88.
        Prizes workers' new housing with drains and water systems and without fire hazards.
1257   [Morley, Henry]. "Beef." 8 (1853-54): 385-88.
        Brackets cattle feed and breeding with beef quality.
1258   [Morley, Henry]. "An Ugly Nursling." 8 (1853-54): 406-08.
        Compares symptoms of a cold to those of influenza and allergies.
1259   [Morley, Henry]. "Your Very Good Health." 8 (1853-54): 524-26.
        Paraphrases *Results of Sanitary Improvement*, by Dr. T. Southwood Smith, on how changes in sewage disposal, air quality, and water supply have slowed cholera.
1260   [Morley, Henry]. "Modern Human Sacrifices." 8 (1853-54): 561-64.
        Indicts captains for nonfeasance and owners for malfeasance, with respect to crews and equipment, in deaths from shipwreck.
1261   [Morley, Henry]. "Change of Air." 8 (1853-54): 570-72.
        Ties wellness to pure air.
1262   [Morley, Henry]. "Preventible Accidents." 9 (1854): 105-06.
        Lists several job-related accidents.

1263 [Martineau, Harriet]. "Deaf Mutes." 9 (1854): 134-38.
Ponders problems of diagnosing infantile hearing loss and of the education and occupations of the hearing impaired.

1264 [Martineau, Harriet]. "Idiots Again." 9 (1854): 197-200.
Proposes how to train and to live with the mentally challenged. See #1250.

1265 [Morley, Henry]. "Ground in the Mill." 9 (1854): 224-27.
Faults employer non-compliance with Factory Acts for employee mishaps. See #1281, #1282, #1283, #1284, #1287, and #1291.

1266 [Martineau, Harriet]. "Three Graces." 9 (1854): 317-20.
Discourses on difficulties of teaching the mentally challenged.

1267 [Morley, Henry]. "Death's Doors." 9 (1854): 398-402.
Hinges residential ventilation, drainage, and water to the health of poor urbanites.

1268 [Martineau, Harriet]. "Blindness." 9 (1854): 421-25.
Realizes that reasons for vision loss and capabilities of the vision impaired are yet unfathomed.

1269 [Morley, Henry]. "The War with Fever." 9 (1854): 447-49.
Yokes overcrowding, stale air, and cesspools of lodging houses to fevers of lodgers.

1270 "Smoke or No Smoke." 9 (1854): 464-66.
Anchors lung ailments of Londoners to air pollution.

1271 [Sala, George A.]. "The Faculty." 9 (1854): 588-93.
Spotlights medical practitioners.

1272 [Dickens, Charles]. "To Working Men." 10 (1854-55): 169-70.
Solicits official action on dwellings for laborers.

1273 [Morley, Henry]. "Piping Days." 10 (1854-55): 196-99.
Centers on the deleteriousness of improper sewage disposal.

1274 [Morley, Henry]. "Medical Practice among the Poor." 10 (1854-55): 217-21.
Grumbles that doctors of the impoverished minister for long hours, often at their own expense.

1275 [Morley, Henry]. "A Home Question." 10 (1854-55): 292-96.
Points to problems in housing, water, and sewerage together with nuisances and vocational accidents as major impediments to wellness. See #1240.

1276 [Morley, Henry]. "Commission and Omission." 10 (1854-55): 319-24.
Couples ineffective sewers and illness.

1277 [Capper, John]. "During Her Majesty's Pleasure." 10 (1854-55): 344.
Ruminates about constraint of the criminally insane. See #1279.

1278   [Morley, Henry]. "Conversion of a Heathen Court." 10 (1854-55): 409-13.
        Depicts one tenement as a sample of how such abodes abet disease. See #1286.

1279   [Wills, W.H.]. "Criminal Lunatics." 10 (1854-55): 453.
        Counters, to #1277, that insane criminals are always released when cured.

1280   [Morley, Henry]. "Houses in Flats." 11 (1855): 182-86.
        Prioritizes apartments conducive to salubrity.

1281   [Morley, Henry]. "Fencing with Humanity." 11 (1855): 241-44.
        Expects safety devices in factories to limit employee mishaps. See #1265, #1282, #1283, #1284, #1287, and #1291.

1282   [Morley, Henry]. "Death's Cyphering Book." 11 (1855): 337-41.
        Accuses manufacturers of downplaying factory accidents in order to avoid costs of safety equipment. See #1265, #1281, #1283, #1284, #1287, and #1291.

1283   [Morley, Henry]. "Deadly Shafts." 11 (1855): 494-95.
        Reiterates ideas of #1281 and #1282. See #1265, #1284, #1287, and #1291.

1284   [Morley, Henry]. "More Grist to the Mill." 11 (1855): 605-06.
        Expands on dangers of unfenced machines. See #1265, #1281, #1282, #1283, #1287, and #1291.

1285   [Sala, George A.]. "Doctoring Begins at Home." 12 (1855-56): 68-72.
        Abridges opinions of Francois Vincent Raspail on health maintenance with respect to diet, clothing, and hygiene.

1286   [Morley, Henry]. "Wild Court Tamed." 12 (1855-56): 85-87.
        Returns to the tenement in #1278 after amelioration.

1287   [Morley, Henry]. "Two Shillings Per Horse-Power." 12 (1855-56): 130-31.
        Echoes #1281, #1282, #1283, and #1284. See #1265 and #1291.

1288   [Morley, Henry]. "An Enemy's Charge." 12 (1855-56): 265-70.
        Alerts about health hazards of burying the dead.

1289   [Morley, Henry]. "Hospitals." 12 (1855-56): 457-61.
        Overview of hospitals would raise salaries of nurses.

1290   [Morley, Henry]. "Colours and Eyes." 12 (1855-56): 521-24.
        From cases on color blindness, expounds on its symptoms. See #1255.

1291   [Morley, Henry]. "Our Wicked Mis-Statements." 13 (1856): 13-19.
        Booster of factory safety laws rebuts a pamphlet by Harriet Martineau. See #1265, #1281, #1282, #1283, #1284, and #1287.

1292 [Lynn-Linton, Eliza and W.H. Wills]. "Common Cookery." 13 (1856): 42-46.
Markets nutritious menus.
1293 [Sala, George A.]. "Houseless and Hungry." 13 (1856): 121-26.
Mourns because many homeless die of starvation or exposure.
1294 [Morley, Henry]. "One Cure More." 13 (1856): 191-92.
Brands as nonsense reliance exclusively on exercise as a restorative.
1295 [Morley, Henry]. "Poison." 13 (1856): 220-24.
Worries about herbs, drugs, and food handled by the ignorant.
1296 [Dixon, Edmund Saul]. "Horse-Eating." 13 (1856): 313-18.
Estimates that horseflesh is nourishing.
1297 [Thompson, ?]. "Sick Railway Clerks." 13 (1856): 325.
Prods railroad clerks to initiate a fund for future sickness and disability.
1298 [Lynn-Linton, Eliza]. "Epidemics." 13 (1856): 397-400.
Determines that some diseases, as cholera, rage because of uncleanliness and air pollution.
1299 [Harvey, ?]. "Strychnine." 13 (1856): 420-24.
Stamps patent medicines with strychnine lethal.
1300 [Hart, Ernest]. "Minerals That We Eat." 13 (1856): 437-42, 486-90.
Interests are salt, iron, and potatoes. Articles cited are not relevant to health.
1301 [Morley, Henry]. "Our Poisonous Wild Flowers." 14 (1856): 234-36.
Flags the harm from accidently eating poisonous plants.
1302 [Carter, R. Brudenell]. "Health and Education." 14 (1856): 313-17.
Denounces, as unsalutary, teaching styles, furnishings, and inattention to physical exercise in girls' schools.
1303 [Morley, Henry]. "Lost in the Pit." 14 (1856): 361-66.
Indicts management for negligence in miners' deaths.
1304 [Mann, Christopher Wharton]. "The Nerves." 15 (1857): 522-25.
Elaborates on the structure and functions of the nerves.
1305 [Lynn-Linton, Eliza]. "Disinfectants." 16 (1857): 9-12.
Puffs sundry disinfectants, some to retard communicable diseases.
1306 [Morley, Henry]. "Doctors' Bills." 16 (1857): 25-28.
Prefers medical profession self-regulated, with high standards, to intervention by Parliament.
1307 [Morley, Henry]. "A Healthy Year in London." 16 (1857): 193-97.
Posits that air, food, and abodes make parts of London salubrious.

1308   [Morley, Henry]. "Lord W. Tyler." 16 (1857): 333-36.
Decrees more state supervision of lodging houses in order to curtail such diseases as cholera.

1309   [Morley, Henry]. "Within Dr. Conolly's Remembrance." 16 (1857): 518-23.
Synopsizes a book by Dr. John Conolly on the progress in care of the insane.

1310   [Morley, Henry]. "A Piece of Work." 16 (1857): 564-68.
Supposes that people will understand health maintenance if schools teach physiology.

1311   [?Robertson, John]. "The Vital Point." 17 (1857-58): 125-26.
Speculates that disturbing a spot between spine and brain means instant death.

1312   [Collins, Wilkie]. "Strike!" 17 (1857-58): 169-72.
Story on public toleration of modern inconveniences glances at risks on railroads without communication between drivers and passengers.

1313   [Lynn-Linton, Eliza]. "Wine, No Mystery." 17 (1857-58): 321-25.
Entry on the composition of wine nods to its adulteration.

1314   [Morley, Henry]. "Use and Abuse of the Dead." 17 (1857-58): 361-65.
Votes for Anatomy Act, which provides for legal acquisition of bodies for dissection.

1315   [Morley, Henry]. "Turpin's Corner." 17 (1857-58): 493-96.
Traces ailments of the indigent in Southwark to substandard food, apparel, and domiciles.

1316   [Morley, Henry]. "A Way to Clean Rivers." 18 (1858): 79-82.
Submits ideas for sewage disposal that will not contaminate river water.

1317   [Dixon, Edmund Saul]. "Dirty Cleanliness." 18 (1858): 121-23.
Would fertilize with sewage, not dump it in the Thames.

1318   [Dixon, Edmund Saul]. "Ozone." 18 (1858): 169-73.
Earmarks ozone as a barrier to dangerous Thames vapors.

1319   [Morley, Henry]. "One Other Hospital for Children." 18 (1858): 379-80.
Would add, to those in London and Liverpool, more hospitals for pauper sick juniors.

1320   [Morley, Henry]. "Three Years Older." 18 (1858): 566-69.
From statistics of the kingdom, 1854-1856, infers that the major causes of death of the English are lung diseases, such as tuberculosis, bronchitis, and pneumonia, which may be offset by adequate sleep, exercise, meat, and cold water when young.

1321 [Morley, Henry]. "Britannia's Figures." 19 (1958-59): 13-16.
Banners numbers of the insane poor reputedly ill because of circumstances of their class.

1322 [Priestley, William Overend]. "Chloroform." 19 (1858-59): 249-52.
Licenses chloroform for surgery and intense pain.

1323 [Morley, Henry]. "At Work in the Dark." 19 (1858-59): 321-24.
Avers that trades for which the vision impaired are trained are filled.

1324 [Morley; Henry]. "The Cure of Sick Minds." 19 (1858-59): 415-19.
Pleads for better care for insane paupers.

HOWITT'S JOURNAL, 1847-1848

Inaugurated by Mary and William Howitt and soon associated with the *People's Journal, Howitt's* disclaimed class bonds, but its essays explored the debility of workers.

1325 Smith, [T.] Southwood. "An Address to the Working Classes of the United Kingdom, on Their Duty in the Present State of the Sanatory [sic] Question." 1 (1847): 3-4.
Assigns high mortality rate of laborers to air and water quality and sewage in their abodes.

1326 Carpenter, Philip P., B.A. "Indirect Advantages Resulting from the Temperance Movement." 1 (1847): 76-78.
Postulates that abstainers from alcohol are less susceptible to sickness than are drinkers.

1327 Amigo. "Common Lodging-Houses, and a Model Lodging-House for the Poor." 1 (1847): 82-83.
Asserts that the housing of the itinerant poor is conducive to the spread of disease.

1328 Carpenter, William B[enjamin], M.D., F.R.S. "Physiology for the People." 1 (1847): 100-02, 132-34, 159-61, 198-201, 226-29, 276-79, 296-98, 341-43, 355-58; 2 (1847): 56-58, 102-05, 138-40, 182-85, 232-36.
Underscores light, ventilation, food, and water for wellness.

1329 A Man of No Party. "Penny Wisdom: Poisoned Peas." 1 (1847): 107-08.
Despises the exploitation of the physically challenged.

1330   "Lord Morpeth's Sanitary Bill." 1 (1847): 212-13; followup, on
        Health of Towns' Association Meeting: 234-38.
        Endorses broad legislation on sewerage and water for towns.

1331   Wallace, Rev. T. "Notes on the Present Condition of the People."
        1 (1847): 321-22.
        Hitches workers' worsening health to their menus.

1332   "Signor Sarti's Anatomical Exhibition." 2 (1847): 30.
        Assumes that wax exhibit by (?Paolo) Sarti will convey enough
        knowledge of anatomy for viewers to identify their ills.

1333   Macleod, W., F.R.C.P., Edinburgh. "Simple and Effectual Method
        of Curing Typhus Fever." 2 (1847): 55.
        Prescribes cold water for typhus.

1334   "Account of the New and Important Discovery of a Disinfecting
        Fluid." 2 (1847): 58-60.
        Promotes, for homes and hospitals, Jean Ledoyen's disinfectant.

1335   Bowring, John. "Free Trade Recollections: Quarantines." 2 (1847):
        362-65, 376-79.
        Enemy of quarantine, as befouling sites, intruding on citizens'
        rights, and expensive, whispers about town sanitation.

1336   "Corporation Resistance to the Well-Being of the Working Class."
        3 (1848): 253-54.
        Roars that poorer sections of towns are unsanitary because
        municipal governors frequently own nuisances or authorize
        inferior sewerage and water supply.

THE IRISH QUARTERLY REVIEW, 1851-1860

Vowing to assess legislation and to advance literature, the *Irish
Quarterly* paid attention to water as beverage and boon.

1337   "The Garret, the Cabin, and the Gaol." 3 (1853): 299-381.
        Tract on crime has a few words on folk remedies.

1338   "The Dublin Hospital and the Blunders of the Census." 4 (1854):
        635-70.
        Contemplates activities of Irish hospitals in relation to their
        funding. See #1339.

1339   "The Census, Part III v. the Dublin Hospitals." 4 (1854): 1161-88.
        Complains that the Census overcounted Dublin beds and
        undercounted Dublin sick, adversely affecting hospital funding.
        See #1338.

1340   "Suicide; Its Motives and Mysteries." 7 (1857-58): 49-87.
        Hypothesizes that some suicides derived from insanity.
1341   "Dr. Madden's *Phantasmata*." 7 (1857-58): 860-99.
        Transmits categories of insanity created by R.R. Madden.
1342   "Life in a Tub." 8 (1858-59): 589-608.
        Features hydropathy and drugs as treatments.
1343   "Fat and Lean." 8 (1858-59): 865-84.
        Enunciates origins of and therapy for obesity and emaciation.
1344   "Eating and Feeding - Living and Existing." 8 (1858-59): 1103-42.
        Discloses the nexus between fitness and diet and sleep.
1345   "The Deaf and Dumb." 8 (1858-59): 1273-1324.
        Reports ideas of John Kitto about the hearing impaired who do not
        speak, many of them Irish children.
1346   "The Blind." 9 (1859-60): 63-103.
        States abilities of the vision impaired.
1347   "Free Public Drinking Fountains." 9 (1859-60): 821-33.
        Emphasizes problems in introducing titled fountains, but marks
        their positive impact on health.
1348   "Poor Law Reform." 9 (1859-60): 860-904.
        Frowns because the poor law does not serve the needy.

THE LONDON QUARTERLY REVIEW, 1853-1900

Backed by Methodists but not bound to religious texts, the *London
Quarterly* inspected especially epidemics and the evolution of women's
role in community vigor.

1349   [Williamson, W.C.]. "Modern and Medieval Hygiene." 1 (1853):
        131-45.
        Speculates that medical knowledge, diet, and personal and public
        cleanliness results in fewer deaths from communicable diseases.
1350   [Williamson, W.C.]. "Anatomical Science: Its History and
        Progress." 2 (1854): 412-40.
        Tracks the study of anatomy and physiology from Hippocrates
        through the seventeenth century.
1351   "Life in Lunatic Asylums." 3 (1854-55): 457-83.
        Scans causes of insanity and the behavior and care of the insane
        in and out of asylums.
1352   [Williamson, W.C.]. "Animal Organization." 4 (1855): 351-77.
        Peruses recent research in anatomy and physiology.

1353   [Leifchild, J.R.]. "Life and Death in Coal Mines." 5 (1855-56): 30-70.
        Records reasons for mortal accidents in coal mines.

1354   [Leach, Henry]. "Baths and Washhouses." 7 (1856-57): 182-200.
        Connects wellness to establishments for bathing and laundering.

1355   [Arthur, William]. "City and Town Missions." 7 (1856-57): 359-80.
        Observes that urban missionaries encounter many ill, mainly from communicable diseases.

1356   "Human Longevity." 7 (1856-57): 501-19.
        Recommends health maintenance and rapid treatment of disorders to secure longevity.

1357   "Insanity, Disease, and Religion." 8 (1857): 145-65.
        Surveys sources of insanity.

1358   [Leach, Henry]. "The Dwellings of the Poor." 9 (1857-58): 459-82.
        Moors maladies of the impoverished to their teeming, dirty, and stuffy residences.

1359   [Rigg, J.H.]. "Births, Marriages, and Deaths." 10 (1858): 188-212.
        Analyzes statistics of the Registrar-General on diseases, noting cholera in relation to sanitation and water quality, and on deaths in several jobs.

1360   "Ragged Homes and Ministering Women." 14 (1860): 416-33.
        Item on women as social reformers joins domestic sanitation and ventilation to illness abatement.

1361   "Dr. Laycock on *Mind and Brain*." 14 (1860): 433-51.
        Abridges notions of Thomas Laycock on consciousness, with some lines on insanity.

1362   [Rigg, J.H.]. "Law and Labour." 26 (1866): 316-39.
        Enlightens readers about the deleteriousness of various occupations.

1363   [Rigg, J.H.]. "*Report of the Registrar-General*." 27 (1866-67): 38-71.
        Pivot is causes of death drawn from the Twenty-Seventh Annual Report of the Registrar-General.

1364   "Notes on Cholera." 27 (1866-67): 218-40.
        Parades roots and symptoms of and preventives and remedies for cholera.

1365   [Williamson, W.C.]. "Reports of the Registrar-General." 32 (1869): 379-92.
        Reflects on official records of the extent of infant mortality and of perils of smoke pollution and improper sewage disposal.

1366   "The Contagious Diseases Act." 35 (1870-71): 128-44.
       Subject is legislation dealing with alleged carriers of venereal
       diseases.
1367   "The Great Social War." 46 (1876): 452-83.
       Account of Contagious Diseases Acts talks about the scope of
       venereal diseases.
1368   "The Science of Health." 50 (1878): 392-408.
       Advises proper food, exercise, and fresh air for salubrity.
1369   "Ladies' Work among the Poor." 53 (1879-80): 53-70.
       Praises female philanthropic efforts to improve hygiene, fare, and
       nursing of paupers.
1370   "Mind and Brain." 54 (1880): 124-53.
       Muses about functions and some malfunctions of the brain and
       nerves.
1371   "The Literature of the Health Exhibition." 2d ser., 3, o.s., 63
       (1884-85): 264-79.
       Assays wholesomeness of exercise.
1372   [Forbes, Urquhart A.]. "The State 'In Loco Parentis'." 2d ser., 15,
       o.s., 75 (1890-91): 256-75.
       Centers on laws to ensure children's wellness, primarily at work.
1373   [Crespi, Alfred J.H.]. "The Rewards and Responsibilities of
       Medical Practice." 2d ser., 16, o.s., 76 (1891): 111-36.
       Informs about the training, fees, and practices of doctors.
1374   "Water Supply." 2d ser., 22, o.s., 82 (1894): 311-27.
       Investigates schemes to obtain pure water.

THE LONDON REVIEW, 1829-1830

Advocating intellectual analysis, the short-lived *London Review* reserved
space for interpretations of wellness.

1375   [Granville, A.B.]. "Diet." 1 (1829): 139-53.
       Excerpt from *A Treatise of Diet*, by J.A. Paris, M.D., offers
       opinions about the process of digestion and its disruption and
       about a salubrious diet.
1376   [Mayo, Thomas]. "Insanity and Its Moral Preventives." 1 (1829):
       198-222.
       Extract from *Commentaries on the Causes, Forms, Symptoms,
       and Treatment, Moral and Medical, of Insanity*, by George Man
       Burrows, M.D., has thoughts on causes and cures of insanity.

1377   "Human Physiology." 1 (1829): 486-502.
        Gleans from *Outlines of Human Physiology*, by Herbert Mayo,
        F.R.S., the effect of physical injury on the blood.

LONGMAN'S MAGAZINE, 1882-1900

Founded by Charles J. Longman to appeal to a mass market, *Longman's*
alternated between the unwholesome conditions of urban areas and the
urgency for undertaking measures for health maintenance.

1378   Richardson, Benjamin Ward, M.D., F.R.S. "Health in a Health
        Resort." 1 (1882-83): 529-50.
        Story on sanitation sets sewerage and uncontaminated air, food,
        and water as goals for towns designated health resorts.
1379   Richardson, Benjamin Ward. "Cycling as an Intellectual Pursuit."
        2 (1883): 593-607.
        Sanctions cycling for physical and mental vigor.
1380   The Author of *Charles Lowder* [Maria Trench]. "A Garden Party
        at Rotherhithe." 5 (1884-85): 67-76.
        Honors cottage hospital where many patients are dockworkers.
1381   Richardson, Benjamin Ward. "Woman's Work in Creation." 8
        (1886): 604-19.
        Stresses risks to health of intensive study by women. See #1382.
1382   Orme, Eliza. "Woman's Work in Creation: A Reply." 9 (1886-87):
        149-58.
        Refutes #1381.
1383   Parker, Robert William. "The Emigration of Young People by the
        State." 9 (1886-87): 378-85.
        Favors officially sponsored emigration of youths starving because
        of poverty.
1384   Scott, Robert H. "London Fogs." 9 (1886-87): 607-14.
        Mates dirty air and respiratory ailments in London.
1385   Richardson, Benjamin Ward. "Toxicopolis." 10 (1887): 361-78.
        Campaigns against heavy alcohol drinking as unhealthy.
1386   Richardson, Benjamin Ward. "Foods for Man - Animal and
        Vegetable: A Comparison." 12 (1888): 26-45.
        Elects vegetarianism for wellness.
1387   Richardson, Benjamin Ward. "The Storage of Life as a Sanitary
        Study." 12 (1888): 381-400.
        Counsels how to stay well so as to live long.

1388 Richardson, Benjamin Ward. "The Health of the Mind." 14 (1889): 145-63.
Remarks on trauma in a mental context.

1389 Richardson, B[enjamin] W[ard]. "Working Hours and Working Men." 16 (1890): 611-31.
Would adjust working hours to job demands for employee vitality.

1390 Richardson, Benjamin Ward. "The Mastery of Pain: A Triumph of the Nineteenth Century." 19 (1891-92): 489-510.
Talks about sundry anesthetics.

1391 Dalby, Sir William B. "Dr. Chesterfield's Letters to His Son on Medicine as a Career." 22 (1893): 556-67; 23 (1893-94): 56-65.
Illustrates the life of a doctor.

1392 Frankland, G.C. "Water Bacteriology and Cholera." 23 (1893-94): 171-75.
Taps polluted water for the spread of cholera and typhoid fever.

1393 Richardson, Benjamin Ward. "The Athletic Life." 23 (1893-94): 251-69.
Prints regimens for athletes' robustness.

1394 Richardson, Sir Benjamin Ward, M.D., F.R.S. " 'How to Make the Most of Life'." 25 (1894-95): 39-54.
Announces physical and mental ways to extend health.

1395 Richardson, Sir Benjamin Ward, M.D., F.R.S. "Past and Ideal Sanitation." 26 (1895): 274-94.
Affiliates sanitary progress and public health.

1396 Richardson, Sir Benjamin Ward, M.D., F.R.S. "The Physical Foundations of Temperance." 27 (1895-96): 141-57.
Rejects alcohol as a deterrent of and restorative after illness.

1397 Frankland, G.C. "The Pasteur Institute." 27 (1895-96): 363-70.
Lauds scientists at Pasteur Institute, notably for their vaccines.

1398 Richardson, Sir Benjamin Ward, M.D., F.R.S. "The Sick Nurse." 28 (1896): 30-46.
Accents duties and difficulties of nursing.

1399 Frankland, G.C. "Milk Dangers and Remedies." 29 (1896-97): 464-76.
Unmasks dangers from bacteria in milk and milk containers.

1400 Frankland, G.C. "Bacteriology in the Queen's Reign." 30 (1897): 213-22.
Memorializes successes of bacteriologists against disease.

1401 Dalby, [Sir] William B. "The Preservation of Hearing." 32 (1898): 218-26.
Probes harms to the ear, and consequently hearing, from sickness, blows, and external objects.

1402   Frankland, G.C. "Some Poisons and Their Prevention." 33 (1898-99): 68-79.
        Illuminates hazards of tetanus, snakebite, and eating eels.

MACMILLAN'S MAGAZINE, 1859-1900

Begun by Alexander Macmillan as a monthly, *Macmillan's* contained abundant appraisals of illness. Central were those on metropolitan citizens and the institutions that served them.

1403   Spencer, Herbert. "The Physiology of Laughter." 1 (1859-60): 395-402.
        Singles out muscles and nerves of laughter.
1404   Maclaren, Archibald. "Systematized Exercise: Expansion and Development of the Chest." 3 (1860-61): 35-40.
        Reports on the nature and outcomes of some exercises.
1405   By the Author of 'John Halifax, Gentleman' [Dinah Maria Mulock]. "Blind!" 3 (1860-61): 53-57.
        Tours a site for training the vision impaired for employment.
1406   Cobbe, Frances Power. "Workhouse Sketches." 3 (1860-61): 448-61.
        Text on the poor law deprecates its treatment of the sick.
1407   [Howman, G.A. Knightley]. "The Fauna of the Streets." 5 (1861-62): 225-29.
        Biography of street urchins broods about their care when ailing.
1408   Greg, Percy. "Homes of the London Workmen." 6 (1862): 63-70.
        Bewails artisans' lodgings in London that speed illness.
1409   By the Author of 'John Halifax, Gentleman' [Dinah Maria Mulock]. "The History of a Hospital." 6 (1862): 252-60.
        Looks at advantages for young patients and the management of Children's Hospital, London.
1410   Macmillan, Rev. Hugh, F.R.S.E. "Human Vegetation." 6 (1862): 459-67.
        Inventories skin diseases.
1411   Maclaren, Archibald. "National Systems of Bodily Exercise." 7 (1862-63): 277-86.
        Pontificates about motives for and methods of exercise.
1412   A Man on the Shady Side of Fifty [A.V. Kirwan]. "Physicians and Surgeons of the Last Generation." 8 (1863): 18-25.
        Spotlights famous physicians and surgeons.

1413   Anstie, Francis E., M.D. "On Physical Pain." 8 (1863): 457-63.
Prompts research on the nature and treatment, as with chloroform, of pain.

1414   Maclaren, Archibald. "Private Schools for Boys: Their Management." 9 (1863-64): 384-92.
Orders regular exercise for boys in private schools.

1415   Maclaren, Archibald. "Girls' Schools." 10 (1864): 409-16.
Detests female dress that inhibits exercise by schoolgirls.

1416   Anstie, Francis E., M.D. "State Medicine." 11 (1864-65): 306-16.
Topic is the interaction between government and doctors, as in certification of insanity and cooperation with local health officers.

1417   Bastian, H. Charlton, M.B., F.L.S. "The Human Brain." 13 (1865-66): 63-71.
Familiarizes audience with the shape and functions of the brain.

1418   Whitehead, Rev. H. "The Broad Street Pump: An Episode in the Cholera Epidemic of 1854." 13 (1865-66): 113-22.
Gauges the role of water pumps in cholera outbreak. See #1422.

1419   [Mulock, Dinah Maria]. "Death on the Seas." 13 (1865-66): 349-52.
Mourns those who died when the ship *London* sank.

1420   Simon, T. Collyns. "Can We See Distance?" 13 (1865-66): 429-42.
Core is vision capability.

1421   Anstie, Francis E., M.D., F.R.C.P. "Workhouse Infirmary Reform." 13 (1865-66): 477-83.
Calls for better facilities for and staffs in poor law infirmaries.

1422   Whitehead, Rev. H. "The Influence of Impure Water on the Spread of Cholera." 14 (1866): 182-90.
Allies polluted water and diffusion of cholera. See #1418.

1423   Heaton, Professor [Charles W.]. "A Hard Day's Work." 15 (1866-67): 432-40.
Fashions ideal menus for the active.

1424   [Anderson], Elizabeth Garrett, L.S.A. "Volunteer and Hospital Nursing." 15 (1866-67): 494-99.
Declares that female volunteer nurses help their sex and themselves in addition to their patients.

1425   Lorimer, James. "Personal Statistics." 16 (1867): 365-72.
Documents effects of education, marriage, and jobs on men's health.

1426   Bain, Professor [Alexander]. "On the Correlation of Force in Its Bearing on Mind." 16 (1867): 372-83.
Chapter on mental activity has some prose on the brain.

1427   "Women Physicians." 18 (1868): 369-80; with note: 528.
        Insists that, because women have a right to enter medicine, they
        should have the same education and standards of practice as men.
1428   Chester, Harry. "The Food of the People." 18 (1868): 476-85; 19
        (1868-69): 13-23.
        Capsulizes sources of food, its preparation, preservation, and sale.
1429   Morison, J. Cotter. "Physical Education." 19 (1868-69): 511-16.
        Agrees with Archibald Maclaren that physical exercise sustains
        vigor.
1430   S., F.R. "On Sleep." 20 (1869): 23-29.
        Dissertation on sleep does not miss its salubriousness.
1431   "On the Rational Treatment of Drunkards." 22 (1870): 309-15.
        Traverses asylums for alcoholics, purportedly akin to those for the
        insane.
1432   Cobbe,   Frances   Power.   "Unconscious   Cerebration: A
        Psychological Study." 23 (1870-71): 24-37.
        Demonstrates how alcohol and anesthetics acts on the brain. See
        #1434.
1433   Day, George E., M.D., F.R.S. "Louise Lateau: A Biographical
        Study." 23 (1870-71): 488-98.
        Fixes on symptoms and treatment of a Belgian woman for quasi-
        religious trauma.
1434   Cobbe, Frances Power. "Dreams as Illustrations of Unconscious
        Cerebration." 23 (1870-71): 512-23.
        Penetrates the link between dreams and the brain. See #1432.
1435   Clarke, W. Fairlie, M.A., M.B. "The Use and Abuse of Hospitals."
        25 (1871-72): 448-54; 28 (1873): 341-47.
        Growls that many patients who can pay for hospital stays do not
        and that some take up staff time with trivial matters.
1436   Dalrymple, D., M.P. "Asylums for Drunkards." 26 (1872): 110-16.
        Scrutinizes United States shelters for alcoholics.
1437   "An Hour with Some Old People." 26 (1872): 461-69.
        Interviews elderly in a workhouse about problems of aging and
        medical care.
1438   O[ldfield], L[aura]. "The Children of the Poor." 27 (1872-73):
        335-44.
        Contends that indigent waifs are susceptible to illness because they
        are undernourished.
1439   Young, John. "Medical Reform." 28 (1873): 278-88.
        Recounts government role in educating and licensing doctors.
1440   Foster, Michael, [Jun.]. "Vivisection." 29 (1873-74): 367-76.
        Accepts vivisection to forward medical knowledge. See #2507.

1441 Stevenson, Robert Louis. "Ordered South." 30 (1874): 68-73.
Estimates merits of Mediterranean climate for invalids.

1442 Hill, Octavia. "The Homes of the London Poor." 30 (1874): 131-38.
Attaches the prevalence of communicable diseases in London to insufficient residential cleanliness and ventilation.

1443 Smedley, M.B. "Workhouse Schools for Girls." 31 (1874-75): 27-36.
Reveals high incidence of ophthalmia among workhouse girls.

1444 Hill, Joanna M. "Homes for the Homeless." 32 (1875): 133-40.
Articulates health benefits of sending orphans to boarding homes.

1445 Whittaker, Thomas P. "The Drinking System; Its Effect on National Prosperity and the Rate of Wages." 33 (1875-76): 147-54.
Aligns alcoholism and insanity.

1446 Simpson, William, M.A. "Pure Water and Pure Rivers - Experiences." 34 (1876): 79-84.
Blames impure water for typhoid fever numbers.

1447 Trench, M[aria]. "Sick-Nurses." 34 (1876): 422-29.
Discusses the training, salary, and duties of nurses.

1448 Macquoid, Katharine S. "The Little Hospital by the River." 36 (1877): 43-46.
Blesses London hospital for children with incurable maladies. See #1459.

1449 Tuke, D. Hack. "Modern Life and Insanity." 37 (1877-78): 130-40.
Weighs causes of insanity in terms of class, age, and sex.

1450 Tuke, D. Hack, M.D. "Broadmoor, and Our Criminal Lunatics." 38 (1878): 137-42.
Pictures an institution for and activities of the criminally insane.

1451 "Methods of Sick Relief." 39 (1878-79): 211-19.
Theme is how dispensaries, free and provident, and friendly societies assisted the ailing poor.

1452 Torrens, W.[T.]M. "What Is to be Done with the Slums?" 39 (1878-79): 533-45.
Paints many London homes as unsanitary and unsafe.

1453 Greenwood, George. "Vivisection." 40 (1879): 523-30.
Affirms vivisection to improve medical knowledge.

1454 Torrens, W.[T.]M. "The Water Supply of London." 41 (1879-80): 183-91.
Earmarks perils of London's polluted water.

1455 Blaikie, W.G. "Life at High Pressure." 41 (1879-80): 225-30.
Predicts heart attacks for people with stressful lives.

1456   Almond, Hely Hutchinson. "Athletics and Education." 43 (1880-81): 283-94.
         Foresees robustness for schoolboys who exercise.
1457   Lane-Poole, Stanley. "Workhouse Infirmaries." 44 (1881): 219-26.
         Decries nursing in poor law infirmaries, especially extortion by staff for services.
1458   Harberton, Florence W. [Pomeroy, Viscountess]. "Rational Dress Reform." 45 (1881-82): 456-61.
         Campaigns for clothes that do not inhibit wellness.
1459   Macquoid, Katharine S. and M.W. Moggridge. "Two Good Institutions." 46 (1882): 54-61.
         Part I repeats opinions of #1448. Part II compliments convalescent homes.
1460   Hubbard, Henry W. "The Poisons of the Day; A New Social Evil." 46 (1882): 238-44.
         Points out dangers of many drugs and patent medicines.
1461   Holland, B. "London Playgrounds." 46 (1882): 321-24.
         Boasts that London playgrounds are salubrious for youthful clients and their female supervisors.
1462   Kerr, F.G. " 'Ephphatha': A Visit to the Deaf and Dumb Asylum at Siena." 46 (1882): 447-55.
         Incorporates United States and Italian programs for the hearing impaired who do not speak.
1463   Paul, S. Casson. "London Evictions." 46 (1882): 498-504.
         Bares inadequacies of slum lighting, ventilation, and drainage and problems that displacement for urban renewal creates for Londoners.
1464   Hubbard, Henry W. "Patent Medicines." 47 (1882-83): 499-504.
         Rages about the availability of patent medicines too often toxic.
1465   [Phillips, John Rowland]. "London Landowners, London Improvements, and the Housing of the Poor." 49 (1883-84): 1-9.
         Chronicles how London domiciliary overcrowding and sewage abet communicable diseases.
1466   Norris, F. "A Note on a Good Work." 49 (1883-84): 309-11.
         Boosts country sojourns for city children's vigor.
1467   Martin, Frances. "Holidays for Working Women." 49 (1883-84): 363-67.
         Counts on rural vacations, with rest and clean air, to restore the vitality of working women.
1468   Foster, H.E. "A Voyage to Australia for Health." 49 (1883-84): 412-18.
         Advocates sea voyages to Australia for those with tuberculosis.

1469   Verney, F.P. "In a Great Town Hospital." 50 (1884): 14-22.
       Etches hospital life from individual cases.
1470   [Morris, Mowbray]. "The Philosophy of Diet; by a Layman." 54
       (1886): 206-112.
       Preaches moderation with respect to diet, alcohol, and tobacco.
1471   [Morris, Mowbray]. "On the Ministry of the Interior." 60 (1889):
       224-29.
       Banks on self-restraint for health maintenance. See #841.
1472   Carpenter, Edward. "The Smoke-Plague and Its Remedy." 62
       (1890): 204-13.
       Plans how to eliminate air pollution.
1473   A Son of the Marshes [Denham Jordon and Jean A. Owen]. "How
       the Cholera Came to Marshton." 63 (1890-91): 45-48.
       Revisits the impact of cholera on villages in Kent.
1474   Torrens, W.[T.]M. "Pure Water and Plenty of It." 63 (1890-91):
       106-11.
       Features the bureaucracy behind clean water supply.
1475   Street, Arthur Edmund. "The Education of the Deaf." 63 (1890-
       91): 364-69.
       Grades British methods of educating hearing impaired juniors as
       inferior to German methods.
1476   Carter, Lorance W. "Types for the Blind." 64 (1891): 51-55.
       Disputes anti-braille essay in the *Edinburgh Review*. See #730.
1477   Bourne, H. Clarence. "Hungry Children." 65 (1891-92): 186-93.
       Tickets charity to waifs unnecessary and socially harmful.
1478   Bourne, H. Clarence. "The Metropolitan Hospitals." 66 (1892):
       362-68.
       Would restrict medical benefits for the poor in London hospitals.
1479   Loch, C.S. "The Prince of Wales's Hospital-Fund." 75 (1896-97):
       401-09.
       Would reorganize London hospitals because of their proliferation
       and that of patients.
1480   Yonge, Eugene S. "The Insanity of the Criminal." 79 (1898-99):
       50-55.
       Correlates behavior of criminals and the insane.

MELIORA, 1858-1869

Devoted to the elimination of societal evils, *Meliora* was always alert to
the risks of alcohol abuse and of juvenile jobs.

1481   "Meliora." 1 (1858-59): 1-16.
        Tract on social problems has some paragraphs on unsalutary
        housing and liquor-induced insanity.
1482   "The Place of Temperance in Society." 1 (1858-59): 56-70.
        Sermonizes about the injuriousness of alcohol.
1483   "The Vices of the Streets." 1 (1858-59): 70-79.
        Entry on prostitution alludes to venereal diseases.
1484   "How Shall We Dispose of Our Dead?" 1 (1858-59): 125-36.
        Blasts burial as a ground pollutant.
1485   "Temperance in History." 1 (1858-59): 176-92.
        Decides, based on English alcohol consumption over centuries,
        that alcoholism is a disease.
1486   "The British Workman." 2 (1860): 38-56.
        Treatise on workers ascribes their unhealthiness to enfeebled
        mothers and unclean homes.
1487   "Types of Disease and Crime." 2 (1860): 142-52.
        Parallels lack of sanitation and crime.
1488   "Death in the Coal-Pits." 2 (1860): 154-68.
        Announces dangers of coal mining for miners.
1489   "Union Surgeons." 2 (1860): 181-89.
        Portrays Poor Law Boards as miserly about doctors' fees and
        patients' relief.
1490   "The Blind." 3 (1861): 1-15.
        Meditates on the training and successes of the vision impaired.
1491   "Causes and Cures of Drunkenness." 3 (1861): 39-48.
        Message on alcoholism does not omit drink's damage to the body.
1492   "The Treatment of Our Lunatics." 3 (1861): 48-63.
        Circulates standards on care of the insane in asylums.
1493   "Tobacco." 3 (1861): 201-12.
        Denominates tobacco deleterious.
1494   "Temperance Reformers." 3 (1861): 348-53.
        Transcribes physical and mental symptoms of sufferers from
        alcoholism.
1495   "The New Discoveries on the Action of Alcohol." 4 (1862): 34-53.
        Divulges recent research on the perniciousness of alcohol.
1496   "The Social Science Congress." 4 (1862): 267-90.
        Relates, from annual meeting of the National Association for the
        Promotion of the Social Sciences, ideas about nutrition, smallpox,
        alcoholism, and infant mortality.
1497   "Ragged London." 4 (1862): 297-312.
        Segment on London paupers prefaces their illnesses with dirt in
        and out of their abodes.

1498   "Is Alcohol Food or Physic?" 4 (1862): 345-58.
       Denies any worth to liquor. See #1499 and #1502.
1499   "Is Alcohol Food or Physic?" 5 (1863): 21-32.
       Restates notions of #1498. See #1502.
1500   "Bread and Bakers." 5 (1863): 239-59.
       Rants about the adulteration of bread and filth of bakeries.
1501   "Obscure Diseases." 5 (1863): 297-323.
       Joins some brain diseases to insanity.
1502   "Is It Food or Poison." 5 (1863): 367-81.
       Rephrases the thesis of #1498 and #1499.
1503   "Idiots and Idiot Life." 6 (1864): 97-117.
       Characterizes the mentally challenged.
1504   "The Employment of Children." 6 (1864): 224-50.
       Enumerates occupations where juveniles are in jeopardy. See
       #1506 and #1510.
1505   "Life and Its Renewal." 6 (1864): 315-29.
       Mulls over various contemporary remedies.
1506   "The Children's Employment Commission." 8 (1865): 102-20.
       Continues #1504. See #1510.
1507   "Stimulants and Narcotics." 8 (1865): 132-46.
       Relays toxicity of alcohol.
1508   "Sudden Dangers; or, Accidents and Emergencies." 8 (1865): 224-
       34.
       Delves into railroad, drowning, and gun accidents.
1509   "Sale of Drugs and Poisons." 8 (1865): 297-307.
       Inculpates ignorant or negligent preparers for adulteration of
       prescriptions.
1510   "What Are the Boys About?" 8 (1865): 307-22.
       Classifies job-related ailments of juniors. See #1504 and #1506.
1511   "Is Medicine a Science?" 9 (1866): 19-29.
       Answers that, because of vast array of illnesses, the medical
       profession cannot invariably restore health to the ill.
1512   "The Amateur Female Casual." 10 (1867): 52-64.
       Deems workhouses noxious environments for women and
       children.
1513   "Light and Health." 10 (1867): 125-38.
       Extols light as a factor in fitness.
1514   "Sound and Sense." 10 (1867): 306-21.
       Discerns a link between hearing and the brain.
1515   "Life in Lunatic Asylums." 10 (1867): 321-31.
       Deliberates about the quality and appropriateness of care of
       individuals in shelters for the insane.

1516   "The Education of Women." 11 (1868): 97-113.
        Piece on women's education has some discourse on female
        doctors.
1517   "Increased Pauperism, and Its Remedy." 11 (1868): 304-16.
        Conjectures that parental temperance would lessen the tally of
        insane or mentally challenged progeny.
1518   "Civilization and Health." 12 (1869): 193-207.
        Testifies that unsanitary cities and sedentary citizens translates into
        an enervated population.
1519   "Report of Convocation on Intemperance." 12 (1869): 219-317.
        Moors mental disabilities at birth and insanity after to progenitors'
        alcoholism.
1520   "The Contagious Diseases Acts." 12 (1869): 336-54.
        Vetoes captioned legislation dealing with venereal diseases.
1521   "Underground Life." 12 (1869): 354-68.
        Tale of mining does not overlook its perils.

THE MODERN REVIEW, 1880-1884

   Born of the *Theological Review*, the *Modern* broadcast a major
controversy on medical care.

1522   [Cobbe, Frances Power]. "The Medical Profession and Its
        Morality." 2 (1881): 296-326; with editorial note: 326-28.
        Inquires into the background and motives of medical students.
        Scolds doctors for their disinterest in patients as people, protracted
        treatment of the rich, mistreatment of women and animals, and
        conspiracy of silence. See #1523, #1524, and #1525.
1523   Carpenter, William B[enjamin]. "The Morality of the Medical
        Profession: A Reply." 2 (1881): 489-532.
        Challenges views in #1522. See #1524 and #1525.
1524   "The Morality of the Medical Profession, II: By Two of the
        Profession." 2 (1881): 533-47.
        Vindicates the medical profession from general attack in #1522.
        Concedes that some specific accusations were accurate. See #1523
        and #1525.
1525   Blackwell, Elizabeth, M.D. "Medicine and Morality." 2 (1881):
        750-61; with editorial note: 761-64.
        Separates reality from rhetoric in the debate about doctors. See
        #1522, #1523, and #1524.

1526   Gardner, Alice. "A Transition Period in Female Education." 5
        (1884): 70-90.
        Warns that improper education can undermine the health of
        women.

THE MONTHLY CHRONICLE, 1838-1841

Acquainting late literates with current achievements, the *Monthly
Chronicle* merely mentioned wellness.

1527   [Lardner, Dionysius and E.L. Bulwer]. "Animal Magnetism." 1
        (1838): 289-306; 2 (1838): 11-30.
        Recites cases of hypnosis as therapy.
1528   "Progress of the Deaf and Dumb." 2 (1838): 154-60.
        Motif is how to communicate with the hearing impaired who do
        not speak.
1529   [Stone, Thomas]. "Treatment of Insanity in England." 2 (1838):
        489-507.
        Contemplates the diagnosis and care of the insane, mainly in
        asylums.
1530   [Stone, Thomas]. "Pathology of the Human Mind." 3 (1839): 302-
        16.
        Abbreviates theories of Thomas Mayo, M.D., on insanity. See
        #1531.
1531   Mayo, Thomas. "Physiology of Mind." 5 (1840): 134-37.
        Supplements #1530.

MURRAY'S MAGAZINE, 1887-1891

Determined to be detached and deliberative, *Murray's* monitored
mishaps and care management as publisher John preserved the family's
Quarterly Review.

1532   Acworth, W.M. "Scarlet Fever in the Metropolis." 2 (1887): 433-
        46.
        Targets tending victims of scarlet fever in London.
1533   Quarter Sessions, Chairmen and Deputy Chairmen of the. "The
        County Government Bill." 3 (1888): 738-60.
        Has some language on insane asylums and on other subjects.

1534   Shaw, Eyre M. "The Protection of Dwelling Houses from Fire."
        4 (1888): 50-58.
        Promulgates procedures to erect residences with fewer fire
        hazards.

1535   A., F. "On Being Ordered Abroad for the Winter." 5 (1889): 238-
        49.
        Observes a bond between climate and health.

1536   Jones, C. Percy. "A Blind, Deaf Mute." 5 (1889): 365-72.
        Protaganist is a wealthy vision and hearing impaired person who
        does not speak.

1537   Covington, William. "Is the Hospital Sunday Fund a Failure?" 6
        (1889): 205-16.
        Indexes sources of hospital revenues.

1538   Tweedie, Ethel B. "A Visit to the 'Institute Pasteur'." 6 (1889):
        503-10.
        Congratulates Louis Pasteur for his rabies vaccine.

1539   Myers, Frederic W.H. "An International Census of
        Hallucinations." 6 (1889): 746-58.
        Comments on studies of hallucination.

1540   Shaw, Eyre M. "Theatre Fires in 1889." 7 (1890): 352-66.
        From statistics, declares that deaths from theatre fires were down
        between 1886 and 1889 and that injuries were the same in 1886
        and 1889 but up in 1887 and 1888. Roots these figures in
        substandard building and audience panic.

1541   Loch, C.S. "Medical Relief in London." 7 (1890): 433-49.
        Lectures on the training of doctors and hospitals and their services
        in London.

1542   Swinton, A.A. Campbell. "The Present Position of Electric
        Lighting." 7 (1890): 525-33.
        Survey of London lighting tabs evils of improper electrical wiring.

1543   Morgan, John H. "Our Hospitals: (1) The House Surgeon." 8
        (1890): 145-62.
        Covers surgeons in hospitals. See #1544.

1544   Stewart, Isla. "Our Hospitals: (2) A Practical View of Nursing."
        8 (1890): 162-69.
        Complements #1543 with words on nurses in hospitals.

1545   Crespi, Alfred J.H. "The Practical Value of Cycling." 8 (1890):
        385-96.
        Hymn to cycling idealizes it as exercise.

1546   Colles, W. Morris. "How the Poor Live." 10 (1891): 180-93.
        Reminds local authorities of their obligation to construct housing
        that is sanitary and spacious.

THE NATIONAL REVIEW, 1855-1864

Heir of the *Prospective Review*, the *National* placed few paragraphs on wellness but these were deftly drafted.

1547 [Patmore, Coventry]. "Hashish." 6 (1858): 91-111.
Explores physical and psychological effects of using cannabis.
1548 "The Blind." 10 (1860): 75-106.
History of the vision impaired notes the physiology of vision loss.
1549 [Greg, Percy]. "Intemperance; Its Causes and Cures." 10 (1860): 107-43.
Censures teetotalers for hyperbole about alcohol's destructiveness.
1550 [Martineau, James]. "Cerebral Psychology: Bain." 10 (1860): 500-21.
Synopsizes concepts of Alexander Bain on comprehending the brain and sensation.
1551 "The Devils of Loudun." 11 (1860): 70-93.
Returns to seventeenth-century French nuns with physical symptoms reputedly from demonic possession.

THE NATIONAL REVIEW, 1883-1900

Preferring Conservative politics, this *National* scouted the salubrity of the poor at length. Rabies and precarious employments also enthralled writers.

1552 Tirard, Nestor, M.D. Lond. "Hospital Problems: The Children of the Poor." 3 (1884): 113-24.
Considers how hospitals attend impoverished young urbanites.
1553 Mott, Albert J. "Alcohol and Total Abstinence." 3 (1884): 293-312.
Proclaims that moderate liquor drinking is not harmful.
1554 Campbell, C.M., M.D. "Medical Relief of the Rural Poor." 4 (1884-85): 403-09.
Would amplify medical care for the agricultural poor.
1555 Greg, Percy. "Stimulants and Narcotics." 4 (1884-85): 776-95.
Stamps alcohol and drugs potent and safe restoratives if utilized wisely.
1556 Johns, B.G. "How the Blind Dream." 5 (1885): 309-19.
Anchors dreams of the vision impaired in their tactile experiences.

1557   Gurney, Edmund and Frederic W.H. Myers. "Some Higher Aspects of Mesmerism." 5 (1885): 681-703.
       Denies the value of hypnosis for medicine.

1558   Author of 'Vera' [Charlotte Dempster]. "Pasteur and Hydrophobia." 7 (1887): 781-93.
       Topic is rabies vaccine developed by Louis Pasteur.

1559   Brabazon, Reginald, [12th Earl Meath]. "Open Spaces and Physical Exercise." 8 (1886-87): 483-90.
       Would stimulate youthful vigor by opening playgrounds and gymnasiums.

1560   Fothergill, J. Milner. "The Effects of Town Life upon the Human Body." 10 (1887-88): 166-72.
       Represents the diet of city dwellers as bad for the stomach and other organs.

1561   Floris, Cha[rle]s L. "Comfort and Safety in London Theatres." 10 (1887-88): 313-25.
       Would safeguard audiences by installing fire escapes and vents for gas lamps in theatres.

1562   Onslow, [William Hillier]. "Dogs in Disgrace." 10 (1887-88): 335-40.
       Would license rather than muzzle dogs to halt rabies.

1563   Carter, R. B[rudenell]. "Medical Science in Relation to Homeopathy." 11 (1888): 14-30.
       Questions merits of homeopathy.

1564   Baumann, Arthur A. "The Lords' Committee on the Sweating System." 12 (1888-89): 145-59.
       Reprehends sweatshops for their multiple health hazards. See #1566.

1565   Norris, Edward S. "As to an Ancient Royal Foundation." 12 (1888-89): 202-07.
       Peers at the past and present of St. Katherine's Hospital, London.

1566   Baumann, Arthur A. "Possible Remedies for the Sweating System." 12 (1888-89): 289-307.
       Propounds ways to curb abuses cited in #1564.

1567   Roy, C.S. and J.G. Adami. "The Physiological Bearing of Waist-Belts and Stays." 12 (1888-89): 341-49.
       Postulates that women's corsets are salubrious if worn neither tightly bound nor during exercise.

1568   Bartholeyns, A. O'D[onnel]. "The Great Hospitals of London." 12 (1888-89): 524-32.
       Names twelve London hospitals as the best for patient care and medical training.

1569   Bartholeyns, A. O'D[onnel]. "The Sick Poor of the Metropolis."
        12 (1888-89): 818-29.
        Monitors medical facilities for impoverished Londoners.

1570   Lymington, [Newton Wallop, Viscount]. "The Housing of the
        Poor." 12 (1888-89): 830-41.
        Rules that urban tenements are teeming and filthy.

1571   Preston-Thomas, H. "Vaccination and the *Encyclopedia
        Britannica*." 13 (1889): 433-55.
        Fan of smallpox vaccination responds to a foe in the *Encyclopedia
        Britannica*. Also has sentences on syphilis and erysipelas. See
        #1572.

1572   Creighton, C[harles], M.D. " 'Vaccination' in the *Encyclopedia
        Britannica*." 13 (1889): 605-16.
        Author of *Encyclopedia Britannica* article on smallpox vaccination
        retorts to #1571.

1573   Twining, Louisa. "Poor Law Infirmaries and Their Needs." 13
        (1889): 630-42.
        Propagandizes about the administration of and care in poor law
        infirmaries.

1574   Black, Charles E.D. "The Education of the Blind and Deaf in the
        United Kingdom." 14 (1889-90): 256-69.
        Encapsulates opinions, held by a Royal Commission, on the
        instruction of the vision and hearing impaired, including those in
        the latter group who do not speak.

1575   Papillon, E.C. "Teplitz." 14 (1889-90): 392-400.
        Puffs Bohemian spa as restorative for many maladies.

1576   Herring, Geo[rge]. "Hydrophobia: Its Treatment by Pasteur." 14
        (1889-90): 538-46.
        Picks sweating over vaccination of Louis Pasteur as a remedy for
        rabies.

1577   Hall, G. Rome. "Public Health and Politics." 14 (1889-90): 598-
        615.
        Backs statutory extension of housing and recreation for health.

1578   Baumann, Arthur A. "Needed Amendments of the Factory Act."
        15 (1890): 145-52.
        Sponsors legislation for more salutary factories.

1579   Parkinson, C. "Colliery Explosions and Their Prevention." 15
        (1890): 167-73.
        Magnifies dangers of coal mining.

1580   Shadwell, Arthur. "Rabies and Muzzling." 15 (1890): 219-31.
        To check rabies, would not muzzle, but would register all dogs and
        confine, then kill any with symptoms of the disease.

1581   Paget, Wally [Walburga]. "A Visit to Count Mattei." 15 (1890): 348-55.
        Favors the treatment developed by Mario Mattei for cancer. See #1582, #1584, #1585, and #1587.

1582   Snow, Herbert, M.D. "Count Mattei and His Treatment of Cancer: A Reply to Lady Paget." 15 (1890): 606-13.
        Rebuttal of #1581 opts for surgery in cancer cases. See #1584, #1585, #1587, and #1810.

1583   Taylor, Charles Bell, M.D. "Pasteur's Prophylactic." 15 (1890): 654-66.
        Suspects the efficacy of rabies vaccination of Louis Pasteur.

1584   Paget, Wally [Walburga]. "Count Mattei's System." 15 (1890): 741-47; with a further challenge by T.R. Allinson, L.R.C.P., 16 (1890-91): 10.
        Reasserts notions of #1581. See #1582, #1585, and #1587.

1585   Kennedy, Samuel, F.R.C.S.E. "Mattei v. The Knife: The Rational Treatment of Cancer." 16 (1890-91): 1-9.
        Justifies methods of Mario Mattei for treating cancer. See #1581, #1582, #1584, and #1587.

1586   Hubbard, Henry W. "Homicide, as a Misadventure." 16 (1890-91): 183-89.
        Fears that many patent medicines are worse than any ailment.

1587   Snow, Herbert. "The Knife v. Mattei." 16 (1890-91): 252-58.
        Replies to #1585. See #1581, #1582, and #1584.

1588   Clark, A. Campbell, M.D. "The History and Nature of Hypnotism." 16 (1890-91): 759-80.
        Story on hypnosis glances at it as therapy. Reference to the *Nineteenth Century* is irrelevant.

1589   Wilkins, W.H. "The London Hospital and Its Nurses." 17 (1891): 118-29.
        Dislikes nurses' training and employment practices in this hospital.

1590   Keneally, Arabella. "The Physical Conscience." 17 (1891): 477-93.
        Themes are awareness of illness by pain and appreciation of good health.

1591   Granville, J. Mortimer. " 'Drink': Ethical Considerations, and Physiological." 18 (1891-92): 160-76.
        Defends moderate liquor drinking as a deterrent to sickness.

1592   Dunraven [W.T. Quin, 4th Earl]. "A Word with the Physicians." 19 (1892): 32-43; with letters: 278-84.
        Chides doctors who voice medical views in the general press. See #1824.

1593   Thwaite, B.H. "London Fog: A Scheme to Abolish It." 20 (1892-93): 360-67.
        Plans to rid London of unsalutary fogs.

1594   Meath [Reginald Brabazon, 12th Earl]. "Physical Education." 20 (1892-93): 461-68.
        Favors exercise to attain and sustain vitality. See #1721.

1595   Mallock, M.M. "Restaurants for the Labouring Classes." 21 (1893): 62-70.
        Would establish "Peoples' Kitchens" with nutritious food at low cost. See #495.

1596   Greville, Violet. "Victims of Vanity." 21 (1893): 71-79.
        Tags tight corsets as the source of myriad ailments of women.

1597   Jeune, M[ary]. "Amusements of the Poor." 21 (1893): 303-14.
        Predicates popular robustness on exercise and recreation.

1598   Eccles, A. Symons. "*Fin de Siecle* Medicine." 21 (1893): 785-91.
        Ranks muscles and nerves as important to wellness.

1599   Eccles, A. Symons. "Sleeplessness." 23 (1894): 797-805.
        Explicates reasons for insomnia and its deleteriousness.

1600   Dendy, H. "The Position of Women in Industry." 23 (1894): 806-14.
        Posts perils of numerous jobs of females.

1601   Atkinson, W.N. "Colliery Explosions and Coal-Dust." 23 (1894): 836-46.
        Underscores dangers of mining.

1602   Chamberlain, J. "Old-Age Pensions and Friendly Societies." 24 (1894-95): 592-615.
        Fan of pensions paints aged as in deteriorating health. See #1603.

1603   Stead, J. Lister. "Friendly Societies and Old-Age Pensions: A Reply to Mr. Chamberlain." 25 (1895): 59-71.
        Responds to #1602.

1604   Eccles, A. Symons. "Headache." 25 (1895): 328-36.
        Pertains to origins and symptoms of headaches.

1605   Shadwell, Arthur. "Intemperance Past and Present." 26 (1895-96): 189-201.
        Has some language on alcohol's damage to the body.

1606   Farrer, [T.H.]. "Taking Stock of Employers' Liability." 26 (1895-96): 356-66.
        Scans statutes on employee accidents.

1607   Diggle, Joseph R. "Child Distress and State Socialism." 26 (1895-96): 519-28.
        Personifies the progeny of workers as inadequately and improperly fed.

1608   Granville, [J.] Mortimer. "A New Theory of Gout, What It Is Not, What It Is, and How to Avoid It." 26 (1895-96): 529-44.

Hypothecates that too many leukocytes in blood, not overproduction of uric acid, causes gout.

1609   Robinson, Louis. "The Science of Change of Air." 27 (1896): 663-72.

Promises that a different climate would be restorative for those with respiratory disorders.

1610   Holland, Lionel. "The Metropolitan Water Question." 28 (1896-97): 406-28.

Contends that the disorganization of London's water supply is a menace to health.

1611   Watson, Emma L. "Some Remarks on Modern Nurses." 28 (1896-97): 567-72.

Nurse addresses characteristics and payment of professionals. See #1612.

1612   Paul, Nancy. "Modern Nurses: A Reply." 28 (1896-97): 701-06.

Contrasts hospital and private nurses. See #1611.

1613   Shadwell, A[rthur]. "The Hidden Dangers of Cycling." 28 (1896-97): 787-96.

Forecasts injuries from cycling. See #1614.

1614   Pollock, Frederick. " 'Hidden Dangers': A Reply." 29 (1897): 113-17.

Contradicts #1613.

1615   Shadwell, A[rthur]. "Suicide by Typhoid Fever." 30 (1897-98): 715-27.

Dubs local government negligence about water supplies the genesis of typhoid fever.

1616   Coryn, Herbert. "Mind as Disease-Producer." 30 (1897-98): 918-28.

Unmasks instances of psychosomatic disturbances.

1617   Shadwell, A[rthur]. "Should Inebriates Be Imprisoned?" 31 (1898): 280-91.

Prophesizes that the incarceration of alcoholics in reformatories will be ineffective.

1618   Vane, Margaret. "The Autocrat of the Sick-Room." 31 (1898): 418-21.

Typifies private nurses as tyrants over patients and their households.

1619   White, Arnold. "The Cult of Infirmity." 34 (1899-1900): 236-45.

Mandates official restriction of reproduction by those ruled unfit physically or mentally.

1620 Morten, Honnor. "Hospital Chaos." 34 (1899-1900): 734-48.
Equates decentralized organization of hospitals and inefficiency.

THE NEW MONTHLY MAGAZINE, 1821-1854

Linked to *Ainsworth's Magazine* and *Bentley's Miscellany*, the *New
Monthly* under Henry Colburn contemplated cholera and insanity in its
forays on fitness.

1621 M[organ, T.C.]. "On Madness." 2 (1821): 113-17.
Clamors for laws to shield the property of those certified insane.
1622 "The Physician." 5 (1822): 254-58, 362-68, 563-70; 7 (1823): 108-
12, 356-63, 420-27, 533-38; 8 (1823): 53-59, 153-60, 326-34, 505-
12; 10 (1824): 181-86, 437-41; 11 (1824): 250-56, 455-60.
Heralds nexus between food, sleep, water, air, exercise, instincts,
imagination, habits, and wellness; and symptoms of and remedies
for the cold, toothache, obesity, fever, and heatstroke.
1623 "On Plague." 11 (1824): 113-20.
Distinguishes roots and variations of plague.
1624 "Insubordination of Modern Stomachs." 13 (1825): 35-39.
Clarifies causes of stomach ailments.
1625 [Sheil, R.L.]. "The Last Wexford Assize." 16 (1826): 296-304.
Magnifies Irish murders by and subsequent trial of person judged
insane.
1626 Marshall, John. "Vaccination Rightly and Popularly Considered."
26 (1829): 61-68.
District Vaccinator hails smallpox vaccination.
1627 "Londoniana." 26 (1829): 68-75, 157-62, 266-74; 28 (1830): 177-
82.
Disquisition on London life excoriates urban sanitation.
1628 "The Metropolis in Danger." 26 (1829): 284-90.
Despairs about impure water of London.
1629 M[organ, T.C.]. "On Fashions in Medicine." 28 (1830): 413-18.
Rants that too many correctives are spurious yet acclaimed by
inept doctors. Demands standards for practitioners.
1630 [Hazlitt, William]. "The Sick Chamber." 29 (1830): 156-60.
Remembers conduct while sick and feelings while recuperating.
1631 Uwins, David, M.D. "Cholera Morbus." 32 (1831): 13-19.
Queries whether cholera is infectious and hence capable of being
an epidemic disease.

1632   M[ac]f[arlane], C[harles]. "The Quarantine." 32 (1831): 37-49.
Retrospective on Mediterranean quarantine subscribes to the policy in order to stop diseases from Asia.

1633   Uccelli, Alessandro. "Cholera Morbus Disarmed." Trans. by John Robert Steuart. 32 (1831): 468-72.
Recapitulates procedures for coping with cholera.

1634   A Physician. "A Few Plain and Practical Remarks on Cholera." 34 (1832): 277-79.
Designs a diet against cholera and remedies for it.

1635   Uwins, David, M.D. "Phrenology." 34 (1832): 445-55.
Trusts phrenology to unlock functions of the brain and factors for insanity.

1636   "The State of the Poor in a Manufacturing Town." 35 (1832): 53-57.
Accepts the thesis of J.J. Kay, M.D., that disease is rampant among the poor in Manchester because sanitation is not.

1637   M[organ, T.C.]. "Private Hints to a Juvenile Physician." 35 (1832): 359-64.
Satirizes, with words on dress, demeanor, office locale, and patient relations, how to become a successful physician.

1638   [Bulwer, E.L.]. "On Ill Health, and Its Consolations." 37 (1833): 24-30.
Expresses patient's perspective on illness.

1639   "Letters on the Condition of the Working Classes in Various Parts of England: The Sheffield Grinders." 38 (1833): 46-56.
Examines maladies of grinders.

1640   W[ebbe], C[ornelius]. "Hints on Hypochondria." 41 (1834): 212-17.
Prefaces hypochondria with no exercise, inadequate rest, and unsuitable menu.

1641   Carne, John. "Lunacy in France." 50 (1837): 15-22, 167-76, 455-62; 51 (1837): 13-19; 53 (1838): 60-67; 56 (1839): 550-56.
Tract on French shelter for the insane discovers that inmates have more to read than have the insane in comparable English establishments.

1642   "On Nervous Influence." 53 (1838): 319-25.
Condenses theories of C. Carleton on effects of nerves on physiology and psyche.

1643   u. [T.C. Morgan]. "The Morality of the Stomach." 56 (1839): 379-87.
Says that a healthy stomach is central to physical and mental well-being.

1644 T[homson], A.T. "Extracts from the Note-Book of a Physician."
57 (1839): 193-200; 58 (1840): 260-71; 59 (1840): 108-18, 227-39, 506-16.
Skims seeds and signs of and treament for hypochondria, insanity, dyspepsia, and tuberculosis.

1645 u. [T.C. Morgan]. "Monomaniacs and Monomania." 68 (1843): 43-51.
Pores over captioned mental disorder.

1646 "Anti-Mathew; or, A Case of Hydrophobia." 69 (1843): 145-51.
Reckons that excessive drinking of water is morbid.

1647 [Bulwer, E.L.]. "Confessions of a Water Patient." 75 (1845): 1-16.
Avows that water is a safe and easy cure for afflictions. See #1136.

THE NEW REVIEW, 1889-1897

Shifting course sporadically, the *New Review* nevertheless routinely bruited the baneful effects of London life.

1648 Compton, [W.G.S.S.]. "The Homes of the People." 1 (1889): 47-61.
Fumes that lodgings of the poor are so dirty as to be deleterious.

1649 Pasteur, Louis. "Rabies." Trans. by [M.] Armand Ruffer. 1 (1889): 505-12, 619-30.
Louis Pasteur avouches merits of his vaccine against rabies.

1650 Mackenzie, Morell. "The Effect of Smoking on the Voice." 2 (1890): 315-28.
Confirms hazards of tobacco.

1651 Roose, Robson. "Fasting and Its Physiology." 2 (1890): 409-17.
Corroborates the harm of food deprivation.

1652 Meath [Reginald Brabazon, 12th Earl]. "Lungs for Our Great Cities." 2 (1890): 423-43.
Envies United States urban parks for their air quality.

1653 Jeune, Mary. "Holidays for Poor Children." 2 (1890): 455-65.
Lobbies for country holidays to strengthen city youths.

1654 "Sweating: The Two Reports." 2 (1890): 483-92.
Interprets reports by Lord Dunraven and the Lords' Committee on the Sweating System. Opts for Dunraven's draft with its greater state action to abolish hazards in such occupations as boot, nail, and chain making.

1655   Bramwell, Milne and Lloyd Storr-Best. "Hypnotism." 2 (1890): 534-45.
       Appraises hypnosis as a medical treatment.

1656   Luckes, Eva C.E. "Trained Nursing at the London Hospital." 3 (1890): 289-304.
       Trumpets the diet and domicile of nurses in the 1880s at London Hospital.

1657   Kerr, Norman. "Ether Drinking." 3 (1890): 536-46.
       Rues, because of consequent harm, the custom of ingesting ether.

1658   Sidgwick, Henry. "A Census of Hallucinations." 4 (1891): 52-59.
       Reprints own and others' research on cases of hallucination.

1659   Farrer, T.H. "A Model City: I. The Water Supply." 4 (1891): 213-28.
       Notices that London water is sometimes contaminated and its supply is currently low. See #1660, #1662, #1663, and #1665.

1660   Arnold, [R.] Arthur. "A Model City: II. The Drainage." 4 (1891): 342-54.
       Details how London sewage disposal pollutes the Thames. See #1659, #1662, #1663, and #1665.

1661   Mackenzie, Morell. "Exercise and Training: Exercise." 4 (1891): 372-78, 450-60.
       Enthusiast of exercise pens regimens appropriate to age and sex. See #1666.

1662   Shaw-Lefevre, G[eorge]. "A Model City; Or, Reformed London: III. A Bird's Eye View." 4 (1891): 432-43.
       Narrative on London streets requests better housing. See #1659, #1660, #1663, and #1665.

1663   Rayleigh [J.W. Strutt, 3d Baron]. "A Model City; Or, Reformed London: IV. Lighting - Electricity." 5 (1891), 31-37; Edmund Vincent. "Gas." 5 (1891): 37-44.
       Thinks that light is as crucial as water to wellness. See #1659, #1660, #1662, and #1665.

1664   Shaw, Eyre M. "Theatre Fires: Their Causes and Remedies." 5 (1891): 146-54.
       Promulgates ways to minimize casualties in theatre blazes.

1665   Ward, H. Marshall. "A Model City; Or, Reformed London: V. Trees and Flowers." 5 (1891): 182-92.
       Notes London's impure air. See #1659, #1660, #1662, and #1663.

1666   Mackenzie, Morell. "Training: Its Bearing on Health." 5 (1891): 222-33, 367-74, 454-62.
       Names food, sleep, and apt apparel as prerequisites of exercise. See #1661.

1667   Roose, Robson. "A Contribution to the Alcohol Question." 7 (1892): 66-79.
        Weighs the impact of drinking on health. See #2553.

1668   Cornish, W. Robert, Surgeon-General. "The Origin and Diffusion of Cholera." 7 (1892): 158-66.
        Pontificates about causes and range of and reactions to cholera.

1669   Williams, James Leon. "Degeneration of Human Teeth; Its Cause and Its Cure." 7 (1892): 466-80.
        Accentuates the structure and decay of teeth.

1670   Meath [Reginald Brabazon, 12th Earl]. "The London County Council and Open Spaces." 7 (1892): 701-07.
        Presses for urban playgrounds where children can breathe clean air and do calisthenics.

1671   Hart, Ernest. "Women, Clergymen, and Doctors." 7 (1892): 708-18.
        Upholds vivisection for medical knowledge after diatribes by Frances Power Cobbe and others. See #1674.

1672   Charcot, J.M. "The Faith-Cure." 8 (1893): 18-31.
        Dissertation on seemingly miraculous cures of breast cancer wonders if original symptoms may have been the byproduct of hysteria.

1673   Wilkinson, J. Frome. "A New Poor Law." 8 (1893): 59-72.
        Underwrites state stipends for paupers during epidemics and in old age.

1674   Wilberforce, Basil. " 'Women, Clergymen, and Doctors': A Reply." 8 (1893): 85-95.
        Negates the opinion on vivisection in #1671.

1675   Jeune, M[ary]. "In Defence of the Crinoline." 8 (1893): 190-200.
        Admits the combustibility of crinolines, but says that recent ones are less perilous and more cleanly.

1676   Law, John [Margaret Elise Harkness]. "The Children of the Unemployed." 8 (1893): 228-36.
        Begs for food and clothing for waifs in London's East End.

1677   Hart, Ernest. "The Coming Cholera." 8 (1893): 290-305.
        Simplifies sources and spread of and solutions for cholera.

1678   Storr-Best, Lloyd. "The Common Sense of Hypnotism." 8 (1893): 363-73.
        Treatise on hypnosis has some sentences on it as therapy.

1679   Roose, Robson. "The Propagation and Prevention of Cholera." 8 (1893): 504-16.
        Apprehends why cholera flourishes sporadically and how to circumscribe it.

1680   Richardson, Benjamin Ward. "Public Slaughter-Houses: A Suggestion for Farmers." 8 (1893): 631-44.
        Would adjust abattoir processing so as not to befoul meat.

1681   [Headingly], Adolphe Smith. "Are We Prepared to Resist a Cholera Epidemic?" 9 (1893): 353-61.
        Argues that improper sewerage and impure water are widespread enough for a cholera episode to be an epidemic.

1682   Dunn, Hugh Percy. "The Increase of Cancer." 9 (1893): 393-408.
        Survey of cancer has statistics on its increase and intelligence about its most prevalent forms and their treatment.

1683   Bayley, E.H. "Is Our Lifeboat System Effectual?" 10 (1894): 71-76.
        Grieves about deaths from shipwreck because lifeboat organization is inadequate and inefficient. See #1684.

1684   Macara, Charles W. "The Royal National Lifeboat Institution and Its Critics." 10 (1894): 232-41.
        Contests #1683.

1685   Waugh, Benjamin. "Our New Protectorate for Children." 10 (1894): 458-67.
        Discusses several cases of extreme child abuse.

1686   Editor, *Bakers' Times* [Charles C. Lee]. "The Truth about the London Bakeries." 10 (1894): 607-14.
        Warrants that London bakeries are sanitary and comply with public health laws.

1687   Dolman, Frederick. "Municipalities at Work." 11 (1894): 74-86.
        Respects, as salubrious, Birmingham's improvements of its water, housing, and food and inauguration of parks.

1688   Meath [Reginald Brabazon, 12th Earl]. "The Possibilities of Metropolitan Parks." 11 (1894): 201-08.
        Fosters parks, with their fresh air and space to exercise, to invigorate city residents.

1689   Beck, S. William. "The Great Underclothing Question." 11 (1894): 534-42.
        Focuses on underwear, partly for reasons of health. See #1690.

1690   Tomlin, Lewis R.S. "The Great Underclothing Question." 11 (1894): 606-11.
        Expands #1689.

1691   Donkin, H.B. "The New Cure." 12 (1895): 191-200.
        Would test an antitoxin for diphtheria on humans.

1692   Mitchell, P. Chalmers. "Pasteur." 13 (1895): 537-44.
        Lionizes Louis Pasteur for his research and his influence on others, as Joseph Lister.

1693 Wells, H.G. "Under the Knife." 14 (1896): 1-13.
Describes surgery from a patient's vantage.
1694 Sellers, Edith. "Depauperised." 14 (1896): 429-35.
Blesses cottage homes that provide food and exercise to pauper children otherwise consigned to institutions.
1695 H., L. "The Privilege of the Patient." 14 (1896): 524-30.
Would bind, by either oath or statute, doctors to protect patient confidentiality.
1696 Carfrae, George M. "The Drift of Modern Medicine." 15 (1896): 182-92.
Congratulates contemporaries for recent discoveries of cures and preventives.

THE NINETEENTH CENTURY, 1877-1900

Displaying breadth and depth in disquisitions, the *Nineteenth Century* of James Knowles, previously of the *Contemporary Review*, dissected health. Occupations and nutrition were foremost. Exercise and environment shared space with diverse diseases.

1697 Watson, Thomas. "The Abolition of Zymotic Disease." 1 (1877): 380-96.
Audits smallpox, typhus, measles, and typhoid fever.
1698 Fowler, John. "Railway Accidents." 1 (1877): 646-64.
Disbelieves that further legislation can brake railroad mishaps.
1699 Stansfeld, James. "Medical Women." 1 (1877): 888-901.
Glorifies women's victory over legal impediments to their becoming doctors. See #1784.
1700 Watson, Thomas. "Hydrophobia and Rabies." 2 (1877): 717-36.
Itemizes symptoms of and treatments for rabies.
1701 Watson, Thomas. "Small-Pox and Compulsory Vaccination." 3 (1878): 1001-09.
Thanks Edward Jenner for his smallpox vaccine. See #2534.
1702 Blackley, William Lewery. "National Insurance." 4 (1878): 834-57.
Would initiate employee contribution scheme for expenses of sickness. See #1708 and #1715.
1703 Granville, J. Mortimer. "Is Insanity Increasing?" 5 (1879): 523-33.
From statistics, infers that insanity is down. Would supervise public asylums more closely for a correspondence in costs.

1704   Thompson, Henry. "Food and Feeding." 5 (1879): 971-91; 6 (1879): 99-118.
Guides readers about nutrition, meal planning, and alcohol and tobacco use.

1705   Romanes, George J[ohn]. "Recreation." 6 (1879): 401-24.
Story on leisure activities adverts to their salubrity and that of exercise and fresh air.

1706   Maclagan, T.J. "Is Typhoid Fever Contagious?" 6 (1879): 809-18.
Treatise on communicable diseases lingers on typhoid fever.

1707   Midleton [William Broderick, 8th Viscount]. "The Noxious Gasses Bill." 6 (1879): 854-68.
Importunes for laws regulating industrial air pollution and waste disposal.

1708   Edwards, W. Walter. "Compulsory Providence: A Reply to Blackley." 6 (1879): 893-903.
Battles compulsory insurance for illness. See #1702 and #1715.

1709   Althaus, Julius. "The Functions of the Brain." 6 (1879): 1021-32.
Analyzes the brain.

1710   Paget, James. "Escape from Pain: The History of a Discovery." 6 (1879): 1119-32.
Surmises that ether, chloroform, and nitrous oxide are valuable pain suppressants in surgery and in childbirth.

1711   Lyttelton, Edward. "Athletics in Public Schools." 7 (1880): 43-57.
Discourages excessive school athletics as damaging physically and intellectually for boys.

1712   Lonsdale, Margaret. "The Present Crisis at Guy's Hospital." 7 (1880): 677-84.
Patron of "new" nurses testifies that they are thoroughly trained and have high moral standards but have met resistance in Guy's Hospital. See #1713 and #1714.

1713   Gull, William W., S.O. Habershon, and Alfred G. Henriques. "On the Nursing Crisis at Guy's Hospital." 7 (1880): 884-904.
Retorts to #1712 by stereotyping "new" nurses as intruders in doctor-patient relationships. See #974 and #1714.

1714   Sturges, Octavius, Seymour J. Sharkey, and Margaret Lonsdale. "Doctors and Nurses." 7 (1880): 1089-1108.
Subjects of individual papers are the doctor-nurse relationship and the traits and training of nurses. See #387, #1712, and #1713.

1715   Tremenheere, Hugh Seymour. "State Aid and Control in Industrial Insurance." 8 (1880): 275-93.
Proffers administrative program for obligatory insurance for sickness, aging, and burial. See #1702 and #1708.

1716 Romanes, G[eorge] J[ohn]. "Hypnotism." 8 (1880): 474-80.
Records study by Dr. R. Heidenhain on hypnosis and the body.
1717 Plimsoll, Samuel. "Explosions in Collieries, and Their Cure." 8 (1880): 895-920.
Expatiates on means to stem gas explosions in coal mines. See #1718 and #1719.
1718 Merivale, J.H. "Explosions in Collieries and Their Cure." 9 (1881): 237-44.
Augments #1717. See #1719.
1719 Shakespear, J.D. "Fire-Damp." 9 (1881): 245-48.
Touches on Samuel Plimsoll's script in #1717. See #1718.
1720 Pollock, W.F. "Smoke Prevention." 9 (1881): 478-90.
Understands risks to health from air pollution.
1721 Brabazon, [Reginald, 12th Earl Meath]. "Health and Physique of Our City Populations." 10 (1881): 80-89.
Gleans wellness from exercise and clean clothing, housing and air, all unavailable to impoverished urbanites. See #1594.
1722 Bevington, L.S. "How to Eat Bread." 10 (1881): 341-56.
Sorts breads according to nutritional worth.
1723 Granville, J. Mortimer. "Worry." 10 (1881): 423-29.
Aligns anxiety and ailing.
1724 Carpenter, W[illiam] B[enjamin]. "Disease-Germs." 10 (1881): 538-54.
Credits a knowledge of microbes for antiseptic surgery, smallpox vaccination, and research on tuberculosis. See #1749.
1725 Rossiter, Elizabeth. "Child Life for Children." 10 (1881): 567-72.
Advocates country sojourns for the mental and physical well-being of city juveniles.
1726 Paget, James, Richard Owen, and Samuel Wilks. "Vivisection: Its Pains and Its Uses." 10 (1881): 920-48.
Welcomes vivisection for medical progress. See #793, #794, #796, #1727, #1728, #1729, and #1730.
1727 Hutton, R[ichard] H[olt]. "The Biologists of Vivisection." 11 (1882): 29-39.
Anti-vivisectionist places animal pain ahead of medical advance. See #1726, #1728, #1729, and #1730.
1728 Kingsford, Anna. "The Uselessness of Vivisection." 11 (1882): 171-83.
Controverts #1726. See #1727, #1729, and #1730.
1729 Gull, William W. "The Ethics of Vivisection." 11 (1882): 456-67.
Adopts thesis of #1726 as a rejoinder to #1728. See #390, #1727, and #1730.

1730   Brunton, T. Lauder. "Vivisection and the Use of Remedies." 11 (1882): 479-87.
        Mirrors the motif of #1726. See #390, #1727, #1728, and #1729.

1731   Carpenter, William B[enjamin]. "Small-Pox Vaccination in 1871-1881." 11 (1882): 526-46.
        With data, defends the worth of smallpox vaccination. See #1732.

1732   Taylor, P.A. "Anti-Vaccination." 11 (1882): 782-802.
        Opponent of #1731 would end mandatory smallpox vaccination.

1733   Frankland, E. "The Climate of Town and Country." 12 (1882): 35-50.
        Dramatizes dangers of urban air contamination.

1734   Cross, Richard Assheton. "Homes of the Poor in London." 12 (1882): 231-41.
        Asseverates that more sanitary and better ventilated domiciles will cut disease among impoverished Londoners.

1735   Brabazon, [Reginald, 12th Earl Meath]. "The Early Closing Movement." 12 (1882): 517-32.
        Juxtaposes overwork and debility.

1736   Harkness, Margaret E[lise]. "Railway Labour." 12 (1882): 721-32.
        Logs harm to railroad employees from exhaustion and accidents.

1737   Watts, G.F. "Our Taste in Dress." 13 (1883): 45-57.
        Guarantees that corsets were bad for female muscles.

1738   Burdett, Henry C. "Our Hospitals." 13 (1883): 359-84.
        Would modify hospital administration, patient care, and education of doctors.

1739   Paget, W[alburga]. "Common Sense in Dress and Fashion." 13 (1883): 458-64.
        Maligns corsets and many cosmetics.

1740   Craven, Florence. "Servants of the Sick Poor." 13 (1883): 667-78.
        Esteems district nurses.

1741   Plimsoll, Samuel. "Cheap Fish for London." 14 (1883): 145-64.
        Orchestrates vending cheap wholesome fish in London.

1742   Frankland, Percy Faraday. "The Cholera and Our Water Supply." 14 (1883): 346-55.
        Determines that polluted water is the carrier of cholera and typhoid fever.

1743   Hodges, Sydney. "After-Images." 14 (1883): 622-38.
        Examines color retention and the physiology of the eye.

1744   Brabazon, [Reginald, 12th Earl Meath] and Samuel A. Barnett. "Great Cities and Social Reform." 14 (1883): 798-818.
        Outlines public health issues, as sanitation, smallpox vaccination, housing, and air quality, of cities.

1745   Hill, Octavia, [Antony Ashley Cooper, 7th Earl] Shaftesbury, H.O. Arnold-Forster, and William Glazier. "Common Sense and the Dwellings of the Poor." 14 (1883): 925-33.
Series of papers decode problems in erecting clean and safe lodgings for the needy.

1746   Paget, James. "Recreation." 14 (1883): 977-88.
Upholds the salubriousness, mental and physical, of recreation.

1747   Cross, Richard Assheton. "Homes of the Poor." 15 (1884): 150-66.
Publicizes how to build and sustain sanitary residences for the impoverished. See #573, not *National Review* article cited.

1748   Huxley, T.H. "The State and the Medical Profession." 15 (1884): 228-38.
Appeals for new medical education curriculum and more institutional interest in medical research.

1749   Carpenter, W[illiam] B[enjamin]. "The Germ-Theory of Zymotic Diseases Considered from the Natural History Point of View." 15 (1884): 317-36.
Reenforces ideas in #1724 with other evidence on microbes.

1750   Brassey, Thomas. "Ship Insurances and Loss of Life at Sea." 15 (1884): 445-54.
Deduces that negligence, and then accidents, can be offshoots of excessive insurance bought by shipowners.

1751   Marryat, Rosalind. " 'Sanitary Aid'." 15 (1884): 840-48.
Grounds rapid communication of diseases in congested abodes and vile water.

1752   Blackburn, Elizabeth J.M. "Our Deaf and Dumb." 16 (1884): 576-97.
Thrust is how to teach, in Great Britain and elsewhere, the hearing impaired who do not speak.

1753   Keppel, W.C. "Cycling and Cyclists." 17 (1885): 92-108.
Tale of cycling hints that it abets health.

1754   Bucknill, John Charles. "Abolition of Proprietary Madhouses." 17 (1885): 263-79.
Would shut private insane asylums because of their laxity toward patients. See #1756.

1755   Thompson, Henry. "Diet in Relation to Age and Activity." 17 (1885): 777-99.
Ordains dairy-vegetable diet after delving into origins of dyspepsia.

1756   Gasquet, J.R. "Lunacy Law Reform." 17 (1885): 857-68.
Defends the validity of certification of the insane for commitment. Opposes #1754.

1757   Farrar, Frederic W. "Lord Bramwell on Drink: A Reply." 17
        (1885): 869-78.
        Disagrees with notions about alcohol of G.W.W. Bramwell in a
        pamphlet reprinted as #1758. See #1761 and #1763.
1758   Bramwell, Lord [G.W.W.]. "Drink." 17 (1885): 878-82.
        Vindicates drinking liquor as freedom of choice. See #1757,
        #1761, and #1763.
1759   Cross, Richard Assheton. "Housing the Poor." 17 (1885): 926-47.
        Parrots perils of unsanitary abodes to the wellness of paupers.
1760   Sully, James. "Genius and Insanity." 17 (1885): 948-69.
        Pens genres of mental illness.
1761   Bramwell, [G.W.W.]. "Drink: A Rejoinder." 17 (1885): 1021-30.
        Prolongs debate, in #1757 and #1758, on alcohol. See #1763.
1762   Foster, J.R. "Mining Inspection a Sham - By a Miner." 17 (1885):
        1055-63.
        Characterizes mining inspectors as few and unqualified. See
        #1765.
1763   Farrar, Frederic W. "Drink: A Last Word to Lord Bramwell." 18
        (1885): 78-87.
        Protracts squabble, in #1757, #1758, and #1761, about merits of
        drinking.
1764   Lankester, E. Ray. "Recent Progress in Biology." 18 (1885): 101-
        10.
        Glimpses, among other matters, the genesis of cholera.
1765   Walker, George Blake. "Mine Inspection - A Reply." 18 (1885):
        124-29.
        Friend of mining inspectors contradicts #1762. Incriminates
        miners, because of their negligence or rulebreaking, in numerous
        accidents.
1766   Cameron, Charles. "Anti-Cholera Inoculation." 18 (1885): 338-52.
        Reproduces the evidence of Dr. Jaime Ferran that cholera could be
        arrested by a vaccine. See #1767.
1767   Willoughby, Edward F. "The Cholera-Inoculation Fallacy." 18
        (1885): 398-407.
        Disbelieves #1766.
1768   Cowper, Katie. "Some Experiences of Work in an East-End
        District." 18 (1885): 783-93.
        Slates overcrowded homes, early marriages, puny progeny, scant
        recreational facilities, and mediocre meat for the debility of the
        London poor.
1769   Furley, John. "The Red Cross." 18 (1885): 879-92.
        Reveres the Red Cross.

1770   Bramwell, [G.W.W.]. "Insanity and Crime." 18 (1885): 893-99.
        Core is the kinship between varieties of insanity and criminal behavior.

1771   Fox, Fortescue. "Stimulants and Narcotics: Their Use and Abuse." 18 (1885): 923-39.
        Prose is principally on tobacco, opium, and cocaine.

1772   DeMauley [C.F.A.C. Ponsonby, 2d Baron]. "A Court of Lunacy." 19 (1886): 257-63.
        Figures that insanity, except hereditary, was up. Would shut inferior private asylums and have doctors certify commitments.

1773   Yeo, J. [I.] Burney. "Food Accessories: Their Influence on Digestion." 19 (1886): 271-79.
        Peers at effects of alcohol, mineral water, coffee, tea, cocoa, and vinegar on digestion.

1774   Lankester, E. Ray. "Pasteur and Hydrophobia." 20 (1886): 149-70.
        Theme is the search by Louis Pasteur for a rabies vaccine.

1775   Yeo, J. [I.] Burney. "English and Foreign Spas." 20 (1886): 201-14.
        Grades European spas for salubriousness.

1776   Myers, Frederic W.H. "Multiple Personality." 20 (1886): 648-66.
        Message on multiple personality disorder adverts to its roots and to hypnosis as therapy.

1777   Twining, Louisa. "Workhouse Cruelties." 20 (1886): 709-14.
        Despairs that workhouse inmates die because of the malfeasance or nonfeasance of their guardians.

1778   Manners, Janetta. "Massage." 20 (1886): 824-28.
        Extols massage as a relaxant and exercise for vitality.

1779   Brabazon, [Reginald, 12 Earl Meath]. "Decay of Bodily Strength in Towns." 21 (1887): 673-76.
        Avouches that impure air, unsanitary housing, and little exercise translate into infirmity for urbanites.

1780   Gordon-Cumming, C.F. "Strange Medicines." 21 (1887): 901-18.
        Subject is folk remedies, British and foreign.

1781   Frankland, Percy Faraday. "The Creatures We Breathe." 22 (1887): 242-47.
        Features air contaminated by dust and microbes.

1782   Sharkey, Seymour J. "Morphinomania." 22 (1887): 335-42.
        Fathoms morphine addiction.

1783   Howie, James Muir. "The Nerve-Rest Cure: A Plea for the Nervous." 22 (1887): 659-66.
        Samples restoratives, such as exercise, rest, and alcohol, to dilute stress.

1784   Jex-Blake, Sophia, M.D. "Medical Women." 22 (1887): 692-707.
        Recalls women's attempts to become doctors. See #1699.
1785   Thompson, Henry. "The Progress of Cremation." 23 (1888): 1-17.
        Directs cremation for public health. See #357.
1786   Hill, Octavia. "More Air for London." 23 (1888): 181-88.
        Terms open spaces beneficial to Londoners.
1787   Millican, Kenneth. "The Present Position of the Medical Schism."
        23 (1888): 258-75.
        Demarcates the division between traditional practitioners and
        homeopaths.
1788   Yeo, J. [I.] Burney. "Long Life and How to Attain It." 23 (1888):
        370-93.
        Piece on longevity banks on diet, exercise, and absence of stress.
        See #2178.
1789   Meath [Reginald Brabazon, 12th Earl]. "A Model Factory." 23
        (1888): 536-40.
        Eulogizes a factory with a healthy environment and pensions for
        illness, accident, and age.
1790   Priestley, Eliza. "Pasteur." 23 (1888): 838-57.
        Admires Louis Pasteur's research, chiefly on rabies.
1791   Yeo, J. [I.] Burney. "The New Cure for 'Growing Too Fat'." 24
        (1888): 196-206.
        Dictates new menus for those who are overweight.
1792   Tuckey, C. Lloyd. "Faith-Healing as a Medical Treatment." 24
        (1888): 839-50.
        Briefs readers on maladies treated by hypnosis. See #439 and
        #1836.
1793   Meath [Reginald Brabazon, 12th Earl]. "A Thousand More
        Mouths Every Day." 25 (1889): 57-72.
        Keys youthful vigor to nourishing food and physical exercise.
1794   Plimsoll, Samuel. "Twelve Millions Wasted in the Sea." 25
        (1889): 325-50.
        Rebukes owners who hire sailors for old or unsafe but insured
        ships. See #1795 and #1798.
1795   Scrutton, Thomas. "Are Twelve Millions Wasted in the Sea?" 25
        (1889): 539-51.
        Reverses #1794. See #1798.
1796   Tuke, John Batty. "Lunatics as Patients, Not Prisoners." 25 (1889):
        595-607.
        Aims for recovery, not merely good care for the insane.
1797   Priestley, Eliza. "The Mysteries of Malaria." 25 (1889): 852-67.
        Unveils the cause and incidence of malaria.

1798 Plimsoll, Samuel. "Twelve Millions Per Annum Wasted in the Sea - A Rejoinder." 25 (1889): 881-93.
Reiterates the thesis of #1794. See #1795.

1799 Cox, Harold. "The Eight Hours Question." 26 (1889): 21-34.
Crusades for the eight-hour day, enforcement of all laws on employee health, and application to men of the safety and hours guidelines in the Factory and Workshop Act (1878).

1800 Mackenzie, Morell. "Health-Seeking in Madeira." 26 (1889): 120-35.
Would settle those with respiratory ailments on South Atlantic islands because of their climate.

1801 Yeo, J. [I.] Burney, M.D. "On Change of Air." 26 (1889): 194-207.
Predicates fitness on clean air in the country or at sea.

1802 Behrend, Henry, M.R.C.P. "Diseases Caught from Butcher's Meat." 26 (1889): 409-22.
Singles out tuberculosis as the major disease in meat. See #1812.

1803 Waller, Jessie Oriana. "Mental and Physical Training for Children." 26 (1889): 659-67.
Urges parents to attend more carefully to the food and clothing of infants.

1804 Mackenzie, Morell. "The Dreadful Revival of Leprosy." 26 (1889): 925-41.
Prods doctors to find a cure for leprosy.

1805 Jersey, M[argaret] E. [Child-Villiers, Countess of]. "Ourselves and Our Foremothers." 27 (1890): 56-64.
Entry on women in the 1890s and earlier generations gathers that the former were healthier because of greater, but not excessive exercise.

1806 Vincent, Charles W. "The Dangers of Electric Lighting." 27 (1890): 145-49.
Petitions for government safety regulations on handling electric wires in order to retard accidents.

1807 Fleming, George. "The Suppression of Rabies in the United Kingdom." 27 (1890): 497-512.
Would muzzle licensed dogs and destroy others to foil rabies.

1808 Knowles, Lees. "Horseflesh." 27 (1890): 592-607.
Endorses statute on the sale of horsemeat as food.

1809 [Webb], Beatrice Potter. "The Lords and the Sweating System." 27 (1890): 885-905.
Defines "sweating trades" as those done in unsanitary conditions by the overworked.

1810   Snow, Herbert. "Increase of Cancer: Its Probable Cause." 28 (1890): 80-88.
        Spans types of malignancies and their origins. See #1582.

1811   Ewart, C. Theodore. "The Power of 'Suggestion'." 28 (1890): 252-59.
        Linchpin is hypnosis as a medical treatment.

1812   Behrend, Henry, M.R.C.P. "Tuberculous Meat and Its Consequence." 28 (1890): 545-62.
        Guesses that diseased cattle cause tuberculosis. See #1802.

1813   Twining, Louisa. "Women as Public Servants." 28 (1890): 950-58.
        Would install women as superintendents of workhouse infirmaries because females reputedly know more about nursing than do males and of insane asylums where staffs typically have no systematic training.

1814   Kingsbury, George C. "Hypnotism, Crime, and the Doctors." 29 (1891): 145-53.
        Disdains hypnosis in "sideshows" but not its study by doctors. See #421.

1815   Berdoe, Edward. "Slum-Mothers and Death-Clubs." 29 (1891): 560-63.
        Insists that destitute mothers tend sick offspring, notwithstanding death insurance.

1816   Russell, [F.A.] Rollo. "A Department of Health." 29 (1891): 615-23.
        Would create a national department to control such diseases as rabies, typhoid fever, diphtheria, and scarlet fever.

1817   Meath [Reginald Brabazon, 12th Earl]. "A Model Dairy." 29 (1891): 624-27.
        Sojourner at a dairy targets its sanitary arrangments with an aside on the value of milk for the young.

1818   Elsdale, Henry. "Resuscitation by Oxygen." 29 (1891): 719-26.
        Would have oxygen readily available in hospitals and with life-saving brigades.

1819   Priestley, Eliza. "The Realm of the Microbe." 29 (1891): 811-31.
        Comments on bacteria as a source of such diseases as tuberculosis.

1820   Horsley, Victor. "The Analysis of Voluntary Movement." 29 (1891): 857-70.
        Motif is voluntary muscles and illnesses affecting them.

1821   Heather-Bigg, Ada. "Women and the Glove Trade." 30 (1891): 939-50.
        Tale of glove trade lists its detrimental effects, such as neuralgia and tuberculosis, on female employees.

1822 Ruffer, M. Armand. "The New Science - Preventive Medicine." 30 (1891): 975-93.
Stimulates research on antiseptics and vaccines in order to slow disease.

1823 Lubbock, John. "The London Water Supply." 31 (1892): 224-32. Would augment water reserves proportionate to London's population.

1824 Maclagan, T.J. "Influenza and Salicin." 31 (1892): 329-39.
Nominates microbes as bearers of all fevers and salicin as therapy for influenza, allegedly akin to malaria. See #1592.

1825 Paget, Walburga. "Vegetable Diet." 31 (1892): 577-85.
Champions vegetarianism for wellness.

1826 Wright, A.E. "Colour-Blindness, Its Pathology and Its Possible Practical Remedy." 31 (1892): 648-60.
Article on the nature of color blindness would pare accidents by having yellow and blue signals.

1827 Dunraven [W.T. Quin, 4th Earl]. "The Invasion of Destitute Aliens." 31 (1892): 985-1000.
Rumors that indigent immigrants willing to toil in any surroundings delay salutary reforms in the "sweated trades."

1828 Loch, C.S. "The Confusion in Medical Charities." 32 (1892): 298-310.
Regrets the tension between general practitioners and dispensaries.

1829 Russell, T.W. "The Lessons of a Decade." 32 (1892): 581-93.
Disquisition on Irish milieu grants that the population is healthier because of better fare and abodes, but confides that insanity is increasing.

1830 Hart, Ernest. "Cholera, and Our Protection Against It." 32 (1892): 632-51.
Ties the burgeoning of cholera to uncleanliness, primarily of water and individuals. Would stem it at ports and send its victims to hospitals. See #1852.

1831 Chamberlain, J. "The Labour Question." 32 (1892): 677-710.
Pores over such issues as employee compensation for accidents and fewer hours for risky employments. See #1833.

1832 Horsley, Victor and M. Armand Ruffer. "The Morality of 'Vivisection'." 32 (1892): 804-17.
Assents to medical experiments on animals. See #1834.

1833 Burns, John, Thomas Burt, H.H. Champion, J. Keir Hardie, and Sam Woods. "Labour Leaders on the Labour Question." 32 (1892): 845-98.
Appendix to #1831 inflates the jeopardy of some jobs.

1834   Manchester, J[ames Moorhouse, Bishop of]. "The Morality of Vivisection: A Reply." 32 (1892): 980-83.
Presents negatives to the position of #1832.

1835   Jex-Blake, Sophia, M.D. "Medical Women in Fiction." 33 (1893): 261-72.
Validates fictional portrayals of female doctors.

1836   Hart, Ernest. "The Revival of Witchcraft." 33 (1893): 347-68.
Rebukes some doctors for their dependence on hypnosis. See #439 and #1792.

1837   Drayson, A.W., Major-General. "The Art of Breathing." 33 (1893): 611-18.
Tract on respiration has some language on the perniciousness of inhaling polluted air.

1838   Tuke, John Batty. "Habitual Drunkards." 33 (1893): 1009-14.
Would legally confine all alcoholics to cure some.

1839   Meath [Reginald Brabazon, 12th Earl]. "Public Playgrounds for Children." 34 (1893): 267-71.
Rhapsodizes about outdoor recreation for robustness, notably of city youths.

1840   Wilkins, W.H. " 'How Long, O Lord, How Long'?" 34 (1893): 329-36.
Excoriates labor environment of needlewomen in London's East End.

1841   Foster, Michael, Jun. "Weariness." 34 (1893): 337-52.
Thrust is fatigue with reference to muscles and nervous system.

1842   Provand, A.D. "Employers' Liability." 34 (1893): 698-720.
Would impose strict liability on owners for employees' mishaps at their jobs. See #443.

1843   Dunn, Hugh Percy. "What London People Die Of." 34 (1893): 875-98.
Essay on respiratory, digestive, nervous, and circulatory ailments, dysentery, cancer, and alcoholism enters the first two as most significant for Londoners' deaths but the last two as proliferating.

1844   Almond, Hely Hutchinson. "Football as a Moral Agent." 34 (1893): 902-11.
Elevates football and other athletics, done properly, for fitness.

1845   Steeves, G. Walter. "Sanitary Insurance: A Scheme." 35 (1894): 32-43.
Would write insurance against defects in residential sanitation and for habitability.

1846   Galton, Douglas. "Feeble-Minded Children." 35 (1894): 276-83.
Elects teachers to note physically and mentally challenged pupils.

1847   Twining, Louisa. "Women as Official Inspectors." 35 (1894): 489-94.
      Would appoint female inspectors in hospitals, infirmaries, prisons, and workplaces to transcribe more easily problems of their sick sisters.

1848   Dunn, Hugh Percy. "Modern Surgery." 35 (1894): 775-95.
      Paper on surgery has paragraphs on antiseptics and techniques to operate on the brain, nerves, and eyes.

1849   Frankland, Percy [Faraday]. "Sunshine and Microbes." 35 (1894): 838-44.
      Showcases research on bacteria inhibition by light.

1850   Webb, Beatrice [Potter]. "The Failure of the Labour Commission." 36 (1894): 2-22.
      Acknowledges that the titled Commission has heeded some occupational health matters.

1851   Dunn, Hugh Percy. "Is Our Race Degenerating?" 36 (1894): 301-14.
      Asserts that contemporary lifestyle is not siring physical decline.

1852   Hart, Ernest. "Cholera and the Sultan." 36 (1894): 538-54.
      Comprehends how cholera flourishes. See #1830.

1853   Heather-Bigg, Ada. "The Case Against Home Work." 36 (1894): 970-86.
      Confutes the deleteriousness of women's work in their dwellings.

1854   Priestley, Eliza. "Penalties of Ignorance." 37 (1895): 579-92.
      Expresses health hazards of homes, such as casual food handling.

1855   Quilter, Harry. " 'In the Days of Her Youth'." 37 (1895): 940-55.
      Would slot exercise in school time for female vigor.

1856   Benson, E.F. "The Recent 'Witch-Burning' at Clonmel." 37 (1895): 1053-58.
      Relays the death of Irish woman after she was tortured as a technique to cure a nervous disorder.

1857   Gorst, John E. "The Conservative Programme of Social Reform." 38 (1895): 3-16.
      Encompasses job-related injuries, the destitute sick, and the aged.

1858   Yeo, J. [I.] Burney, M.D. "Medicine and Society." 38 (1895): 1025-40.
      Account of doctor-patient relations does not omit expensive specialists or "quacks." Eulogizes the general practitioner. Detests medical "advertising," such as book publishing.

1859   Fenton, W.H. "A Medical View of Cycling for Ladies." 39 (1896): 796-801.
      Would revitalize women by a cycling regimen.

1860   Waldo, F.J., M.D., and David Walsh, M.B. "Murder by Measles."
        39 (1896): 957-63.
        Mourns fatalities, chiefly among the impoverished, from measles.
1861   Frankland, G.C. "Boiling Milk." 40 (1896): 454-60.
        Persuades audience that pasteurization of milk destroys bacteria.
1862   Leigh, [Francis] Dudley. "Horse Ambulances." 40 (1896): 609-18.
        Would emulate United States horse-drawn ambulances for
        emergencies.
1863   Morris, Malcolm. "The Superfluous Vaccination Commission." 40
        (1896): 958-73.
        Impugns captioned Commission for merely seconding that
        vaccination shortens smallpox.
1864   Priestley, Eliza. "Nurses *a la Mode*." 41 (1897): 28-37.
        Concerns goals, traits, and training of nurses. See #1867.
1865   Barnett, Henrietta O. "The Verdict of the Barrack Schools." 41
        (1897): 56-68.
        Would segregate, educationally, pauper children with ophthalmia
        or ringworm and those who are either physically or mentally
        challenged.
1866   Bosanquet, Helen, Louise Creighton, Beatrice [Potter] Webb, and
        Lucy C.F. Cavendish. "Law and the Laundry." 41 (1897): 224-35.
        Turns on ambiguities and omissions in legislation on laundry work
        to the detriment of young employees.
1867   Fenwick, Ethel Gordon. "Nurses *a la Mode*: A Reply to Lady
        Priestley." 41 (1897): 325-34.
        Corrects notions in #1864 with respect to nurses, but hints that
        others, as nannies, undermine the reputation of professionals.
1868   Low, Francis H. "How Poor Ladies Live." 41 (1897): 405-17.
        Commemorates the many gentlewomen on small incomes who
        are constantly anxious about the costs of illness. See #1869,
        #1870, and #1875.
1869   Orme, Eliza. "How Poor Ladies Live: A Reply." 41 (1897): 613-
        19.
        Accepts state pensions only for the protagonists of #1868. See
        #1870 and #1875.
1870   Shaw, Edith M. "How Poor Ladies Might Live: An Answer from
        the Workhouse." 41 (1897): 620-27.
        Critic of #1868 would legislate pensions. See #1869 and #1875.
1871   West, Algernon. "Some Changes in Social Life During the
        Queen's Reign." 41 (1897): 639-55.
        Surveys improvements in medical care, hospitals, sanitation, and
        occupational well-being during Victoria's reign.

1872 Morris, Malcolm. "The Progress of Medicine During the Queen's Reign." 41 (1897): 739-58.
Deems surgery, with anesthetics, antiseptics, and new procedures, and obsterics progressive. Lionizes specialists for their knowledge of the latest treatments.

1873 Heward, Edward Vincent. "Tobacco in Relation to Health and Character." 41 (1897): 808-23.
Fancies that smoking tobacco was not harmful.

1874 Priestley, Eliza. "The French and English Treatment of Research." 42 (1897): 113-23.
Would have Parliament invest more money in health research.

1875 Low, Francis H. "How Poor Ladies Live: A Rejoinder and a 'Jubilee' Suggestion." 42 (1897): 161-68.
Riposte to #1869 and #1870 reaffirms #1868. Welcomes charity for gentlewomen.

1876 Hogg, Edith F. "School Children as Wage Earners." 42 (1897): 235-44.
From statistics, extrapolates that paper and milk delivering and babysitting tired pupils.

1877 Londonderry, Theresa [Vane-Tempest-Stewart, Marchioness of]. "The 'Conservative' Compensation (Workmen's) Bill of 1897." 42 (1897): 349-52.
Inculpates workers for some job mishaps.

1878 Glenesk, Alice [Borthwick, Lady]. "The Increasing Duration of Human Life." 42 (1897): 393-401.
Details effects of diet, occupation, and temperament on longevity.

1879 Long, James. "Consumption in Cattle Conveyable to Man." 42 (1897): 581-93.
Would stifle tuberculosis by monitoring the flesh and milk of cows for disease.

1880 Hogg, Edith F. "The Fur-Pullers of South London." 42 (1897): 734-43.
Maximizes risks to fur-pullers of this residential labor.

1881 King, E. Augusta. "Deaths under Chloroform." 43 (1898): 512-20.
Apprises readers of the danger when chloroform is improperly administered. See #1884 and #1886.

1882 Thompson, Henry. "Why 'Vegetarian'?" 43 (1898): 556-69, 966-76.
Wonders about the salubrity of vegetarianism. See #1887.

1883 Hutton, John. "Cottage Homes for the Aged Poor." 43 (1898): 633-36.
Would tax to support boarding homes for the elderly.

1884   Buxton, Dudley W. and William Ramsay. "Deaths under Chloroform." 43 (1898): 668-78.
        Response to #1881 rehabilitates chloroform if pure and given by experts. See #1886.

1885   Thomson, R.T. "The Workmen's Compensation Act." 43 (1898): 899-914.
        Furnishes main components of titled statute on compulsory employer compensation for employee accidents.

1886   King, E. A[ugusta]. "Death and Torture under Chloroform: A Rejoinder." 43 (1898): 985-93.
        Returns to the theme of #1881, and equates chloroform and suffering. See #1884.

1887   Oldfield, Josiah. "Vegetarian Still: A Reply to Sir Henry Thompson." 44 (1898): 246-52.
        Defends vegetarianism against the attack in #1882.

1888   Tuckwell, Gertrude [M.]. "Commercial Manslaughter." 44 (1898): 253-58.
        Hits hazards to laborers in pottery industry.

1889   Maxwell, Herbert. "Tuberculosis in Man and Beast." 44 (1898): 673-87.
        Would nip tuberculosis by means of cattle inspection and milk sterilization.

1890   Howard, Mabel. "Nursing the Poor in Their Homes." 44 (1898): 835-39.
        Balances assets, as availability and low wages, and liabilities, as short training and ready dispensation of morphine, of district nurses.

1891   Shaw[-]Lefevre, G[eorge]. "The London Water Supply." 44 (1898): 980-90.
        Whines about the unreliability of London's water supply. See #1893.

1892   Gibson, James Arthur. "The Open-Air Cure of Consumption." 45 (1899): 92-101.
        Would combat tuberculosis with the regimen followed in Nordrach, Germany. See #1894 and #1895.

1893   Shadwell, Arthur. "The London Water Supply: An Answer." 45 (1899): 282-94.
        Confutes #1891.

1894   Coghill, J.G. Sinclair, M.D. "The Prevention of Consumption." 45 (1899): 304-14.
        Incorporates alternative treatments to that in #1892 for tuberculosis and deterrents to its diffusion. See #1895.

1895 Gibson, James Arthur. "The Nordrach Cure Practicable in This Country." 45 (1899): 389-403.
Reenforces ideas in #1892 that #1894 downplayed.

1896 Keneally, Arabella, L.R.C.P. "Woman as an Athlete." 45 (1899): 636-45.
Speculates that some exercise is salutary for females whereas too much can diminish femininity. See #1898 and #1900.

1897 Priestley, Eliza. "Winged Carriers of Disease." 45 (1899): 671-80.
Theme is mosquitoes as agents of malaria.

1898 Chant, L. Ormiston. "Woman as an Athlete: A Reply to Dr. Arabella Keneally." 45 (1899): 745-54.
Disputes the opinion of #1896. See #1900.

1899 Jessop, Augustus. "The Cry of the Villages." 45 (1899): 865-79.
Chapter on village life mentions that opportunities for free medical care are few.

1900 Keneally, Arabella, L.R.C.P. "Woman as an Athlete: A Rejoinder." 45 (1899): 915-29.
Restates the thinking in #1896 after a challenge in #1898.

1901 Gabbett, Henry S., M.D. "Beneficient Germs." 45 (1899): 938-43.
Points out the utility of some bacteria, such as to ripen cheese, and the harm to humans of disinfectants.

1902 Gorst, John E. "School Children as Wage-Earners." 46 (1899): 8-17.
Would reserve easy jobs, as caddying, for juveniles and restrict their labor so as not to vitiate vitality.

1903 Collins, E., Editor of 'The Dentist.' "The Teeth of the Schoolboy." 46 (1899): 84-93.
Warns that youthful tooth decay is up and that its neglect will lead to more serious disorders.

1904 Elsdale, H[enry]. "Why Are Our Brains Deteriorating?" 46 (1899): 262-72.
Attributes brain deterioration to modes of education, stress, democracy, and materialism.

1905 Gibson, James Arthur. "The Cry of the Consumptives." 46 (1899): 641-53.
Would thwart tuberculosis with hospitals for the poor, specialized training for doctors, and regulation of cattle.

1906 Sutherland, Alexander. "Woman's Brain." 47 (1900): 802-10.
Hypothesizes that women's brains are smaller than are those of men.

1907 Skelton, Reginald A. "Statistics of Suicide." 48 (1900): 465-82.
Biography of suicides categorizes some of them as insane.

THE NORTH BRITISH REVIEW, 1844-1871

Coming from a Scottish and Free Church background, the *North British* was more ecumenical in its entries on ailments.

1908   [Chalmers, Thomas]. "Report on the Poor Laws of Scotland." 2 (1844-45): 471-514.
        Disparges medical care under Scottish law of the destitute ill, principally the insane.

1909   "Hospitals for the Insane Poor." 3 (1845): 387-405.
        Endorses a bill for better care of the indigent insane. Wishes for a parallel one for Scotland and Ireland.

1910   "Kitto's *Lost Senses*: Instruction of the Deaf and Dumb." 6 (1846-47): 331-64.
        Abridges a book by John Kitto on how to tutor the hearing impaired who do not speak.

1911   "State of Scottish Towns." 7 (1847): 54-71.
        Exaggerates the sanitation and housing of the English town. Claims that those in the Scottish speed communicable diseases.

1912   [Miller, James]. "Painless Operations in Surgery." 7 (1847): 169-206.
        Focuses on ether in surgery and childbirth.

1913   [Raleigh, Samuel]. "What Is Life Assurance?" 12 (1849): 1-20.
        Paper on life insurance nods to mortality tables.

1914   [Brown, John]. "Locke and Sydenham." 12 (1849): 53-85.
        Tribute to Thomas S. Sydenham has some words on his study of epidemics and diagnostics. Would teach doctors science, humor, and judgment in the apprenticeship, with its mechanism for bonding, not in classes.

1915   [Masson, David]. "Edwin Chadwick, C.B." 13 (1850): 40-84.
        Paen to Edwin Chadwick credits him with reducing disease by rallying for sanitary legislation.

1916   [Brown, Samuel]. "Animal Magnetism." 15 (1851): 133-59.
        Approves hypnosis as medical therapy.

1917   [Kingsley, Charles]. "The Water Supply of London." 15 (1851): 228-53.
        Dockets London's polluted water as a source of Londoners' sicknesses.

1918   [Brewster, David]. "Binocular Vision and the Stereoscope." 17 (1852): 165-204.
        Explains binocular vision.

1919   [Brewster, David]. "Sir H. Holland on Mental Physiology, Electro-Biology, Etc." 22 (1854-55): 179-224.
       Inventories many aspects of the interaction between mind and body.

1920   [Brewster, David]. "Dr. George Wilson on Colour-Blindness." 24 (1855-56): 325-58.
       Discusses color blindness and its implications for society.

1921   [Brewster, David]. "The Sight and How to See." 26 (1856-57): 145-84.
       Describes the eye and its diseases.

1922   [Kaye, J.W.]. "The Employment of Women." 26 (1856-57): 291-338.
       Underlines occupational risks to females, as in needlework.

1923   [Lindsay, William Lauder]. "Scottish Lunacy Commission." 27 (1857): 106-26.
       Clamors about the treatment of the insane in Scotland.

1924   [Brewster, David]. "Researches on Light - Sanatory [sic] - Scientific and Aesthetical." 29 (1858): 177-210.
       Links light and salubrity.

1925   [Brewster, David]. "Life-Boats - Lightening Conductors - Lighthouses." 31 (1859): 492-529.
       Ascribes fewer maritime accidents and deaths to recent inventions on ships or on shores.

1926   [Laycock, Thomas]. "Modern Necromancy." 34 (1861): 110-41.
       Classifies as insane those who purportedly contact the dead.

1927   [Brewster, David]. "Railway Accidents." 34 (1861): 399-427.
       Has data on injuries and fatalities in railroad mishaps. Presents such causes as employee and brake fault and track obstruction.

1928   [Skae, David]. "Lunacy Legislation." 36 (1862): 453-84.
       Remonstrates about methods of care of the insane, notably the indigent.

1929   [Laycock, Thomas]. "The Education and Management of the Imbecile." 39 (1863): 120-33.
       Would institutionalize for training the mentally challenged.

1930   [Dasent, G.W.]. "Wildbad and Its Water." n.s., 2, o.s., 41 (1864): 393-436.
       Guest at German spa talks about the experience.

1931   [Foster, Michael, Jun.]. "Sir Benjamin Collins Brodie, Bart." n.s., 4, o.s., 43 (1865): 127-50.
       Treasures medical research of Benjamin Brodie.

1932   [Smith, Robert A.]. "Disinfection." n.s., 5, o.s., 44 (1866): 458-96.
       Pushes disinfectants to stop communicable diseases.

1933   [Playfair, Lyon]. "On the Relation of the Food of Man to His Muscular Power." n.s., 6, o.s., 45 (1866): 189-96.
Hooks health to diet.

1934   [Jenkin, H.C. Fleeming]. "Population." n.s., 8, o.s., 47 (1867): 441-62.
Essay on fertility notes perils of pregnancy.

1935   [Playfair, Lyon]. "On Sleep." n.s., 9, o.s., 48 (1868): 498-512.
Teams sleep and vitality.

1936   [Greenwell, Dora]. "On the Education of the Imbecile." n.s., 10, o.s., 49 (1868): 73-100.
Prays for tutoring of the mentally challenged.

1937   [Mitchell, Arthur]. "The Increase of Lunacy." n.s., 11, o.s., 50 (1869): 123-58.
Because incurably insane paupers were allegedly multiplying, would assign them to private home care.

ONCE A WEEK, 1859-1880

Contracting to amuse and to advise, *Once a Week* tended to instruct on aspects of illness. Employment and nourishment, adulteration and sanitation sustained legions of sentences. The brain and its malfunction further absorbed authors.

1938   Clyne, John. "Dumb Mouths." 1 (1859): 136-38.
Enlightens on how to teach the hearing impaired to speak and sign.

1939   Martineau, Harriet. "Herod in the Nineteenth Century." 1 (1859): 195-98.
Avows that over forty percent of children die before age five from too much or too little food, narcotics, or brain maladies.

1940   Martineau, Harriet. "School for Life or Death." 1 (1859): 254-59.
Would have schools encourage pupil hygiene and exercise and provide students with nutritious meals.

1941   Martineau, Harriet. "Follies in Food." 1 (1859): 299-303.
Situates sickness in personal uncleanliness and improper diet.

1942   Martineau, Harriet. "How to Learn to Swim." 1 (1859): 327-28.
Slates swimming as a salubrious sport.

1943   Martineau, Harriet. "The Cook or the Doctor?" 1 (1859): 331-35.
Catalogs kinds of fare that reenforce robustness.

1944   Martineau, Harriet. "Dress and Its Victims." 1 (1859): 387-91.
Banners harmful apparel, such as slickers and corsets.

1945 Martineau, Harriet. "Home or Hospital." 1 (1859): 419-23.
Marks as deleterious abodes without adequate air, light, and water.

1946 Martineau, Harriet. "Woman's Battle-Field." 1 (1859): 474-79.
Stipulates ideal qualities and real duties of nurses. See #1963.

1947 Martineau, Harriet. "Self-Murder." 1 (1859): 510-14.
Text on suicide has some sentences on alcoholism and insanity.

1948 Salus Populi. "Real and Sham Vaccination." 1 (1859): 523-24.
Strikes at incorrectly administered smallpox vaccinations.

1949 Martineau, Harriet. "The Cost of Cottages." 2 (1859-60): 61-65, 169-70.
Shares the price of healthy rural habitations.

1950 D., M. "Physical Antipathies." 2 (1859-60): 113-15.
Pivot is varieties of allergies.

1951 Adams, W. Bridges. "The Refuse of Towns and Cities." 2 (1859-60): 128-31.
Pairs sewage disposal and polluted waters in municipalities.

1952 Martineau, Harriet. "The Student - His Health." 2 (1859-60): 144-47.
Recommends exercise to male students.

1953 Martineau, Harriet. "The Young Lady in Town and Country - Her Health." 2 (1859-60): 191-95.
Counsels girls to exercise brains and bodies for wellness.

1954 D., M. "Aerated Bread." 2 (1859-60): 235-37.
Broadcasts hazards of badly made bread in questionable bakeries.

1955 E., E. "Blown to Pieces." 2 (1859-60): 255-58.
Highlights dangers of mining.

1956 Scott, Ingelby. "Representative Women - The Free Nurse." 2 (1859-60): 258-62.
Honors Catherine Mompesson, Mary Pickard, and Florence Nightingale for their nursing.

1957 Martineau, Harriet. "The Rural Labourer - His Health." 2 (1859-60): 278-81.
Believes that better health for rustics will parallel better working circumstances.

1958 Martineau, Harriet. "The Statesman - His Health." 2 (1859-60): 347-50.
Decrees sufficient sleep and recreation for statesmen with occupational stress.

1959 Martineau, Harriet. "The Maid of All Work - Her Health." 2 (1859-60): 464-67.
Anchors maladies of maids to lack of sleep and dyspepsia because of frequent calls.

1960   Martineau, Harriet. "The Policeman - His Health." 2 (1859-60): 522-26.
Selects respiratory ills as the main medical problem of policemen.

1961   Scott, Ingelby. "Representative Women - Dr. Elizabeth Blackwell." 2 (1859-60): 577-81.
Accolade to Elizabeth Blackwell petitions for more women doctors, particularly in gynecology, obstetrics, and pediatrics.

1962   W[ynter], A[ndrew]. "Shipwrecks." 2 (1859-60): 588-91.
Blames the ignorance or laxity of seamen for many shipwrecks.

1963   Martineau, Harriet. "The Training of Nurses." 3 (1860): 7-9.
Centers on training nurses for the insane. See #1946.

1964   Martineau, Harriet. "The Steel-Grinder - His Health." 3 (1860): 91-95.
Records risks of steelgrinding.

1965   Martineau, Harriet. "The Governess - Her Health." 3 (1860): 267-72.
Yokes their alcoholism to the overwork and underpayment of governesses.

1966   W[ynter], A[ndrew]. "Morbid Memory." 3 (1860): 285-87.
Postulates that memory disorder may be a sign of brain disease.

1967   "The Helmshore Tragedy." 3 (1860): 335-36.
Deplores the multitude of railroad mishaps.

1968   Martineau, Harriet. "The Artist - His Health." 3 (1860): 370-74.
Distinguishes painters, sculptors, and actors with respect to wellness.

1969   Scott, Ingelby. "Representative Men - Physiological Discoverers." 3 (1860): 483-89.
Salutes Edward Jenner for his smallpox vaccine.

1970   Martineau, Harriet. "The Baker - His Health." 3 (1860): 540-44.
Supposes that bakers die of exhaustion or respiratory afflictions.

1971   Martineau, Harriet. "The Needlewoman - Her Health." 3 (1860): 595-99.
Denominates job milieu as the source of needlewomen's debility.

1972   Martineau, Harriet. "The Aged - Their Health." 4 (1860-61): 119-24.
Article on aging has language about mindset and levels of care.

1973   Turner, Godfrey. "How I Did Not Prevent Sea-Sicknesses." 4 (1860-61): 191-93.
Eliminates stomach pad as a remedy for seasickness.

1974   From the Mountain. "Deaths by Fire." 5 (1861): 63-67.
Speculates that most casualties of fire are the victims of individual accidents.

1975 Adams, W. Bridges. "Railway Risks." 5 (1861): 351-53.
Divulges that a safe wheel is available but not common on railroads.

1976 Adams, W. Bridges. "The Hartley Pit Hecatomb." 6 (1861-62): 184-85.
Appeals on behalf of families of miners killed on the job.

1977 From the Mountain. "The English Boy of the Future." 7 (1862): 203-06.
Depends on more physical exercise for less feeble lads.

1978 From the Mountain. "A New Kind of Wilful Murder." 8 (1862-63): 36-39.
Sketches death by crinoline fire. See #1981.

1979 L., J. "A Destructive Cap." 8 (1862-63): 123-26.
Worries about explosions in gun factories.

1980 Adams, W. Bridges. "The Development of Human Food." 8 (1862-63): 138-39.
Permits chemicals in foods.

1981 From the Mountain. "The Wilful Murder Case - Pleas for the Defence." 8 (1862-63): 287-91.
Claims that crinolines are fire hazards and otherwise detrimental to wearers. See #1978.

1982 "Sympathetic Surgery." 8 (1862-63): 374-77.
Synchronizes patient faith in folk remedies and their potential for cure.

1983 "Tobacco." 8 (1862-63): 499-501.
Fathoms harms of smoking.

1984 W[ynter], A[ndrew]. "The Impurities of the Loaf." 8 (1862-63): 551-53.
Arraigns bakery environments for adulterated bread and ailing bakers.

1985 W[ynter], A[ndrew]. "A Day with the Coroner." 8 (1862-63): 664-67.
Script of coroner's jury converges on accidental deaths.

1986 W[ynter], A[ndrew]. "Smallpox in London." 9 (1863): 36-38.
Analyzes why Londoners resist smallpox vaccination. Authorizes medical officers to advance it.

1987 Browne, C.T. "City Dwellings and City Gardens." 9 (1863): 67-70.
Broods that overcrowded houses without green space are baneful for poor urbanites.

1988 L., J. "My Knife." 9 (1863): 104-06.
Concentrates on the jeopardy to grinders from dust and tools.

1989　From the Mountain. "Our Legacy from Mary Ann Walkley." 9 (1863): 119-23.
　　　Subject is one example of how unhealthy needlework is for needlewomen.

1990　From the Mountain. "The Merits of Half-and-Half Training." 9 (1863): 357-61.
　　　Rages about the exertion and surroundings of children in the pottery, match, paper-staining, and other trades.

1991　"Our Meat." 9 (1863): 426-27.
　　　Swears that one-fifth of meat for sale is from diseased animals.

1992　W[ynter], A[ndrew]. "Death in a Match-Box." 9 (1863): 556-58.
　　　Headlines how phosphorus in the manufacture and nonchalence in the use of matches result in fatalities.

1993　W[ynter], A[ndrew]. "Dipsomania, or Thirst-Madness." 10 (1863-64): 209-10.
　　　Would treat alcoholism as an illness similar to insanity.

1994　"Body-Snatching and Burking." 10 (1863-64): 261-66.
　　　Remembers how anatomists once acquired bodies for dissection.

1995　W[ynter], A[ndrew]. "Sweets for the Million." 10 (1863-64): 318-21.
　　　Authenticates that most candy is no longer adulterated.

1996　"Ear for Eye." 11 (1864): 80-83.
　　　Vaunts the stethoscope for differentiating respiratory disorders.

1997　Wynter, Dr. Andrew. "Human Wasters." 11 (1864): 174-79.
　　　Tours an asylum, supervised by Dr. John L.H. Down, that tutors mentally challenged children.

1998　Plummer, John. "A Real Social Evil." 11 (1864): 278-80.
　　　Peers at physical and moral problems of women in the mining industry.

1999　Clare. "How to Deal with Our London Poor." 11 (1864): 315-20.
　　　Grieves that London paupers eat badly, allow their offspring to play with tools, and buy the apparel of neighbors dead from smallpox and typhus.

2000　"Dangerous Dresses." 11 (1864): 719-22.
　　　Segregates female victims of crinoline fires.

2001　"Preserved Meats and Vegetables." 12 (1864-65): 157-60.
　　　Summarizes methods of preserving meat and vegetables.

2002　Plummer, John. "Straw-Plait and Bonnet Makers." 12 (1864-65): 464-67.
　　　Silhouettes youthful straw workers exhausted by their jobs.

2003　W[ynter], A[ndrew]. "Our Lifeboats." 12 (1864-65): 537-43.
　　　Trails lifeboats from shore in shipwreck rescues.

2004   Arnold, R. Arthur. " 'Typhus-Nesting'." 12 (1864-65): 677-82.
Lists crowded lodgings with inadequate ventilation and drains, improper diet, and impure water as important in the proliferation of typhus.

2005   M. "The Country Doctor." 13 (1865): 52-54.
Profiles rural general practitioner.

2006   King, Harold. "Invalids' and Children's Dinner Tables." 13 (1865): 176-79; with letter by G.M. Hicks: 238.
Hails those who bring meals to convalescent adults and chronically ill juveniles.

2007   Rose, H. Cooper, M.D. "Nature's Marvels: The Eye, What Is It?" 13 (1865): 180-82.
Scope is the anatomy of the eye.

2008   King, Harold. "Foundlings and Infanticide." 13 (1865): 332-36.
Visits London Foundling Hospital.

2009   Adams, W. Bridges. "The Gas Poisons of Our Dwellings." 13 (1865): 433-34.
Chronicles how garbage and solid human waste befoul residential air.

2010   L., G. "Prolonged Sleep." 13 (1865): 560.
Presents cases of coma and narcolepsy.

2011   Bevan, G[eorge] Phillips. "Things to be Altered." n.s., 1 (1866): 137-39.
Expects better sewerage to abate communicable maladies in villages.

2012   W. "The Flesh-Worm Disease." n.s., 1 (1866): 384-88.
Mulls over the cause and symptoms of trichinosis.

2013   Arnold, R. Arthur. "Pure Air." n.s., 2 (1866): 149-54.
Theme is varieties of sewerage.

2014   Steinmetz, Andrew. "More and Better Water for London." n.s., 2 (1866): 274-76.
Labels London water disease-laden.

2015   W[ynter], A[ndrew]. "Metropolitan Improvements: Artistic and Structural." n.s., 2 (1866): 542-46.
Rhapsodizes about the nexus between urban open spaces, with clean air and recreation opportunities, and the wellness of urbanites.

2016   Adams, W. Bridges. "Aeriform Sewage and Captain Liernur's System." n.s., 3 (1867): 46-49.
Would implement air-valve scheme of Charles T. Liernur in order to remove human waste efficiently and to halt water contamination.

2017   W[ynter], A[ndrew]. "Adulterations of Food." n.s., 4 (1867): 322-24.
       Reveals that numerous foods, among them sugar, pepper, and milk, are deliberately adulterated.
2018   Plummer, John. "Dinners on the Cheap." n.s., 4 (1867): 517-19.
       Wants more cheap urban restaurants that serve nutritious fare.
2019   "Through a Match Factory." 3d ser., 1 (1868): 80-82.
       Presumes that new mode of match production no longer leads to jaw ailments.
2020   "Cholera." 3d ser., 2 (1868): 33-36.
       Opposes opiates and astringents as remedies for cholera.
2021   "On the Preservation of Meat." 3d ser., 3 (1869): 101-05, 126-29.
       Features several techniques to prevent meat spoilage.
2022   "Gheel." 3d ser., 3 (1869): 167-70.
       Heralds Belgian program of boarding the insane with country families.
2023   "Preserving Life at Sea." 3d ser., 3 (1869): 233-38.
       Counts on buoys and rafts to save lives in shipwrecks.
2024   "Trade Tricks." 3d ser., 3 (1869): 280-84.
       Proposes legislation to punish those who adulterate food.
2025   "A Few Words on Chloral." 3d ser., 4 (1869-70): 305-07.
       Subject is chloral hydrate as an anesthetic.
2026   A Lady. "More about Tobacco." 3d ser., 4 (1869-70): 424-27, 455-58.
       Exegesis on tobacco does not miss the jeopardy of smoking or chewing it.
2027   An Old Physician. "On Sleep and Dreams." 3d ser., 5 (1870): 467-72, 544-48.
       Values undisturbed sleep for vitality. Has a note on narcolepsy.
2028   "Our Alcoholic Drinks." 3d ser., 6 (1870): 253-56.
       Balances assets and liabilities of liquor drinking.
2029   "On Wakefulness." 3d ser., 8 (1871): 8-11.
       Grasps how unsalutary lack of sleep is.
2030   "Are Our Pipes to be Put Out?" 3d ser., 8 (1871): 89-93.
       Fancies that tobacco is not pernicious except for juniors.
2031   "Bachelor Invalids and Male Nurses." 3d ser., 8 (1871): 317-21.
       Prods men to become nurses in order to tend men.
2032   An Old Physician. "Hits on the Head." 3d ser., 8 (1871): 475-79.
       Interest is brain injuries from falls or blows.
2033   "Peat Charcoal as a Filtering and Deodorizing Agent." 3d ser., 9 (1872): 383-87.
       Would try peat charcoal to filter drinking water.

2034 "Dust and Smoke." 3d ser., 10 (1872): 276-81.
      Alerts that the air is full of microbes.
2035 Hopkins, John Baker. "An Hour with the Outcasts." 3d ser., 10
      (1872): 338-45.
      Accompanies medical volunteers in London slum.
2036 "The Operation of the Adulteration Act." 3d ser., 10 (1872): 416-
      18.
      Complains that food adulteration is regular irrespective of laws.
2037 "The Casual Observer - Among the Little Ones." 3d ser., 13
      (1874): 544-45.
      Taps country holidays to energize city children.
2038 "The Casual Observer - At a London Hospital." 3d ser., 13 (1874):
      654-56.
      Wanders through several wards of a London hospital.
2039 Fenn, George Manville. "On the Rail." 4th ser., 1 (1874-75): 183-
      85.
      Logs occupational accidents of railroad employees.
2040 Fenn, George Manville. "Seeing a Tragedy." 4th ser., 2 (1875): 7-
      9.
      Recollects dangers during a theatre fire.
2041 Fenn, George Manville. "Shadowed Lives." 4th ser., 2 (1875):
      156-58.
      Deals with the insane in institutions.
2042 Fenn, George Manville. "A Knotty Point." 4th ser., 2 (1875): 189-
      90.
      Crusades for quality meat for the impoverished.
2043 "The Croyden Sewage Farm." 4th ser., 2 (1875): 210-11.
      Banks on efficient sewage disposal to slow some diseases.
2044 Fenn, George Manville. "In Our Midst." 4th ser., 2 (1875): 214-
      17.
      Lauds London hospitals.
2045 "The Boy O'Connor." 4th ser., 2 (1875): 223-25.
      Protagonist is allegedly insane criminal, Arthur O'Connor.
2046 "The Bursting of Boilers." 4th ser., 2 (1875): 255.
      Indicts boilermakers for negligence in factory deaths.
2047 "Teeth and the Toothsome." 4th ser., 3 (1875-76): 143-44.
      Diet for those without teeth downplays meat lozenges and juices
      but not beef and turtle soups.
2048 "Effects of the Sun on Lunatics." 4th ser., 4 (1876): 83.
      Hinges moods of the insane to colors.
2049 "Life-Saving at Sea." 4th ser., 4 (1876): 180.
      Enthuses about the life raft of George F. Parratt.

2050   "The Best Pabulum [sic]." 4th ser., 4 (1876): 263-64.
Exaggerates benefits for babies of the milk powder marketed by Henri Nestle.

2051   "Colour Blindness." 4th ser., 6 (1877): 298.
Bruits symptoms of color blindness.

2052   "Life Without Meat." 4th ser., 9 (1878-79): 63-64.
Assesses vegetarianism as a menu for health.

2053   "Planting for Health." 4th ser., 9 (1878-79): 198-99.
Would plant shrubs to drain disease-ridden marshes.

2054   "Drowning and Swimming." 4th ser., 9 (1878-79): 238-39.
Slots drownings as mishap, suicide, or occupational hazard.

2055   "Noxious Vapours." 4th ser., 10/11 (1879): 135.
Grumbles about the toxicity of chemical fumes in workplaces.

2056   "Life Saving." 4th ser., 10/11 (1879): 195.
Puffs portable inflatable hat as life preserver at sea.

2057   "Prevention of Seasickness." 4th ser., 10/11 (1879): 195.
Stars a cot that will purportedly thwart seasickness.

2058   "Poison." 4th ser., 10/11 (1879): 206.
Warns of the danger to children of arsenic in wallpaper.

2059   "Life Saving Floats." 4th ser., 10/11 (1879): 386.
Notices new float designed by a Capt. Warren, R.N.

2060   "Substitutes for Potatoes." 4th ser., 10/11 (1879): 410.
Prefers legumes to potatoes for nutrition.

2061   M., W.T. "Among the Sanitarians - By Our Own Hygeist [sic]." 4th ser., 10/11 (1879): 460-61.
Proponent of educating the poor about health maintenance glances at disinfectants and mineral waters.

2062   "The South London Medical Aid Institute." 5th ser., 1 (1880): 94-95.
Praises titled Institute where impoverished South Londoners can consult a specialist for a small fee.

THE OXFORD AND CAMBRIDGE MAGAZINE, 1856

Standing for no party but for principled leadership, the *Oxford and Cambridge* had little time to talk about afflictions.

2063   [Faulkner, C.J. and Cormell Price]. "Unhealthy Employments." 1 (1856): 265-71.
Represents inherent and preventible perils at labor sites.

THE PEOPLE'S (AND HOWITT'S) JOURNAL, 1846-1851

Supervised by John Saunders, the *People's Journal*, joined by *Howitt's* in 1849, was a weekly priced for workers and thus scrutinized their injurious work and inadequate medical resources.

2064 Fox, W.J. "On the Progress of Science in Its Influence upon the Condition of the People." 1 (1846): 30-35.
Dissertation on science in society has some prose on sanitation and medical knowledge.

2065 "Dr. Southwood Smith." 1 (1846): 99-101.
Commends T. Southwood Smith for his interest in sanitation and factory youths.

2066 Smiles, S. "What is Doing for the People in Leeds?" 1 (1846): 136-38.
Favors benefit associations that offer sickness funds.

2067 "Progress of the Sanatory [sic] Movement." 1 (1846): 181-82.
Illuminates groups that sponsor broad improvements in towns' sewerage.

2068 M. "Our Sister Island." 1 (1846): 184-85.
Groans that the Famine in Ireland exacerbates peasant starvation.

2069 Martineau, Harriet. "Survey from the Mountain." 1 (1846): 303-05.
Vends hygiene, moderation, and smallpox vaccination for wellness.

2070 Winter, Andrew. "Country Houses for the Working Classes." 2 (1846): 134-36.
Avouches that metropolitan slum abodes accelerate communicable diseases.

2071 Howitt, William. "Increasing Obstructions to Bathing, and Misuse of the Police." 2 (1846): 221-23.
Objects to prohibitions by water companies on bathing in their canals.

2072 Haughton, James. "What is Doing for the People in Dublin?" 2 (1846): 233-36.
Would concentrate on health maintenance of the Irish because of the Famine.

2073 Rogerson, John Bolton. "What is Doing for the Poor in Manchester?" 2 (1846): 270-72, 319-22.
Registers hospitals for the indigent in Manchester.

2074   Howitt, William. "Condition of the Poor in London." 2 (1846): 283-85.
        Decries insufficient drainage, light, and air in domiciles of destitute Londoners.

2075   Martineau, Harriet. "Household Education: Care of the Frame." 3 (1847): 23-25.
        Advocates hygiene, exercise, and suitable fare to have sturdy infants.

2076   Beard, Dr. "Benefit Societies." 3 (1847): 250-51, 327-29; 4 (1847): 41-42, 97-98.
        Doubts that benefit societies defrayed costs of effective health care.

2077   W., J.M. "The New Consumption Hospital at Brompton." 3 (1847): 341-43.
        Welcomes Brompton Hospital because tuberculosis is pervasive in Great Britain.

2078   Winter, Andrew. "A Visit to the Model Lodging House, at St. Giles's." 4 (1847): 132-34.
        Observes salubrious ventilation and sanitation in London lodging house.

2079   Mill, John. "Are Our Large Towns in a State to Receive the Cholera?" 4 (1847): 342-44.
        Reckons that, because of their sewage and stale quarters, towns are likely to have cholera epidemics.

2080   Philp, R. Kemp. "The Philosophy of Exercise." 5 (1848): 76-79.
        Sponsors exercise, principally by juveniles outdoors, for robustness.

2081   "Out-of-Door Recreation for the People." 5 (1848): 319-20.
        Flaunts recreation in fresh air for vitality.

2082   "Births, Deaths, and Marriages." 6 (1848): 194-96, 208-10; 7 (1849): 280.
        Extrapolates, from a report of the Registrar-General, 1842-45, that many deaths are from such diseases as cholera, that spread in unsanitary milieus, but that citizens are generally well.

2083   Saunders, John. "The True Mission of Cholera." 6 (1848): 211-14.
        Posits that cholera is not airborne so, because its origin is unclear, sewerage, ventilation, and clean attire may prevent it.

2084   "Cholera Not Contagious." 6 (1848): 236-38.
        Professes that friends and medical personnel are not at risk from those with cholera, since it is not airborne.

2085   "Consumption." 6 (1848): 251-52.
        Reviews study by Dr. T.H. Yeoman of tuberculosis.

2086 Alison, S. Scott, Esq., M.D. "On Epidemic Indian Cholera, Its
Treatment and Sanitary Requirements." 6 (1848): 254-57, 289-92.
Lectures on symptoms, treatment, and contagiousness of cholera.
2087 "Consideration of the Means Serving to the Maintenance of a
Healthy Life." 7 (1849): 21-22.
Informs about elements of health maintenance, as housing, diet,
marital status, job, and recreation.
2088 Yeoman, T.H., M.D. "On the Healthy Discipline of Home." 7
(1849): 204-05, 221-22, 231-32, 243-44, 259-60.
Hitches physical well-being to mental and emotional states.
2089 "Appetite, and the Heat of the Body." n.s., 1 (1849): 46-47.
Repeats John Dyer that being fat and lethargic is unhealthy.
2090 "The Structure of Skin." n.s., 1 (1849): 57-58.
Paraphrases Thomes Innis, M.D., about the nexus of skin and
salubrity.
2091 "Baths and Bathers." n.s., 1 (1849): 84.
Repeats notions of Thomas Embling about when and how to bathe,
namely never after eating and never in cold water after a "night of
profligacy."
2092 "Health Made Easy." n.s., 1 (1849): 112.
Growls that hospitalized indigents cost taxpayers too much money.
2093 "Exercise and Sleep." n.s., 1 (1849): 155-56.
Conveys the message of Thomas Innis about the profit to wellness
from moderate exercise, as walking or dancing, and sleep.
2094 "Hints to Householders." n.s., 2 (1850): 123.
Prints words of Francis Cross on merits of good ventilation and
pure water in homes.
2095 Usher, Rufus. "Physical and Mental Suffering." n.s., 2 (1850):
181-82.
Hypothesizes that the mind can sire epilepsy and insanity, chiefly
in the rank above workers, the "struggling"; and that smallpox
vaccination and medical knowledge guarantee a more vigorous
population.
2096 "Smithfield Market." n.s., 3 (1850): 11-13.
Tags Smithfield Market a health hazard.
2097 "Opium and Its Effects." n.s., 3 (1850): 24-25.
Borrows from Nathan Allen, M.D., ideas about the evil of opium
for body and mind.
2098 "Explosions in Mines: Causes, and Means to be Adopted for Their
Prevention." n.s., 3 (1850): 26-28.
Would install better ventilation systems and Davy lamps
underground and stronger cages in shafts to protect miners.

2099   H. "The Pleasures of Illness!" n.s., 3 (1850): 97-98.
       Envies those with minor maladies who enjoy sympathy and leisure.
2100   "Diseases of the Ear." n.s., 3 (1850): 139-40.
       Publicizes cases from the Report of the Royal Dispensary for Diseases of the Ear. Derives loss of hearing from lack of hygiene, neglect of symptoms, as from infections, and resort to spurious curatives or curers.
2101   F., J.H. "Life-Risks; and the Means of Providing Against Them." n.s., 3 (1850): 186-87.
       Urges workers to buy insurance for sickness and accidents.
2102   "Henry Clutterbuck, M.D." n.s., 3 (1850): 245-47.
       Memorializes a doctor famous for his efforts to reorganize the College of Physicians and to help the distressed.
2103   D., J. "Medical Men." n.s., 3 (1850): 255-57.
       Stereotypes doctors as silent or talkative, morbid or jolly, skeptical, and learned. Trusts readers to choose a doctor with common sense.
2104   "Hospitals of London." n.s., 3 (1850): 292-93.
       Abridges ideas of Edward Crisp, M.D., on London hospitals. Lobbies for parliamentary committee to investigate their care of the indigent ill and their advancement of medical erudition.
2105   P., G.F. "Andri [sic] Versalius, the First Anatomist." n.s., 3 (1850): 342-43.
       Sanctions the study by doctors of diseased corpses.
2106   White, Mrs. Caroline. "Servitude as We Sometimes See It." n.s., 4 (1851): 91-92.
       Assumes that servants' backgrounds do not include habits of hygiene.
2107   "Trade Association Asylums." n.s., 4 (1851): 202-04.
       Lauds tailors for financing a home for their ailing and aged comrades.
2108   "The Burning Waste of Clackmannan." n.s., 4 (1851): 312-14.
       Delineates how to obviate fire in coal mines from Scottish one.

THE QUARTERLY REVIEW, 1824-1900

Addressed to aristocratic Anglicans, the *Quarterly*, from the same house as *Murray's Magazine*, did not overlook the opportunities for disease in towns. Dangerous jobs and jejune diets were other ongoing motifs.

2109   [Gooch, Robert]. "Plague, a Contagious Disease." 33 (1825-26): 218-57.
        Exhibits many episodes of plague as evidence of its contagiousness. See #242.

2110   [Gooch, Robert]. "Vaccination." 33 (1825-26): 550-60.
        Would stem smallpox by vaccination.

2111   [Ferguson, Robert]. "Gooch on Insanity." 41 (1829): 163-83.
        Circulates notions of Robert Gooch, M.D., about insanity in women.

2112   [Gooch, Robert]. "Unlawful Disinterment of Human Bodies." 42 (1830): 1-17.
        Would permit medical students to dissect bodies of unclaimed decedents lest learning require graverobbing.

2113   [Gooch, Robert]. "Insanity." 42 (1830): 350-77.
        Would amend laws on the commitment and care of the insane.

2114   [Brewster, David]. "Connexion of Intellectual Operations with Organic Actions." 45 (1831): 341-58.
        Shows how afflictions of the body touch the mind.

2115   [Ferguson, Robert]. "The Cholera." 46 (1831-32): 169-202.
        Scrutinizes roots and course of cholera beyond Asia.

2116   [Ferguson, Robert]. "Directions of the Privy Council in Case of Pestilence." 46 (1831-32): 264-73.
        Relays how to cope with a cholera epidemic.

2117   [Scrope, G. Poulett]. "Senior's Letter on the Irish Poor." 46 (1831-32): 390-410.
        Concurs with N.W. Senior that the impoverished ill and aged in Ireland require statutory aid.

2118   [Croker, J.W.]. "Granville's *Catechism of Health*." 47 (1832): 394-407.
        Captures thinking of A.B. Granville, M.D., on cholera.

2119   [Brewster, David]. "Philosophy of Apparitions." 48 (1832): 287-320.
        Connects apparitions and optic functions.

2120   [Scrope, G. Poulett]. "Amendments of the Poor-Laws." 48 (1832): 320-45.
        Ratifies poor relief for the sick and seniors.

2121   [MacMichael, William]. "Salt." 48 (1832): 375-91.
        Offers salt as an antidote for some poisonings and fevers.

2122   [Ferguson, Robert]. "Sir Henry Halford's *Essays* - Death and Madness." 49 (1833): 175-98.
        Skims over scenes of the dying and of the insane, primarily from literature.

2123   [Croker, J.W.]. "Madden on the *Infirmities of Genius*." 50 (1833-34): 34-56.
        Contests the opinion of R.R. Madden about a tie between patients and genius.

2124   [Lockhart, J.G.]. "German Watering-Places." 50 (1833-34): 308-47.
        Voyages to various German health spas.

2125   [Scrope, G. Poulett]. "The Poor-Law Question." 50 (1833-34): 347-73.
        Evaluator of the poor law would retain it for the ailing and old.

2126   [Hayward, Abraham]. "Cookery." 52 (1834): 406-15.
        Story on cooking has some language on nutrition.

2127   [Head, Francis B.]. "English Charity." 53 (1835): 473-539.
        Insert on workhouses in Kent glances at the ill and aged.

2128   [Hayward, Abraham]. "*Physiologie du Gout*: Gastronomy and Gastronomers." 54 (1835): 117-55.
        History of cooking, preeminently French, elaborates on menus.

2129   [Scrope, G. Poulett]. "Foreign Poor-Laws - Irish Poverty." 55 (1835-36): 35-73.
        Criticizes British failure to pass legislation for the destitute in Ireland to the detriment chiefly of the sick, young, and elderly.

2130   [Scrope, G. Poulett]. "Combe's *Outlines of Phrenology*." 57 (1836): 169-82.
        Rejects concepts of George Combe on phrenology.

2131   [Ferguson, Robert]. "Latham on Diseases of the Chest, Investigated by Auscultation." 57 (1836): 199-223.
        Warrants, as did P.M. Latham, M.D., the value of the stethoscope to detect respiratory disturbances.

2132   [Cooper, Antony Ashley, 7th Earl Shaftesbury]. "The Factory System." 57 (1836): 396-443.
        Documents disease and drug use among factory youths.

2133   [Ferguson, Robert]. "Animal Magnetism." 61 (1838): 273-301.
        Ruminates about hypnosis as a treatment for epilepsy and insanity.

2134   [Ferguson, Robert]. "Dr. Holland's *Medical Notes and Reflections*: Diet and Dyspepsy." 65 (1839-40): 315-40.
        Condenses the study of Henry Holland, M.D., on digestion.

2135   [Ferguson, Robert]. "Public Health and Morality." 66 (1840): 115-55.
        Casts official indifference as the source of urban paupers' ills.

2136   [Brodie, Benjamin C.]. "Medical Reform." 67 (1840-41): 53-79.
        Decrees more practical training, then examination and licensing for prospective doctors. See #2140.

2137 [Cooper, Antony Ashley, 7th Earl Shaftesbury]. "Infant Labour." 67 (1840-41): 171-81.
Brands most juvenile jobs deleterious.

2138 [Gregory, William]. "Liebig's *Animal Chemistry*." 70 (1842): 98-128.
Quotes Justus von Liebig, M.D., on digestion in humans and animals. See #596.

2139 [Ferguson, Robert]. "Colliers and Collieries." 70 (1842): 158-95.
Biography of miners bruits occupational perils, mainly for women and children.

2140 [Brodie, Benjamin C.]. "Brandy and Salt - Homeopathy - Hydropathy." 71 (1842-43): 83-106.
Condemns atypical restoratives. Reiterates the need to license doctors. See #2136.

2141 [Head, Francis B.]. "Report on the Sanitary Condition of the Labouring Classes." 71 (1842-43): 417-53.
Assigns the prevalence of disease among metropolitan workers to no sewerage, impure water, and little ventilation indoors.

2142 [Ferguson, Robert]. "Sir Charles Bell." 72 (1843): 192-231.
Recounts accomplishments of a surgeon who studied the nerves.

2143 [Croker, J.W.]. "Railway Legislation." 74 (1844): 224-80.
Finds fewer railroad injuries and deaths between 1840 and 1843 because of legislation.

2144 [Blackwell, J.]. "Report on the Treatment of Lunatics." 74 (1844): 416-47.
Bares conditions in establishments for the insane.

2145 [Brodie, Benjamin C.]. "Sir J. Graham's Medical Bill." 75 (1844-45): 1-31.
Assents to the captioned bill for greater government regulation of medical accreditation.

2146 [Scrope, G. Poulett]. "Poor Laws for Scotland." 75 (1844-45): 125-48.
Supports Scottish poor law because contagions are rampant among paupers.

2147 [Taylor, George]. "Census of 1841." 76 (1845): 11-38.
Essay on the Census of 1841 mentions sanitation.

2148 [Croker, J.W.]. "Reid - Ventilation." 77 (1845-46): 381-404.
Remarks on views of D.B. Reid, M.D., about the worth of ventilation for vigor.

2149 [Cooper, Antony Ashley, 7th Earl Shaftesbury]. "Lodging-Houses." 82 (1847-48): 142-52.
Appreciates efforts for cleanliness in lodging houses.

2150   [Elwin, Whitwell]. "Fontenelle on the Signs of Death." 85 (1849): 346-99.
       Pirates from J. Fontenelle, J.A. Symonds, and Z. Buchat concepts on the physiology and psychology of dying.

2151   [Elwin, Whitwell]. "Spectacles." 87 (1850): 45-59.
       Mulls over the fit and utility of eyeglasses.

2152   [Ward, F.O.]. "Metroplitan Water Supply - The New Sources." 87 (1850): 468-502.
       Details how London water is polluted.

2153   [Ward, F.O.]. "Sanitary Consolidation - Centralization - Local Self-Government." 88 (1850-51): 435-92.
       Presses for more official action on sanitation, especially sewerage.

2154   [Armstrong, John]. "Vauxhall Factory Schools." 92 (1852-53): 1-18.
       Salutes the recreation of titled schools as salubrious for pupils.

2155   [Wynter, Andrew]. "Human Hair." 92 (1852-53): 305-28.
       Entry on hair has some correctives for baldness.

2156   [Ferguson, Robert]. "The Two Systems at Pentonville." 92 (1852-53): 487-506.
       Declares that "separate system" in prison does not beget insanity.

2157   [Wynter, Andrew]. "The London Commissariat." 95 (1854): 271-308.
       Includes foods in London and their distribution.

2158   [Wynter, Andrew]. "Fires and Fire-Insurance." 96 (1854-55): 1-43.
       Expounds on harms from fires and the scope of insurance.

2159   [Ferguson, Robert]. "Psychological Inquiries." 96 (1854-55): 86-117.
       Elucidates the physiology of the brain and nerves with words on insanity.

2160   [Tomlinson, Charles]. "The Open Fire-Place." 96 (1854-55): 145-76.
       Plans how to reduce smoke inhalation from open hearths.

2161   [Scrope, G. Poulett]. "Provident Institutions." 96 (1854-55): 176-99.
       Thesis is how workers can finance sick care.

2162   [Wynter, Andrew]. "Food, and Its Adulterations." 96 (1854-55): 460-93.
       Unmasks the adulteration of food.

2163   [Brodie, Benjamin C.]. "The Circulation of the Blood." 97 (1855): 28-41.
       Comments on studies of the blood.

2164 [Cheney, R.H.]. "The Charities and the Poor of London." 97 (1855): 407-50.
Joins poverty with debility in London.

2165 [Wynter, Andrew]. "Lunatic Asylums." 101 (1857): 353-93.
Traverses institutions for the insane.

2166 [Elwin, Whitwell]. "Sense of Pain in Man and Animals." 103 (1858): 180-218.
Explores how humans and animals experience pain.

2167 [Wynter, Andrew]. "Shipwrecks." 104 (1858): 170-200.
Tale of shipwrecks tells of jeopardy to survivors.

2168 [Martineau, Harriet]. "Miss Nightingale's *Notes on Nursing*." 107 (1860): 392-422.
Reviews nursing style of Florence Nightingale.

2169 [Leifchild, J.R.]. "Life, Enterprise, and Peril in Coal-Mines." 110 (1861): 329-67.
Piece on miners verifies hazards of their employment.

2170 Smiles, S. "Workmen's Benefit Societies." 116 (1864): 318-50.
Approves activities, as collecting for sick funds, of legitimate benefit societies.

2171 [Shaw, Benjamin]. "Sanitary Reform in the Metropolis." 118 (1865): 254-80.
Recites statutes on water supply, smallpox vaccination, interment, and sewerage that have decelerated disease in London.

2172 [Johns, B.G.]. "Blind People." 118 (1865): 430-68.
Subjects are the other senses of the vision impaired and their schools.

2173 [Tremenheere, J.H.]. "The Children's Employment Commission." 119 (1866): 364-93.
Rephrases captioned commission about evils in many occupations of juniors. See #2177.

2174 [Percy, John]. "Coal and Smoke." 119 (1866): 435-72.
Treatise on possible coal shortage glimpses danger of smoke inhalation.

2175 [Davies, James]. "Female Education." 119 (1866): 499-515.
Article on women's education accords with others that schools are damaging for females.

2176 [Macpherson, John]. "The Cholera Conference." 122 (1867): 29-55.
Traces the course and curbs of cholera since the sixteenth century.

2177 [Tremenheere, J.H.]. "Agricultural Gangs." 123 (1867): 173-90.
Corroborates the harm to children of field work in gangs far from home. See #2173.

2178   [Davies, James]. "Longevity and Centenarianism." 124 (1868): 179-98.
        Ponders causes and cases of longevity. See #1788.

2179   [Chambers, T.K.]. "Aims of Modern Medicine." 126 (1869): 534-58.
        Recapitulates shifts in medical remedies for illnesses.

2180   [Pole, William]. "The Water-Supply of London." 127 (1869): 444-77.
        Story on London water supply estimates its purity.

2181   [Macpherson, John]. "Baths and Bathing Places, Ancient and Modern." 129 (1870): 151-82.
        Retrospective on spas marks them salutary.

2182   [Clarke, W. Fairlie]. "The Medical Charities of London." 136 (1874): 371-94.
        Queries, in terms of costs, why London has so many hospitals and dispensaries for the impoverished.

2183   [Stanhope, Edward]. "Friendly Societies." 138 (1875): 206-29.
        Scope is insurance for illness, old age, and death, with parenthesis on child neglect by paupers.

2184   [Eastlake, Elizabeth]. "Drink: The Vice and the Disease." 139 (1875): 396-434.
        Tabs alcoholism a sickness.

2185   [Blakesley, Joseph W.]. "Dr. Carpenter's *Mental Physiology*." 143 (1877): 83-104.
        Interprets William Benjamin Carpenter on the interaction of physiology and psychology.

2186   [Lilly, W.S.]. "Railway Accidents." 145 (1878): 163-87.
        Recognizes perils of railroad travel and employment.

2187   [Bennett, James Risdon]. "The College of Physicians." 148 (1879): 351-76.
        Remembers the past of the College of Physicians.

2188   [Creighton, Charles]. "The Progress of Medicine." 156 (1883): 57-89.
        Stars the suppression of malaria and success of medical research.

2189   [Dibdin, Lewis T.]. "Dwellings of the Poor." 157 (1884): 144-68.
        Submits that abodes of London's poor are still filthy. See #807.

2190   [Creighton, Charles]. "Epidemics." 164 (1887): 193-217.
        Essay on epidemics, as cholera, posits why some diseases speed.

2191   [Bear, William E.]. "Our Meat Supply." 165 (1887): 37-59.
        Boosts legislation against meat contamination.

2192   [Bear, William E.]. "Dairy Products." 165 (1887): 298-326.
        Pledges that dairy products are of better quality.

2193   [Brabrook, E.W.]. "Friendly Societies." 166 (1888): 374-406.
       Tract on friendly societies whispers about insurance as a reason for
       child neglect.
2194   [Gregory, Robert]. "The Inhabitants of East London." 169 (1889):
       431-59.
       Picture of East Londoners refers to their job-related afflictions.
2195   [Black, Charles E.D.]. "The Blind and the Deaf." 170 (1890): 59-
       79.
       Familiarizes audience with the instruction and care of the vision
       and hearing impaired.
2196   [Shadwell, Arthur]. "Mesmerism and Hypnotism." 171 (1890):
       234-59.
       Follows hypnosis as a therapy from the days of Friedrich Mesmer.
2197   [Pole, William]. "The Water Supply of London." 174 (1892): 63-
       94.
       Credits London's water quantity for efficient waste disposal.
2198   [Horner, Joseph G.]. "State Pensions for Old Age." 174 (1892):
       505-33.
       Vetoes national pensions as unnecessary because many workers
       die young or need to learn thrift.
2199   [Smith, C. G. F.]. "The Modern Hospital." 177 (1893): 464-94.
       Outlines the management, supplies, nursing, and treatment,
       mostly of indigents, in hospitals.
2200   [Emmett, J.T.]. "Londoners at Home." 182 (1895): 59-82.
       Grumbles that many London residences are still unhealthy.
2201   [Mackay, Thomas]. "Old Age Pensions." 182 (1895): 254-80.
       Would leave the aged to private resources.
2202   [Drage, Geoffrey]. "Poor Law Reform." 191 (1900): 154-73.
       Judgment of the poor law has some sentences on the elderly and
       on contagions passed by tramps.
2203   [Haden, Francis]. "The Ethics of Cremation." 192 (1900): 45-67.
       Disputes that burial of the dead broadens disease.
2204   [Shipley, Arthur E.]. "Malaria and the Mosquito." 192 (1900):
       291-311.
       Magnifies the mosquito that transmits malaria.

THE RAMBLER, 1848-1862

Precursor of the *Home and Foreign Review* and pen of English Roman
Catholics, the *Rambler* had intermittent inserts on wellness.

2205   "The Ideas of the Deaf and Dumb." 3 (1848-49): 94-103.
Reflects on attempts to teach religion to the hearing impaired who do not speak.

2206   "The Water-Cure at Home." 4 (1849): 205-07.
Extrapolates ideas of Edward Johnson, M.D., on hydropathy.

2207   "Catholic Parochial Ministrations: Visitation of the Sick." 4 (1849): 354-57, 432-35; 5 (1850): 19-25.
Enters patients' reactions to visits by priests.

2208   [Capes, J.M.]. "Animal Magnetism." 8 (1851): 296-326.
Footnotes hypnosis as therapy.

2209   "Insanity in Its Relation to Catholicism." 2d ser., 4, o.s., 16 (1855): 108-19.
Transmits theories on insanity of Daniel Noble, M.D.

2210   [Capes, J.M.]. "A Doctor's Opinions on Physic." 2d ser., 7, o.s., 19 (1857): 470-75.
Amplifies the view of Sir John Forbes, M.D., that the body often cures itself, so doctors should devote their time to preventive medicine.

2211   [Capes, J.M.]. "Noble on the Mind and the Brain." 2d ser., 9, o.s., 21 (1858): 353-56.
Scans the research of Daniel Noble, M.D., on the brain.

2212   [Simpson, Richard]. "Mr. George Combe and His Phrenology." 2d ser., 10, o.s., 22 (1858): 373-88.
Attacks phrenology because it is both simplistic and not authenticated.

SAINT PAULS, 1867-1874

Trying to edify and to entertain, *Saint Pauls*, with Anthony Trollope as early editor, pondered the outcomes of health statutes on beneficiaries and bystanders.

2213   [Lewes, George Henry]. "The Dangers and Delights of Tobacco." 3 (1868-69): 172-84.
Argues that tobacco smoking is harmful only in excess.

2214   [?Mariast, Atheni]. "A Lunatic Colony." 4 (1869): 79-83.
Would replicate in England a Belgian plan for care of the insane.

2215   "The Workhouse." 7 (1870-71): 70-87.
Criticizes the medical staff and inattention to patients in workhouse infirmaries.

2216 Pitt, James. "Convivial Pauperism." 7 (1870-71): 435-43.
Tours a workhouse and its wards for the insane.
2217 Pitt, James. "The Paupers' Pension Day." 8 (1871): 119-32.
Castigates poor law boards disinterested in the starving.
2218 Haddon, Charlotte. "Nursing as a Profession for Ladies." 8 (1871): 458-61.
Calls for adequately trained and salaried nurses.
2219 Browne, Matthew [William Brighty Rands]. "Light, Heat, and Air." 12 (1873): 37-41.
Propounds risks of air pollution and merits of light.
2220 Gentles, R.L. "Convalescence." 12 (1873): 459-63.
Represents recovery from patient's perspective.
2221 Browne, Matthew [William Brighty Rands]. "Tea Considered as a Cause of National Demoralization." 12 (1873): 701-05.
Satirizes recent *Lancet* treatise on the hazards of drinking tea.
2222 Blackstone, Samuel. "Paternal Government: Whither Are We Drifting?" 12 (1873): 718-41.
Votes against coercive health laws, as the Contagious Diseases Acts, that undermine order and turn police and sanitary inspectors into spies.

THE SCOTTISH REVIEW, 1882-1900

Loyal to its label, the *Scottish* heeded local ailments and simultaneously scanned national ones.

2223 [?Cameron, Charles or David Caldwell M'Vail]. "Medical Reform." 1 (1882-83): 318-29.
Muses about professional training and certification of doctors in Scotland, Ireland, and England.
2224 [Conder, Francis R.]. "On the Water Circulation of Great Cities." 7 (1886): 264-86.
Overview of urban water systems cautions about their contaminants.
2225 Cameron, Charles. "The Modern Cremation Movement." 10 (1887): 1-38.
Would cremate the dead to stifle disease among the living.
2226 Fournier de Flaix, E. "Alcohol and Alcoholism." 10 (1887): 322-37.
Identifies alcohol as a food whose moderate intake is salutary.

2227   Murray, J. Clark. "The Blind Deaf-Mute, Helen Keller." 14 (1889): 380-98.
        Linchpin is how to educate the vision and hearing impaired who do not speak.

2228   [Robertson, F.L.]. "The Social Condition of the Poor in Glasgow." 20 (1892): 1-29.
        Murmurs that the impoverished of Glasgow are sick because of unsanitary domiciles and improper fare.

2229   Crespi, Alfred J.H. "The Low Death-Rate." 21 (1893): 59-81.
        Teams fewer deaths and more sanitation.

2230   [Clouston, T.S.]. "The Medical Schools of Scotland." 23 (1894): 1-31, 380-86.
        Essay on previous and current medical education generates anonymous letter with information on degrees from St. Andrew's.

2231   Spence, T.W.L. "Pauper Lunacy and Ordinary Pauperism." 25 (1895): 129-41.
        Articulates why insanity among the destitute is burgeoning.

THE SUNDAY MAGAZINE, 1864-1900

Commencing without a preamble, the *Sunday Magazine*, with the same ancestry as the *Contemporary Review* and *Good Words*, clarified in its volumes its views on salubrity. Patients, primarily children, paupers, and elders, and their refuges, were in its spotlight.

2232   A Lady-Superintendent. "Sunday in Hospital." 1 (1864-65): 62-65.
        Watches hospital routines.

2233   Leifchild, J.R. "The Collier's Day of Rest." 1 (1864-65): 78-80.
        Contrasts peace of Sundays with danger of other days for miners.

2234   Thorold, A.W. "On Being Ill." 1 (1864-65): 233-38.
        Peeks at patients through a religious lens.

2235   Ballantyne, R.M. "The Lifeboat." 1 (1864-65): 366-70.
        Applauds rescues from shipwreck by National Lifeboat Institution.

2236   Miller, Professor [?James]. "Design in Disease." 1 (1864-65): 371-77.
        Imagines the body as a mechanism able to repair and protect itself.

2237   DeLiefde, John. "A Very Remarkable Dinner-Table." 2 (1865-66): 114-18.
        Raves about Invalids' Dinner Table, which feeds the sick poor, the aged, and the young in their homes or at its headquarters.

2238 Blaikie, W.G. "The Missionaries' Work in London." 3 (1866-67): 44-49.
Proclaims that cholera outbreak unveils London's problems with sanitation.

2239 "How to Get Rid of an Enemy - Addressed to Working Men by a Doctor's Wife." 3 (1866-67): 406-13, 455-61.
Pens ways to suppress and treat typhus.

2240 Rowe, Richard. "A Morning Amongst Deaf Mutes." 5 (1868-69): 613-16.
Travels to a shelter for the hearing impaired who do not speak.

2241 M. "Some Notes on Nursing and Lady-Superintendence." 7 (1870-71): 606-08.
Holds that women superintendents need not be as strong or as rigorously prepared as nurses.

2242 The Editor [Thomas Guthrie]. "Charity in London." n.s., 1 (1871-72): 17-23, 101-11, 273-84, 345-54, 612-21, 790-97.
Meditates about care of the physically challenged, incurables, and old and ill seamen in London.

2243 Twining, Louisa. "Dress." n.s., 1 (1871-72): 466-67.
Conjectures that some female attire and most cosmetics are deleterious.

2244 Guthrie, Thomas. "Among the Stricken." n.s., 2 (1872-73): 47-54.
Journeys to refuges for infants and youths who are physically challenged.

2245 Page, H.A. "Sunshine in a Shady Place." n.s., 3 (1873-74): 453-59.
Introduces a haven with healthful environment that caters to the progeny of indigents and others.

2246 Page, H.A. "Outside and Inside." n.s., 3 (1873-74): 630-36.
Pertains to homes for destitute juveniles.

2247 The Editor [W.G. Blaikie]. "Miss Macpherson and the 'Home of Industry'." n.s., 3 (1873-74): 669-75.
Extols sanctuaries of Annie Macpherson that instruct the starving young and send them to Canada.

2248 Doherty, F.M. "Children's Dinners." n.s., 3 (1873-74): 774-76.
Thanks groups that feed children as a deterrent to or in recuperation from illness.

2249 The Editor [W.G. Blaikie]. "The Liverpool Seamen's Orphanage." n.s., 3 (1873-74): 805-07.
Tale of orphans has some causes of death of seamen.

2250 Page, H.A. "Orphans and Imbeciles." n.s., 4 (1874-75): 52-58.
Reveres Andrew Reed for his projects to assist mentally challenged juniors.

2251   Beale, Anne. "A Birthday at a Kindergarten." n.s., 4 (1874-75): 302-04.
       Smiles on German home for juvenile paupers.

2252   Blaikie, W.G. "Miss Clugston and Her Work." n.s., 4 (1874-75): 337-42.
       Prizes a private facility for convalescents in Scotland.

2253   Page, H.A. "The Victoria Hospital for Children." n.s., 5 (1875-76): 701-06.
       Warrants the need for captioned London hospital.

2254   Page, H.A. "Errands of Mercy." n.s., 6 (1876-77): 58-61, 118-23, 254-56, 409-12.
       Personifies district nurses and medical missionaries in London, together with other topics.

2255   Gladstone, Mrs. W.E. [Catherine]. "Convalescent Homes." n.s., 7 (1877-78): 171-73.
       Prays for more places for patients in recovery.

2256   Chessar, Miss. "Fearfully and Wonderfully Made: Glimpses of the Marvel of the Human Frame." n.s., 7 (1877-78): 181-85, 388-91, 742-44.
       Illuminates the heart, nerves, and eyes.

2257   Meade, L.T. "Little Sick Children: A Visit to a Hospital for the Incurable." n.s., 7 (1877-78): 464-66.
       Contemplates standards and milieu of London's Cheyne Home for Sick Children whose patients have incurable ailments.

2258   Stephenson, Rev. T. "The Engine-Driver." n.s., 8 (1878-79): 23-27.
       Message on physical and mental health of railwaymen would give them statutory redress for any mishap not from their own negligence.

2259   The Riverside Visitor. "The Hidden Sick." n.s., 8 (1878-79): 170-73.
       Murmurs about the sick poor too proud to seek public relief.

2260   Currie, Sir Edmund Hay. "The Story of the London Hospital." n.s., 8 (1878-79): 176-79.
       Parades patients, many of them accident victims and children, in London Hospital.

2261   Author of 'John Halifax, Gentleman' [Dinah Maria Mulock]. "Save the Children." n.s., 8 (1878-79): 248-54.
       Citing East London Hospital as a precedent, pleads for care, preferably by female nurses, of unwell youths.

2262   The Riverside Visitor. "Nurse Nine." n.s., 8 (1878-79): 843-48.
       Treasures retired nurse who acts as a good neighbor.

2263 Garnett, Mrs. Charles [Elizabeth]. " 'Sister Dora'." n.s., 9 (1879-80): 518-24.
Celebrates the career of Dorothy Pattison, a district nurse.

2264 Turner, Alice Jane. "Once Deaf and Dumb." n.s., 9 (1879-80): 678-80.
Rejoices that hearing impaired children are learning to communicate.

2265 Stretton, Hesba. "Little and Lame." n.s., 10 (1880-81): 241-43.
Ventures to London's Hospital for Hip Disease in Childhood.

2266 Hart, Elizabeth. "The Ealing College and Oral Teaching of the Deaf and Dumb." n.s., 10 (1880-81): 681-86.
Publicizes causes of hearing loss and one method to teach those so affected.

2267 Selbon, Lois. "Two Aspects of an East-End Hospital." n.s., 10 (1880-81): 686-88.
Deems a pleasant environment central for Londoners' recoveries.

2268 Ritchie, J. Ewing. "Rambling among Obscure Charities." n.s., 11 (1881-82): 173-75, 269-70, 390-92, 588-90.
Incorporates rabies, climate and health, and care of the physically challenged young.

2269 Ewart, Henry C. "Charles Lowder." n.s., 12 (1882-83): 19-22.
Appreciates Charles Lowder, who has aided to the indigent ill.

2270 Owen, J[ean] A. "A Beautiful Lancashire Charity: Sea-Breezes for Sick Poor Children." n.s., 12 (1882-83): 238-40.
Trumpets Southport shelter for unwell waifs.

2271 Millin, George F. "London Babies." n.s., 12 (1882-83): 369-71.
Decries the diet and housing of London infants of destitute parents.

2272 Beale, Anne. "The St. Helena Home for Trained Nurses." n.s., 12 (1882-83): 482-84.
Would shorten hours of nurses for efficiency.

2273 Farrar, Abraham, Jun. "Speech for the Deaf and Dumb." n.s., 12 (1882-83): 733-37.
Stamps sign language a barrier that precludes the hearing impaired from intellectual growth and community respect. Would substitute reading and speech.

2274 Writer of 'The Bitter Cry of Outcast London' [William C. Preston]. "What Should Be Done with the Blind?" n.s., 13 (1883-84): 167-71.
Sets forth how to teach the vision impaired.

2275 Carr, Jessie. "A Hospital for Fever." n.s., 13 (1883-84): 298-99.
Core is the London Fever Hospital.

2276　Beale, Anne. "Fresh Air for the Children." n.s., 13 (1883-84): 369-72.
　　　Pumps for rural holidays for metropolitan youths.

2277　Beale, Anne. "The Isle of Wight Flower Mission." n.s., 13 (1883-84): 461-63.
　　　Forwards flowers for rapid convalescence.

2278　Clarke, Benjamin, Superintendent, Gifford Hall Mission. "Penny Dinners for Poor Children." n.s., 13 (1883-84): 603-04.
　　　Campaigns for nutritious fare for young paupers.

2279　Preston, William C. "Heroism at Sea: Tales of Storms." n.s., 13 (1883-84): 656-59.
　　　Protagonists are lifeboat brigades.

2280　Beale, Anne. "Market and Mission." n.s., 13 (1883-84): 715-17.
　　　Raves about London mission that provides nourishing meals and medical care to the poor.

2281　Preston, William C. "Pantomime Waifs." n.s., 13 (1883-84): 764-68.
　　　Fulminates about perils of pantomime for junior performers.

2282　Stretton, Hesba. "The Prevention of Cruelty to Children: The Appeal of the London Society." n.s., 13 (1883-84): 777-79.
　　　Scolds parents guilty of child abuse or neglect.

2283　Dale, A.W.W., M.A. "Professor Fawcett and the Blind." n.s., 14 (1884-85): 96-99.
　　　Salutes the determination of Henry Fawcett to secure training for the vision impaired.

2284　Telford, J. "Dr. Stephenson's Home for Children." n.s., 14 (1884-85): 257-61.
　　　Centers on a refuge run by Dr. (?T.B.) Stephenson with good food for minors in London's East End.

2285　Meade, L.T. "One in a Thousand." n.s., 14 (1884-85): 372-74.
　　　Condemns child abuse.

2286　Reaney, Mrs. G.S. [Isabel]. "Tram-Car Humanity." n.s., 14 (1884-85): 522-25.
　　　Would ameliorate working conditions of tram conductors.

2287　Beale, Anne. "A People's Garden." n.s., 14 (1884-85): 701-03.
　　　Fastens health to clean air.

2288　"Cruelly Treated Children." n.s., 14 (1884-85): 797-99.
　　　Befriends abused offspring.

2289　Preston, William C. "A Home for Little Cripples." n.s., 15 (1885-86): 112-17.
　　　Categorizes juveniles in London haven as physically challenged from birth or parental indifference.

2290 Beale, Anne. "Bright Stars in East London." n.s., 15 (1885-86): 253-55.
Theme is East London hospital for the impoverished pregnant and their issue.

2291 Beale, Anne. "A Morning with a Nurse in East London." n.s., 15 (1885-86): 330-33.
Follows a nurse on stops at abodes of the sick in East London.

2292 Beale, Anne. "From Half-Past Twelve to One at Lisson Grove." n.s., 15 (1885-86): 388-91.
Banks on meals of board schools for nutrition of needy pupils.

2293 Lamb, Ruth. "Manchester Waifs." n.s., 15 (1885-86): 521-25.
Flags Manchester sanctuary for orphans and abused minors.

2294 S., M.S. "A Factory Girl's Life Fifty Years Ago." n.s., 15 (1885-86): 562-65.
Recalls health hazards, as machines, overwork, and tuberculosis, for women employees in early factories.

2295 Pennington, Mrs. "Starving Scholars." n.s., 16 (1886-87): 414, 518-19.
Agonizes that students are often famished or fed badly.

2296 Reaney, Mrs. G.S. [Isabel]. "Homes for Our East-End Poor." n.s., 16 (1886-87): 740-43, 812-15.
Would revamp London residences, particularly those of unwell paupers.

2297 Harrison, Mary. "London's Missions to Its Poor Children." n.s., 17 (1887-88): 21-24, 162-64, 814-16.
Admires London charities that serve meals to the young and deliver them from family abuse or flower vending.

2298 Reaney, Rev. G.S. "City Children at Play." n.s., 17 (1887-88): 40-42.
Hopes for urban sites where children can exercise safely.

2299 Harrison, Mary. "Elizabeth Gilbert." n.s., 17 (1887-88): 90-92.
Respects Elizabeth Gilbert, herself vision impaired, who helps others who do not see.

2300 Holmes, Isabella M. "Green and Grey London." n.s., 17 (1887-88): 268-71.
Prompts more parks in London for cleaner air and exercise space.

2301 Paul, Thomas. "Hospital Ships for the Trawlers." n.s., 17 (1887-88): 300-07.
Pinpoints dangers of deep-sea fishing.

2302 Whiting, Mary B. "Prize Day at the Deaf and Dumb Asylum, Margate." n.s., 17 (1887-88): 310-11.
Thinks about tutoring for the hearing impaired who do not speak.

2303   Beale, Anne. "A Lady's Hospital." n.s., 17 (1887-88): 482-84.
        Voyager to the New Hospital for Women, London, validates
        females as doctors.

2304   Beale, Anne. "A Wing upon the Sea." n.s., 17 (1887-88): 618-21.
        Capsulizes therapies for tuberculosis.

2305   Waugh, Rev. Benjamin. "Our Babies' Colosseum." n.s., 17 (1887-
        88): 770-73.
        Insists that working in pantomimes is detrimental to children.

2306   Harrison, Mary. "Healers and Teachers: A West London Mission."
        n.s., 18 (1888-89): 190-92.
        Blesses those who succor the sick in London.

2307   Preston, William C. "Parliament's Battles for the Children." n.s.,
        18 (1888-89): 300-04, 474-78, 618-22, 706-11.
        Gathers statutes that have improved conditions for juveniles in
        factories, chimneys, and brickyards.

2308   Garnett, Mrs. Charles [Elizabeth]. "In the Evening of Life: A Visit
        to the 'Aged Pilgrims' Asylum'." n.s., 18 (1888-89): 306-09.
        Cheers a home at Hornsey Rise for penniless seniors, many
        unwell. See #2320.

2309   G., H.C. "With the Dock-Sisters in East London." n.s., 18 (1888-
        89): 483-87.
        Pens activities, as bringing food to ailing paupers, of volunteers in
        East London.

2310   The Riverside Visitor. "Free Dinner Children." n.s., 18 (1888-89):
        546-49.
        Seconds meal program for pupils otherwise ill from hunger.

2311   Canterbury, Archbishop of [E.W. Benson], Mrs. [Millicent
        Garrett] Fawcett, and the Editor [Benjamin Waugh]. "Theatre
        Children: Or, Ought Christians to Patronize Performances by
        Young Children?" n.s., 19 (1889-90): 121-31.
        Targets the health of young theatre employees.

2312   Butler, Rev. H. Montagu, D.D., Master of Trinity College and
        Vice Chancellor of the University of Cambridge. "A Christian
        Hospital." n.s., 19 (1889-90): 153-56.
        Perceives that faculties of medical schools have opportunities to
        share skills, do research, and ready new doctors and nurses.

2313   Brewer, Mrs. "A Visit to the Pasteur Institute." n.s., 19 (1889-90):
        167-70.
        Text is the treatment for rabies developed by Louis Pasteur.

2314   Blaikie, Prof. W.G., D.D., LL.D. "Dr. Barnardo." n.s., 19 (1889-
        90): 694-700.
        Hails T.J. Barnardo for his charity to starving and abused minors.

2315 Forster, William J. "Dr. Bowman Stephenson and the Children's Home." n.s., 19 (1889-90): 823-29.
Stars T.B. Stephenson's shelter for destitute youths.

2316 Ede, Rev. W. Moore, M.A. "The Bethlehem of Penny Dinners." n.s., 20 (1890-91): 56-60.
Fixes on a scheme to distribute nutritious fare to impoverished juniors.

2317 Buckland, Rev. A.R., M.A. "The Great Playgrounds of a Great City." n.s., 20 (1890-91): 416-19.
Story on street games assures that, absent more playgrounds, recreation is perilous for the urban young.

2318 Wortley, Hon. Mrs. James Stuart [?Victoria]. "The Shadwell Hospital for Children." n.s., 20 (1890-91): 486-89.
Article on titled children's hospital lobbies for better outpatient departments and convalescent homes for boys.

2319 Jones, Rev. Harry. "A Home Circuit." n.s., 20 (1890-91): 522-25, 607-10.
Notes that refuges for prostitutes usually have some facilities for hygiene.

2320 Pike, G. Holden. "The Aged and Their Claims." n.s., 20 (1890-91): 847-50.
Applauds Aged Pilgrims' Friend Society for its sanctuaries for elderly, frequently ill indigents. See #2308.

2321 Burdett-Coutts, Rt. Hon. the Baroness [Angela]. "Our Children's Shelter." n.s., 21 (1891-92): 42-47, 164-71.
Acclaims London haven of the Society for the Prevention of Cruelty to Children.

2322 Wood, Rev. Theordore, F.E.S. "Natural Chloroform." n.s., 21 (1891-92): 130-32, 189-91.
Conjectures that human pain is more intense than animal and that of whites', especially the educated, greater because their nerves and brains are highly developed.

2323 Preston, William C. "The Night Shelters of the Salvation Army." n.s., 21 (1891-92): 311-18.
Honors the Salvation Army because it houses and feeds the needy.

2324 Preston, William C. " 'Darkest England' Matches." n.s., 21 (1891-92): 447-53.
Segregates captioned company from most others where phosphorus jeopardizes workers' lives.

2325 Mearns, Rev. Andrew. "The Common Lodging-Houses of London." n.s., 22 (1892-93): 16-21, 102-09.
Blasts unsanitary lodging houses in London for abetting disease.

2326   Bowditch, A.M. "The Employment of Cripples." n.s., 22 (1892-93): 686-87.
Would relocate physically challenged children to the country where they may make jam.

2327   Bolton, Mary P., Assistant Secretary of the National Society for the Prevention of Cruelty to Children. "Discipline of Children." n.s., 22 (1892-93): 762-67.
Concentrates on cases of child beating and other abuses.

2328   Pike, G. Holden. "The World of the Blind." n.s., 23 (1893-94): 130-33.
Subjects are causes of vision loss, instruction of the vision impaired, and care of the aged so affected.

2329   Buckland, Rev. A.R., M.A., Morning Preacher at the Foundling Hospital. "Child-Gatherers of Food and Fuel." n.s., 23 (1893-94): 519-24.
Laments that famished youths have to search refuse and bakery discards for something to eat.

2330   Pike, G. Holden. "Facts about the Deaf and Dumb." n.s., 23 (1893-94): 561-65.
Survey of the hearing impaired who do not speak moors the condition in heredity. Faults parents for waiting until progeny are five before enrolling them for sign and oral training.

2331   Bolton, Mary P. "Miss Steer's Homes for Girls." n.s., 23 (1893-94): 678-83.
Gauges the success of Mary Steer's project to domicile girls in salutary surroundings.

2332   Bolton, Mary P. "Miss Parker's 'Home'," n.s., 23 (1893-94): 845-49.
Traverses a haven for female victims of child abuse.

2333   Baring-Gould, Rev. S., M.A. "Country Remedies." n.s., 24 (1894-95): 240-45.
Favors traditional village herbalists to recent charlatans with chemical elixirs.

2334   Lamont, Alexander. "A Glasgow Home for Infirm Children." n.s., 24 (1894-95): 263-67.
Idealizes Scottish shelter for neglected offspring of the impoverished.

2335   Stuart, Mrs. James [?Laura]. "A Home of Peace for the Dying." n.s., 24 (1894-95): 677-82.
Walks through St. Luke's Hospital, London, where "respectable poor," most with tuberculosis or cancer, arrive from other hospitals or drift in to die.

2336 Warren, Kate M. "The Experiences of a Hospital Nurse." n.s., 25 (1895-96): 433-36.
Peruses nurses' training, duties and relations with patients.

2337 Treanor, Rev. T.S. "A Lifeboat Rescue." n.s., 25 (1895-96): 517-20.
Lionizes lifeboat brigades.

2338 Hirst, Alfred. "A Friend and Benefactor of the Blind." n.s., 25 (1895-96): 736-39, 836-41.
Hero is T.R. Armitage, a fan of braille for the vision impaired.

2339 Forbes, Mrs. A.K.H. "The Selfishness of Ill Health." n.s., 26 (1896-97): 163-65.
Imagines that sickness sires self-centeredness.

2340 Faunthorpe, Rev. J.P., M.A., Principal of Whitelands Training College, Chelsea. "Girlhood and Its Chances." n.s., 27 (1897-98): 156-59.
Pontificates that women are born nurses.

2341 Lillingston, Leonard W. "The Red Cross." n.s., 27 (1897-98): 527-31.
Glorifies the Red Cross.

2342 Davidson, Right Rev. Randall Thomas, D.D., Bishop of Winchester. "The Trust Given to Our Doctors - A Sermon Preached to the British Medical Congress, Portsmouth, August 1, 1899." n.s., 28 (1898-99): 804-07.
Acknowledges the increase of medical learning. Reminds doctors of their primary responsibilty to tend the ill.

TAIT'S EDINBURGH MAGAZINE, 1832-1855

Adjusting its style and scope over time, *Tait's*, launched by William, ordinarily noted unwholesome labors and neighborhoods.

2343 [DeQuincey, Thomas]. "Animal Magnetism." 4 (1833-34): 456-74.
Moves from the work of F.A. Mesmer to hypnosis as medical therapy. See #2351.

2344 "The Miseries of Artificial Teeth." 4 (1833-34): 476-82.
Articulates difficulties of false teeth from a wearer's perspective.

2345 Martineau, Harriet. "Letter to the Deaf." n.s., 1, o.s., 5 (1834): 174-79.
Tutors the hearing impaired about appropriate endeavors.

2346   Martineau, Harriet. "The Hanwell Lunatic Asylum." n.s., 1, o.s.,
        5 (1834): 305-10.
        Thesis is that insanity is increasing but that captioned pauper
        asylum clearly demonstrates how an active regimen and any
        companionship profits patients.

2347   "Baines' *History of the Cotton Manufacture.*" n.s., 2, o.s., 6
        (1835): 235-52.
        Review of a study by Edward Baines paints factory milieu as
        damaging to young toilers.

2348   [Johnstone, Christian]. "Pictures of Ireland, from the Life - Report
        of the Poor Law Commissioners." n.s., 3, o.s., 7 (1836): 141-56.
        Gleans from featured document that Irish peasants have inadequate
        sustenance leaving them susceptible to maladies but without
        medical care. See #2349.

2349   [Johnstone, Christian]. "Observations on Miliken's Abridgement
        of the Report of the Poor-Law Commissioners." n.s., 3, o.s., 7
        (1836): 235-39.
        Reprints notions of #2348 based on publisher's edition of the
        Report.

2350   Caius. "Smoke!" n.s., 3, o.s., 7 (1836): 383-87.
        Disbelieves that tobacco smoking is unhealthy.

2351   [Johnstone, Christian]. "*Animal Magnetism.*" n.s., 5, o.s., 9 (1838):
        460-67.
        Abstract of a text by Baron J. Du Potet de Sennevoy has some
        words on hypnosis as a medical treatment. See #2343.

2352   [Johnstone, Christian]. "Madhouses, and the Treatment of the
        Insane." n.s., 6, o.s., 10 (1839): 746-56.
        Extrapolates from one case circumstances in institutions for the
        insane.

2353   [Meysey, Henry Stephen]. "Tee-Total Societies in Ireland." n.s.,
        7, o.s., 11 (1840): 205-10.
        Insists that evidence from Ireland shows greater vigor among those
        abstaining from alcohol.

2354   [Johnstone, Christian]. "*A Lecture on the Management of Lunatic
        Asylums.*" n.s., 7, o.s., 11 (1840): 314-18.
        From the text of Robert Gardiner Hill, House-Surgeon, Lincoln
        Lunatic Asylum, infers that establishments for the insane are not
        humane.

2355   [Chadwick, Edwin]. "Sanatory [sic] Inquiries and Proposed
        Legislation." n.s., 8, o.s., 12 (1841): 705-09.
        Links diseases of the impoverished to personal and household
        uncleanliness, insufficient sewers, and unwholesome fare.

2356 [Johnstone, Christian]. "Statistics of the Retreat Lunatic Asylum near York, Since the Year 1796." n.s., 8, o.s., 12 (1841): 757-60.
Paen to titled facility for its care also penetrates causes of insanity.

2357 [Johnstone, Christian]. "The Glasgow Mortality Bill for 1840." n.s., 9, o.s., 13 (1842): 36-37.
Linchpin is death rate of Glasgow's young poor.

2358 "Colliers and Collieries." n.s., 9, o.s., 13 (1842): 375-79.
Bewails that work in mines destroys workers' health.

2359 [Johnstone, Christian]. *"Hydropathy, or the Cold Water Cure."* n.s., 9, o.s., 13 (1842): 379-84.
Refers to a volume by T. Claridge, Esq., on the treatment initiated by Vincent Priessnitz in Austria.

2360 [Johnstone, Christian]. "Taylor's *Notes of a Tour in the Manufacturing Districts of Lancashire.*" n.s., 9, o.s., 13 (1842): 557-60.
Transcribes experiences of W. Cooke Taylor. Observes that many destitute die from starvation or ail from ingestion of garbage.

2361 [Johnstone, Christian]. *"Report on the Sanitary Condition of the Labouring Population of Great Britain."* n.s., 9, o.s., 13 (1842): 649-60.
Abstracts from cited report the harm of defective sewers, foul water, unventilated abodes, inadequate food, and widespread filth.

2362 Ramsay, George, B.M. "On Poor Laws." n.s., 12, o.s., 16 (1845): 79-84.
Would keep a poor law for the ill and aged.

2363 The English Opium Eater [Thomas DeQuincey]. "On the Temperance Movement of Modern Times." n.s., 12, o.s., 16 (1845): 658-85.
Tickets diet, exercise, and mindset to counter a desire for alcohol.

2364 "The Potato Crop in Ireland." n.s., 12, o.s., 16 (1845): 762-64.
Rumors that famine was debilitating the Irish.

2365 [Johnstone, Christian]. "The Naveys." n.s., 13, o.s., 17 (1846): 323-26.
Highlights job mishaps of railroad employees.

2366 [Dick, Robert]. *"Homeopathy; Its Principal Theory, and Practice."* n.s., 13, o.s., 17 (1846): 390-93.
Features views of M.B. Sampson, a fan of homeopathy.

2367 [Troup, George]. "The Sanatory [sic] Question." n.s., 15, o.s., 19 (1848): 49-53, 126-36, 845-52.
Delineates the damage to urbanites from dirty air and water, little light, few sewers, and unsanitary interments. Lists statistics from deaths, chiefly from cholera and fevers.

2368   [Troup, George]. "Life Assurance." n.s., 15, o.s., 19 (1848): 191-
        94, 251-55, 343-46, 414-17.
        Piece on insurance mentions that women, mainly wives, live long
        and that offspring are sometimes victims of parental abuse.

2369   [Troup, George]. "Nautical Blunders and Manslaughters." n.s., 15,
        o.s., 19 (1848): 620-26.
        Logs (as hazards of sea work or travel) unsafe fishing boats,
        hurricanes, ship fires, and inept liner crews.

2370   [Troup, George]. "The Pestilence and Sanatory [sic] Measures."
        n.s., 16, o.s., 20 (1849): 118-22.
        Avers that cholera is not contagious but comes principally from
        sewage.

2371   [Troup, George]. "Scottish Drunkenness." n.s., 17, o.s., 21 (1850):
        547-56.
        Measures alcohol in excess as unsalutary for all, not merely Scots.

2372   "Colds and Cold Water." n.s., 17, o.s., 21 (1850): 705-08.
        Professes that sponge baths are the best prophylactic for colds.
        Offers remedies for sufferers.

2373   [Taylor, Tom]. "The Siege of Smithfield." n.s., 18, o.s., 22 (1851):
        245-46.
        Would situate meat market outside London in quarters appropriate
        for public health.

2374   [Leifchild, J.R.]. "Coal Mine Explosions." n.s., 18, o.s., 22 (1851):
        370-73.
        Reckons that more inspectors will guarantee enough ventilation,
        and therefore fewer explosions, in mines.

2375   [Leifchild, J.R.]. "How to Put in Air and Put out Fire in Coal-
        Mines." n.s., 18, o.s., 22 (1851): 660-66.
        Discloses the technology to secure against explosions in mines.

2376   Thaler, Dr. Kein [G.F. Collier]. "On Homeopathy." n.s., 18, o.s.,
        22 (1851): 732-38.
        Dubs the homeopath a quack whose patients either recover
        naturally, not from minute doses of drugs, or die from failure to
        undergo recognized surgical procedures.

2377   [Taylor, Tom]. "The Water Question." n.s., 19, o.s., 23 (1852): 52-
        57.
        Depicts the Thames as unfit to drink.

2378   The Author of 'The Philospher's Mite' [G.F. Collier]. "The Health
        of the Metropolis During the Year of the Great Exhibition." n.s.,
        19, o.s., 23 (1852): 99-107.
        Denounces London hospitals, water, sewerage, and cemeteries.
        Pleads for new legislation to transform the metropolis.

2379 Thaler, Dr. Kein [G.F. Collier]. "On Preventible Death." n.s., 19, o.s., 23 (1852): 129-35.
Would stall disease by modifying ventilation, light, and drains in domiciles; adjusting burial arrangements; and ending nuisances.

2380 "A Psychological Study." n.s., 21, o.s., 25 (1854): 33-38.
Biography of Mary Elizabeth Squirrel, Shottisham, encapsulates her diverse maladies revealed under hypnosis.

2381 "Ages and Occupations of the People." n.s., 21, o.s., 25 (1854): 548-53.
Spells out how occupations can affect wellness.

2382 [Troup, George]. "Our Social Morality." n.s., 21, o.s., 25 (1854): 603-10.
Despises Englishmen for their habits of beating wives and exposing them to venereal diseases by patronizing prostitutes.

2383 "The Perils of Industry." n.s., 21, o.s., 25 (1854): 705-12.
Concentrates on accidents in the workplace, whether from employer negligence or employee ignorance.

2384 "The Copper Works of Swansea." n.s., 22, o.s., 26 (1855): 149-57.
Maximizes perils from tasks and environment of copper plant in Wales.

2385 [Mansfield, Horatio]. "The Diggings and Diggers of the West Country." n.s., 22, o.s., 26 (1855): 193-200.
Profile of Cornish miners has some language about the jeopardy of their job.

2386 [Ritchie, J. Ewing]. "The Poor Man's Market in London." n.s., 22, o.s., 26 (1855): 337-42.
Account of London markets protests that foodstuffs available to the poor are often tainted.

TEMPLE BAR, 1860-1900

Aspiring to enlighten effortlessly the recently rich, *Temple Bar* showed variety in its spasmodic versions of sickness.

2387 [Browne, C.T.]. "Criminal Lunatics." 1 (1860-61): 135-43.
Spotlights problems in dealing with the criminally insane.

2388 [Yates, Edmund]. "The Houseless Poor." 1 (1860-61): 225-29.
Postulates that many without homes are likewise without health.

2389 [Ansted, D.T.]. "What Our Coal Costs Us." 1 (1860-61): 258-67.
Grasps risks of coal mining.

2390   "On the Causes of Railway Accidents." 1 (1860-61): 344-55.
        Looks at railroad accidents with injuries.

2391   "Muscular Education." 4 (1861-62): 47-62.
        Models exercises for robust boys and girls.

2392   W[raxall], L[ascelles]. " 'De Lunatico'." 5 (1862): 528-41.
        Compares public and private establishments for the insane.

2393   "The Blackburn Sewing Schools." 7 (1862-63): 339-48.
        Prefaces the debility of Lancashire citizens with destitution
        because of unemployment resulting from cotton shortage.

2394   "What to Do and How to Do It." 7 (1862-63): 419-26.
        Spurs official action for public health.

2395   "Forty Per Cent." 8 (1863): 513-20.
        Attributes deaths of forty percent of infants under one year to
        communicable diseases, insufficient fare, and unsanitary abodes.

2396   "Wanted: Apartments." 13 (1864-65): 85-88.
        Espouses clean and airy lodgings, similar to those of artisans, for
        gentlemen.

2397   [Bushnan, John S.]. "Medical Education." 13 (1864-65): 215-28.
        Summarizes goals and subjects of university medical education
        and degrees conferred.

2398   [Cazalet, W.W.]. "Hippophagy and Onophagy." 19 (1866-67): 31-
        36.
        Advertises the nutritiousness of horse and ass meat.

2399   [Dodd, George]. "Fires and Fire Brigades." 20 (1867): 135-44.
        Headlines activities of fire squads.

2400   Beale, Annie [Anne]. "The Country Doctor: A Welsh Sketch." 33
        (1871): 385-93.
        Rambles about the routine of a local Welsh doctor.

2401   [Austin, Alfred]. "The Pace That Kills." 44 (1875): 474-83.
        Rues the stress from contemporary living.

2402   [Archdale, George]. "What Shall I Drink?" 70 (1884): 61-69.
        Says that liquor in moderation is not detrimental.

2403   [Wildey, Alexander]. "Dr. Gabriel's Experiment." 87 (1889): 192-
        99.
        Quotes Dr. A. Gabriel, an oculist, on harmful effects of ultraviolet
        light on the retina.

2404   [O'Neill, John]. " 'Centenarianism'." 87 (1889): 338-46.
        Ascribes instances of longevity primarily to lifestyle, then
        heredity.

2405   [Crawford, Virginia M.]. "Life in the London Slums: Extracts
        from the Diary of a District Nurse." 91 (1891): 275-83.
        Witnesses attitudes and actions of a district nurse in London.

2406 [Vaughan, John]. "The Growth of Sanitary Science." 94 (1892): 365-75.
History of sanitation notices its nexus to the spread of communicable diseases, as cholera.

2407 Aikman, C.M. "Louis Pasteur." 109 (1896): 375-95.
Pivot is the research on bacteria by Louis Pasteur.

2408 [Blaikie, J. Lang]. "London Doctors and Their Work." 116 (1899): 548-61.
Surveys London doctors.

THE THEOLOGICAL REVIEW, 1864-1879

Preceding the *Modern Review*, the Unitarian *Theological* all but ignored illness.

2409 B[inns], W[illiam]. "The Homes of the Agricultural Poor." 2 (1865): 406-29.
Pictures hovels of rural poor as crowded and filthy centers of contagions and alcoholism.

2410 Herford, W.H. "Female Education in the Middle Class." 3 (1866): 526-40.
Sermonizes that the education of gentlewomen will improve their mental health but that studying the same subjects as men will culminate in permanent damage to female brains.

2411 [Paul, C. Kegan]. "The Condition of the Agricultural Labourer." 5 (1868): 107-27.
Treatise on agrarian workers has words on the deleteriousness of their dirty dwellings.

TITAN: A MONTHLY MAGAZINE, 1856-1859

Superseding *Hogg's Instructor*, *Titan* did not muse very much about vitality.

2412 W., A.A. "The Evil of the Day." 1 (1856): 405-08.
Minimizes dangers of tobacco.

2413 "Human Hair and Its Restoratives." 6 (1859): 48-57.
Inventories baldness, greying, and illnesses that alter or reduce hair.

THE WESTMINSTER REVIEW, 1824-1900

Bred from Benthamite radicalism, the *Westminster* combined in the 1830s with the *London Review* shaped by John Stuart Mill and in the 1840s with the *Foreign Quarterly Review*. Throughout its history, the periodical adhered to the notion that progress proceeded from considered change. The amplitude and assortment of its probes of health testified to this belief.

2414   [Smith, T. Southwood]. "Use of the Dead to the Living." 2 (1824): 59-97.
        Would legalize dissection of the dead by medical students in order to enhance medical treatment, specifically for aneurism, hernia, and afflictions of the liver and brain. See #2424 and #2434.

2415   [?Smith, T. Southwood]. "Hydrophobia." 2 (1824): 324-34.
        Discusses symptoms of and remedies for rabies.

2416   [Smith, T. Southwood]. "Contagion and Sanitary Laws." 3 (1825): 134-67.
        Distinguishes communicable and epidemic diseases with examples of each. See #2417.

2417   [Smith, T. Southwood]. "Plague - Typhus - Fever - Quarantine." 3 (1825): 499-530.
        Completes #2416. Dismisses sanitary statutes and quarantines as ineffective against epidemic diseases allegedly not communicable.

2418   "Willis on *Mental Derangement*." 5 (1826): 149-56.
        Excerpts ideas of Francis Willis, M.D., on the identification of and treatment for insanity.

2419   [Wakely, Thomas]. "College of Surgeons." 6 (1826): 303-25.
        Records the debate about the attempt by the Court of Examiners of the captioned college to restrict the practice of surgery.

2420   [Smith, T. Southwood]. "Life and Organization." 7 (1827): 208-26.
        Ruminates about human physiology. See #2421.

2421   [Smith, T. Southwood]. "Human and Comparative Physiology." 7 (1827): 416-44.
        Extension of #2420 parenthesizes concepts of Peter M. Roget, M.D., F.R.S.

2422   [Smith, T. Southwood]. "Nervous System." 9 (1828): 172-98, 451-80.
        Illustrates the development and functions of the nervous system in humans and animals.

2423 [Chadwick, Edwin]. "Life Assurances - Diminution of Sickness and Mortality." 9 (1828): 384-421.
Has statistics on rates of death and costs of illness.

2424 [Smith, T. Southwood and Jeremy Bentham]. "Anatomy." 10 (1829): 116-48.
Would provide doctors with cadavers for anatomical study by legislating access to bodies of unclaimed paupers since exhumation is unreliable and perhaps criminal. See #2414 and #2434.

2425 "Wadd's *Comments on Corpulency*." 10 (1829): 169-73.
Tabs obesity more baneful than does W. Wadd.

2426 "Thames Water Question." 12 (1830): 31-42.
Argues that the Thames, notwithstanding sewage, is potable.

2427 "On Continued Fever." 12 (1830): 195-213.
Describes symptoms of and treatments for fevers.

2428 [Smith, T. Southwood]. "*Phenomena of the Human Mind*." 13 (1830): 265-92.
Review of a book by James Mill, Esq., hypothesizes that many forms of insanity have physical roots.

2429 "Hydrophobia." 13 (1830): 415-19.
Investigates the onset of rabies in people.

2430 [Arnott, Neil]. "Professional Morality." 14 (1831): 463-81.
Scorns those who practice medicine without adequate training.

2431 [?Smith, T. Southwood]. "Spasmodic Cholera." 15 (1831): 457-90.
Synopsizes origins, signs, and international outbreaks of, and therapies for cholera in the nineteenth century.

2432 [Arnott, Neil]. "History of Medicine." 16 (1832): 73-89.
Tracks those who have practiced medicine.

2433 [?Chadwick, Edwin]. "Animal Physiology." 16 (1832): 192-203.
Couples attire and diet with wellness.

2434 [Arnott, Neil]. "Regulation of Anatomy." 16 (1832): 482-96.
Echoes #2414 and #2424.

2435 "Esquirol on the Treatment of the Insane." 18 (1833): 129-38.
Abridges opinions of Jean E.D. Esquirol, a French doctor, on the merits of isolating the insane from society.

2436 "Condition of the Working Classes, and the Factory Bill." 18 (1833): 380-404.
Characterizes industrial laborers as enervated because of their unsanitary residences and factories.

2437 "Sinking System at Sea." 19 (1833): 366-72.
Prophesizes that better ship construction will reduce maritime accidents.

2438   [Symonds, Arthur]. "Public Walks." 20 (1834): 496-514.
        Fosters urban public baths for hygiene and parks for clean air and
        exercise.

2439   [?Symonds, Arthur]. "Improvements of the Metropolis." 21
        (1834): 195-203; with a note by T.P. Thompson: 199.
        Booms that London water and roads are filthy.

The London and Westminster Review

2440   H[ickson], W.E. "Local Government of the Metropolis." 25 and
        3 (1836): 71-103.
        Survey of London municipal administration dockets such problems
        as sewerage, street cleaning, and services for the insane.

2441   R., J. [W. Bridges Adams]. "Domestic Arrangements of the
        Working Classes." 25 and 3 (1836): 450-66.
        Concludes that the poor are inefficient toilers because of debility,
        the result of their menus and quarters.

2442   S[mith], D. [T. Southwood]. "Medical Reform." 26 and 4 (1836):
        58-92.
        Chides the College of Physicians, College of Surgeons, and Court
        of Examiners of the Apothecaries' Company for allowing
        incompetents to practice. Seeks uniform educational and
        qualification standards.

2443   S[mith], D. [T. Southwood]. "The Factories." 26 and 4 (1836):
        174-215.
        Dramatizes physical and mental evils of factory labor for the
        young.

2444   J. "Dr. Arnott on Ventilating and Warming." 28 and 6 (1838): 345-
        67.
        Entry on a volume by Neil Arnott, M.D., about stoves envisions
        that they will replace dangerous sweeping and reduce influenza
        because of their effects on heat and ventilation.

The Westminster Review

2445   T[homson], R.W. "Medical Corporations." 35 (1841): 481-95;
        with a note by Ed. [W.E. Hickson]: 495-97.
        Desires a strict canon for doctors and apothecaries to ensure
        quality medical care and discourage charlatans.

2446   [Hickson, W.] E. "The Hand-Loom Inquiry Commission." 36
        (1841): 87-132.
        Shows the impact of low wages on diet and thence health.

2447 O. "Industry and Its Reward in Great Britain and Ireland." 37 (1842): 216-26.
Groans that illness comes to badly paid young workers.

2448 S[ymons], J[elinger] C. "Lunacy: *Statistics of the Retreat*, Etc." 37 (1842): 305-21.
Books on insane asylums are the basis for thoughts about English ones.

2449 "Protection of Children: Mines and Collieries." 38 (1842): 86-139.
Posts perils of mining, notably for women and children.

2450 D[enton], J[ohn] B[ailey]. "Drainage." 39 (1843): 231-66.
Essay on city and country drainage bruits the deleteriousness of insufficient sewerage.

2451 R[oebuck], J.A. "Trial of Macnaughten and the Plea of Insanity." 39 (1843): 457-74.
Subject is insanity defense in a criminal trial.

2452 [Hickson, W.E.]. "Municipal Reform." 39 (1843): 495-586.
Dissertation on London government castigates metropolitan royal hospitals closed to indigents.

2453 G[reg], W.R. "Resources of an Increasing Population: Emigration or Manufactures." 40 (1843): 101-22.
Story on the impoverished whispers that urbanites have improper fare and sanitation.

2454 [?Elliott,] J. [H.]. "London Churchyards." 40 (1843): 149-82.
Fears that London burials are hazardous for gravediggers and neighbors of cemeteries. Would alter coffins, alignments of corpses, and time for interment as antidotes.

2455 [Bayley, Robert S.]. "Working Classes of Sheffield." 40 (1843): 460-70.
Regrets that grinders die young from tuberculosis.

2456 L[amport, W.J.]. "Collision of Ships: The Rules of the Sea." 42 (1844): 117-34.
Would clarify rules on ship traffic and impose new onboard norms in order to obviate mishaps.

2457 G. "Lunatic Asylums." 43 (1845): 162-92.
Intellectualizes about institutions for the insane who are categorized as curable, incurable, or criminal.

2458 L. "The Medical Police of the United Kingdom." 45 (1846): 56-88.
Clamors for legislation on medical practice, public health, and care of the insane or otherwise sick poor.

2459 G[rant, Horace]. "*The Lost Senses*." 45 (1846): 345-54.
Borrows from J. Kitto, D.D., cases of the vision and hearing impaired, many of them Irish.

2460   H[ickson, W.E.]. "Railways and Metropolitan Improvement." 45 (1846): 462-507.
Ordains that better sanitation, housing, water, and burial modes, and less smoke would be salubrious for Londoners.

The Westminster and Foreign Quarterly Review

2461   Z. [?R.W. Thomson]. "The Water Cure." 46 (1846-47): 174-82.
Exegesis on hydropathy labels some variations quackery.

2462   [Hickson, W.E.]. "Patronage of Commissions." 46 (1846-47): 222-45.
Selection on sundry official commissions is for clean air and light and against slaughterhouses in London.

2463   R., J. [W. Bridges Adams]. "Colney Hatch Asylum." 48 (1847): 119-30.
Quotes John Conolly, M.D., on model shelters for the insane.

2464   H., G.A. [W. Bridges Adams]. "Preservation of Food." 48 (1847): 303-14; with response. 50 (1848): 276-78.
Previews techniques of food preservation.

2465   G., L. "The Bicetre Asylum." 49 (1848): 70-84.
Would emulate French program to train the mentally challenged.

2466   [Hickson, W.E.]. "The Corporation of London, and Sanitary Improvement." 49 (1848): 421-40.
Accuses London Sewer Commissioners of negligence.

2467   [Hickson, W.E.]. "Epidemics." 52 (1850): 301-51.
Article on several diseases accents cholera.

2468   [Bain, Alexander]. "Metropolitan Commission of Sewers." 52 (1850): 491-94.
Would use sewage from towns as manure in rural areas.

2469   [Greg, W.R.]. "Prostitution." 53 (1850): 448-506.
Paper on prostitution has paragraphs on syphilis.

2470   [Beardmore, Nathaniel]. "Water Supply." 54 (1850): 368-87.
Balances pure water for citizens and power for industry.

2471   "Electro-Biology." 55 (1851): 312-28.
Thesis is effects of hypnosis.

The Westminster Review

2472   [Brown, Samuel]. "Physical Puritanism." n.s., 1, o.s., 57 (1852): 405-42.
Reconnoiters vegetarianism, homeopathy, hydropathy, hypnosis, and abstinence from alcohol.

2473 [Martineau, Harriet]. "Conditions and Prospects of Ireland." n.s., 3, o.s., 59 (1853): 35-62.
Tale of the Irish Famine realizes how it has enervated individuals.

2474 [Lewes, George Henry]. "The Physiological Errors of Teetotalism." n.s., 8, o.s., 64 (1855): 94-124.
Pronounces liquor in moderation safe. See #2483.

2475 "Drunkenness Not Curable by Legislation." n.s., 8, o.s., 64 (1855): 463-91.
Would cancel statutes against drunkenness and design more parks, with pure air and exercise space, for the wellness of workers.

2476 [Chapman, John]. "Medical Despotism." n.s., 9, o.s., 65 (1856): 530-62.
Opposes legislation on doctors because certification will not end ineptitude.

2477 [Lewes, George Henry]. "Hereditary Influence, Animal and Human." n.s., 10, o.s., 66 (1856): 135-62.
Theme is the inheritance of characteristics and habits and their impact on health.

2478 [Lewes, George Henry]. "Suicide in Life and Literature." n.s., 12, o.s., 68 (1857): 52-78.
Account on causes of suicide has an aside on insanity.

2479 "Spirits and Spirit-Rapping." n.s., 13, o.s., 69 (1858): 29-66.
Delves into the influence of mediums, such as by alleged healings.

2480 [Chapman, John]. "Medical Reform." n.s., 13, o.s., 69 (1858): 478-530.
Differentiates certifications of physicians, surgeons, and apothecaries. Opts for professional rather than parliamentary reform.

2481 [Chapman, John]. "Medical Education." n.s., 14, o.s., 70 (1858): 107-62.
Tract on medical training incorporates such matters as testing, degrees and certification, and cost.

2482 [Chapman, John]. "Chloroform and Other Anesthetics." n.s., 15, o.s., 71 (1859): 99-146.
Nub is the use of chloroform during childbirth.

2483 [Carpenter, William Benjamin]. "Alcohol: What Becomes of It in the Living Body." n.s., 19, o.s., 75 (1861): 33-56.
Catalogs alcohol as an anesthetic and a food. See #633 and #2474.

2484 [Child, Gilbert W.]. "Marriages of Consanguinity." n.s., 24, o.s., 80 (1863): 88-109.
Challenges the view that consanguineous marriages generate feeble offspring. See #778, #2510, and #2513.

2485   "Astrology and Magic." n.s., 25, o.s., 81 (1864): 48-88.
        Postulates that diseases and drugs stimulate symptoms seemingly
        mysterious or magical.
2486   "The Physiology of Sleep." n.s., 25, o.s., 81 (1864): 203-17.
        Calculates that some stages of sleep are salutary.
2487   [Child, Gilbert W.]. "Physiological Experiments: Vivisection."
        n.s., 29, o.s., 85 (1866): 132-55.
        Fan of vivisection points out that in everyday life and many sports
        Victorians express little concern about animal well-being.
2488   "The Royal Hospital of Bethlehem." n.s., 29, o.s., 85 (1866): 331-
        57.
        Regards Bedlam's quality of care and opportunity for the study of
        mental illness as worthwhile.
2489   [Child, Gilbert W.]. "Physiological Psychology." n.s., 33, o.s., 89
        (1868): 37-65.
        Explains functions of the brain and nervous system as they touch
        on behavior.
2490   [Playfair, W.S.]. "Sea-Sickness." n.s., 34, o.s., 90 (1868): 462-86.
        Ruminates about roots and symptoms of and remedies for
        seasickness.
2491   [?Lankester, Edwin]. "The Adulteration of Food and Drugs." n.s.,
        35, o.s., 91 (1869): 185-206.
        Broadcasts the extent of adulteration of food and drugs and
        statutes against it.
2492   "Domestic Fireplaces." n.s., 35, o.s., 91 (1869): 399-410.
        Juxtaposes assets and liabilities for salubriousness of residential
        hearths.
2493   [Chapman, John]. "Prostitution in Relation to the National
        Health." n.s., 36, o.s., 92 (1869): 179-234.
        Details symptoms of syphilis, theorizing that it leads to other
        ailments. See #2495, #2496, #2498, #2511, and #2520.
2494   "Water Supply of London." n.s., 36, o.s., 92 (1869): 388-414.
        Petitions for adequate and unpolluted water for London.
2495   [Simon, John]. "Prostitution: Its Sanitary Superintendence by the
        State." Intro. John Chapman. n.s., 36, o.s., 92 (1869): 556-79.
        Doubts that medical supervision of prostitutes can significantly
        curtail venereal diseases. See #2493, #2496, #2498, #2511, and
        #2520.
2496   [Chapman, John]. "Prostitution: Governmental Experiments in
        Controlling It." n.s., 37, o.s., 93 (1870): 119-79.
        Objects to monitoring prostitutes to stem veneral diseases. See
        #2493, #2495, #2498, #2511, and #2520.

2497 "Pauper Girls." n.s., 37, o.s., 93 (1870): 461-76.
Figures that the boarding system saves poor girls from illness and prostitution and citizens from higher taxes of workhouses. See #350.

2498 [Chapman, John]. "Prostitution: How to Deal with It." n.s., 37, o.s., 93 (1870): 477-535.
Rejects legislation as a tool to curb venereal diseases. See #2493, #2495, #2496, #2511, and #2520.

2499 "A Partial Remedy for the Pressure of 'Local Taxation,' Arising from the Execution of Sanitary Works." n.s., 38, o.s., 94 (1870): 294-306.
Would have Parliament pay for local sewerage.

2500 [Ireland, William W.]. "The Scottish Poor Law." n.s., 38, o.s., 94 (1870): 340-67.
Chapter on Scottish poor law glances at care of the physically and mentally ill.

2501 "Gunpowder." n.s., 38, o.s., 94 (1870): 387-410.
Fathoms dangers of gunpowder manufacturing.

2502 "The Function of Physical Pain: Anesthetics." n.s., 40, o.s., 96 (1871): 198-205.
Analysis of the nature of pain recommends anesthetics to neutralize it.

2503 [Scully, James]. "Recent Experiments with the Senses." n.s., 42, o.s., 98 (1872): 165-98.
Ponders the physiology and psychology of sensation.

2504 [Chapman, John]. "Medical Charity: Its Extent and Abuses." n.s., 45, o.s., 101 (1874): 174-224.
Bemoans the expense and some management of the poor law. See #2505.

2505 [Chapman, John]. "Medical Charity: Methods of Administering It." n.s., 45, o.s., 101 (1874): 464-514.
Would limit medical treatment under the poor law to the truly needy. See #2504.

2506 "American Women: Their Health and Education." n.s., 46, o.s., 102 (1874): 456-99.
Asserts that college, even co-educational, does not damage female health. See #768.

2507 Kingsford, Ninon [Anna]. "The Best Food for Man." n.s., 46, o.s., 102 (1874): 500-14.
Proponent of vegetarianism criticizes those who condemn vivivsection or conditions in slaughterhouses but eat meat. See #770 and #1440.

2508   "Merchant Shipping Legislation." n.s., 47, o.s., 103 (1875): 452-83.
        Records risks of being a seaman.

2509   "House Ventilation and Warming." n.s., 48, o.s., 104 (1875): 160-82.
        Suspects that impure air fills most abodes.

2510   *"The Marriage of Near Kin."* n.s., 48, o.s., 104 (1875): 299-317.
        Misinterprets A. H. Huth about hazards to heirs of consanguineous marriages. See #778, #2484, and #2513.

2511   [Chapman, John]. "Compulsory Medication of Prostitutes by the State." n.s., 50, o.s., 106 (1876): 137-88.
        Worries that prostitutes, leaving areas designated by Contagious Diseases Acts, disseminate venereal disease. See #2493, #2495, #2496, #2498, and #2520.

2512   [Cooke-Taylor, Richard Whately]. "The Factory and Workshop Acts." n.s., 51, o.s., 107 (1877): 36-58, 462-92.
        Scans diverse statutes on wellness in the workplace.

2513   [Huth, A. H.]. "Cross-Fertilization of Plants, and Consanguineous Marriages." n.s., 52, o.s., 108 (1877): 466-85.
        Disputes that marriages between close kin creates frail descendants. See #778, #2484, and #2510.

2514   "The International Medical Congress and the Progress of Medicine." n.s., 60, o.s., 116 (1881): 403-39.
        Exposes tensions between medical researchers and practitioners. Attributes advances to more knowledge of surgery, pathology, and drugs.

2515   "Working-Class Insurance as It Is." n.s., 61, o.s., 117 (1882): 81-98.
        Addresses the insolvency of insurers whose business is sickness expenses of laborers.

2516   "Town Smoke and Town Fog." n.s., 61, o.s., 117 (1882): 136-57.
        Ticketing urban smoke and fog detrimental, offers ways to extirpate them.

2517   "Fires in Theatres." n.s., 61, o.s., 117 (1882): 412-26.
        Outlines how to secure theatres from conflagrations.

2518   Forbes, Urquhart A. "River Pollution." n.s., 62, o.s., 118 (1882): 313-36.
        Roars that many rivers are contaminated by sewage and industrial waste, so edible fish cannot survive.

2519   "The Employers' Liability Act, 1880: Accidents and Accident Assurance." n.s., 63, o.s., 119 (1883): 54-71.
        Has statistics on death or disablement in numerous occupations.

2520 [Chapman, John]. "Prostitution in Paris." n.s., 63, o.s., 119 (1883): 494-521.
Reiterates that legislation does not retard venereal diseases. See #2493, #2495, #2496, #2498, and #2511.

2521 "Dr. Tuck's *History of the Insane in the British Isles.*" n.s., 64, o.s., 120 (1883): 501-10.
Samples the investigation by D. Hack Tuke, M.D., of care of the insane.

2522 "The Dwellings of the Poor." n.s., 65, o.s., 121 (1884): 137-51.
Preaches that too many dwellings of the poor are deleterious to health.

2523 Dudgeon, Henry D. "Compulsory Vaccination." n.s., 65, o.s., 121 (1884): 496-528.
Enemy of compulsory vaccination, as a violation of individual rights, would inhibit smallpox by sanitation.

2524 Chapman, John, M.D. "The Non-Contagiousness, Causation, and Scientific Treatment of Cholera." n.s., 66, o.s., 122 (1884): 472-533.
Covers causes and signs of and treatments for cholera.

2525 "Our Life Assurance Companies." n.s., 68, o.s., 124 (1885): 1-18.
From insurance tables, glimpses mortality rates by occupation.

2526 Salt, H[enry] S. "Food Reform." n.s., 70, o.s., 126 (1886): 483-99.
Noises about the value of vegetarianism.

2527 "The Adulteration of Food." 128 (1887): 1090-99.
Complains of pervasive adulteration of food. See #2528.

2528 "Adulteration of Food and the Remedy." 129 (1888): 22-28.
Expands #2527.

2529 An Habitual Drunkard. "Habitual Drunkenness." 129 (1888): 600-12.
Earmarks alcoholism as dangerous to general health.

2530 "Nurses and Nursing." 130 (1888): 11-16.
Dockets duties of district, hospital, and private nurses.

2531 "Mental Deterioration: Some of Its Avoidable Causes." 130 (1888): 64-81.
Tags overwork and undersleep, liquor, tobacco, and opiates, especially morphine, harmful.

2532 "Life in a London Hospital." 131 (1889): 26-33.
Protagonists are nurses, medical students, and indigent and juvenile patients.

2533 [Tebb, William]. "Vaccination by Act of Parliament." 131 (1889): 96-112.
Asserts that vaccination cannot hinder smallpox. See #2534.

2534   Tebb, William. "What Is the Truth about Vaccination?" 131 (1889): 187-200.
        Enlarges #2533. See #1701.
2535   "The Flaw in the Employers' Liability Bill." 131 (1889): 492-500.
        Plumbs the tie between private insurance and statutory compensation scheme for job injuries.
2536   Jersyd. "The Poor at Home." 131 (1889): 619-25.
        Walks with district nurse to dwellings of the impoverished.
2537   L., E.M. and C.B.L. "Lunacy Law Reform." 134 (1890): 128-42.
        Pushes for a probe of insanity, chiefly its legal definition and its committal standards.
2538   Cox, Harold. "Re-Housing the Poor of London." 134 (1890): 611-23.
        Parrots that homes of London's masses have insufficient light, ventilation, and cleanliness.
2539   Thomson, St. Clair, M.D. "The Dangers of Hypnotism." 134 (1890): 624-31.
        Deems hypnosis as medical therapy inaccurate and possibly perilous.
2540   Ramsey, Laon [Ramsden Balmforth]. "A Plea for an Eight Hours Day." 134 (1890): 642-55.
        Slots factory overwork as physically and mentally baneful.
2541   "A Privileged Profession." 135 (1891): 6-10.
        Proposes that nurses' training parallel that of other professions.
2542   Strahan, S.A.K., M.D. "Consanguinous Marriages." 135 (1891): 258-64.
        Expects descendants of consanguineous marriages to manifest familial weaknesses and diseases.
2543   Ellis, Emily Glode. "The Fetish of Charity." 135 (1891): 301-10, 373-84.
        Diatribe on misuses of charity has hospitals as one example.
2544   Leppington, C.H. d'E. "Side Lights of the Sweating Commission." 136 (1891): 273-88, 504-16.
        Decides, from the text of named commission, that circumstances of sweating trades were detrimental, mainly for females.
2545   McMillan, Margaret. "The Woman's Labour Day." 136 (1891): 517-26.
        Stars women workers, as nurses, miners, and mothers.
2546   Wallace, Lionel John. "Vivisection." 137 (1892): 245-60.
        Votes for vivisection.
2547   Blake, Matilda M. "The Lady and the Law." 137 (1892): 364-70.
        Essay on women's legal position would certify midwives.

2548 Blake, Matilda M. "Women as Poor-Law Guardians." 139 (1893): 12-21.
Sanctions females as poor law agents to ameliorate the care of the sick generally and the young with ophthalmia specifically.

2549 Buckland, E.S.L. *"Suffering London."* 139 (1893): 125-34.
Abstract of notions of A. Egmont Hake on the management and activities of London's voluntary hospitals has some prose on the incidence of accidents at home and in employment.

2550 Hollander, Bernard. "Herbert Spencer as a Phrenologist." 139 (1893): 142-54.
Claims that phrenology has influenced Herbert Spencer's thinking. Offers many perspectives on brain functions.

2551 Bulman, G.W., M.A., B. Sc. "Are Bacilli Causes of Diseases?" 139 (1893): 500-07.
Questions whether bacteria are the source of such diseases as rabies and cholera. See #857.

2552 Newman, Alfred S., M.A. "Cremation." 139 (1893): 654-59.
Would cremate the dead to squelch communicable diseases.

2553 Longhurst, Arthur E.T., M.D. "Scientific Aspect of the Temperance Question." 140 (1893): 8-16.
Labels liquor pernicious. See #1667.

2554 Blatch, H. Stanton. "Another View of Village Life." 140 (1893): 318-24.
Impugns impressions of *Royal Commission on Labour - The Agricultural Labourer* about the wellness of rustics.

2555 "A New Plan of Distributing Fish to Consumers." 140 (1893): 414-24.
Item on cooperatives to sell fish espouses its nutritive worth.

2556 Dix, Gertrude. "Hard Labour in the Hospitals." 140 (1893): 627-34.
Patron of nurses extols their energy in many hospital departments.

2557 Rolleston, Charles. "The Victims of Industry." 141 (1894): 417-27.
Prioritizes job injuries and maladies, primarily those affecting vision.

2558 Corbet, W.J. "How Insanity Is Propagated." 142 (1894): 153-63.
Foresees more insanity, particularly among children of consanguineous marriages. See #854, #2574, and #2576.

2559 DePledge, Josephine L. "The History and Progress of Nursing in Poor-Law Infirmaries." 142 (1894): 173-82.
Scope is patient care and nurses' situation in workhouse infirmaries.

2560   Corbet, W.J., M.R.I.A. "Private Lunatic Asylums." 142 (1894): 369-80.
        Apprehends that statutes on insanity could be manipulated to closet the sane. See #2561 and #2563.

2561   Pieterson, J.F.G. " 'Ought Private Lunatic Asylums to be Abolished?' " 142 (1894): 688-94.
        Medical superintendent of a private establishment for the insane refutes #2560. See #2563.

2562   Davies, Joseph J. "The Struggle for Healthy Schools." 143 (1895): 48-53.
        Would oblige public and grammar schools to meet the same sanitary criteria as do board institutions.

2563   Haslett, W.J. Handfield. "Modern Private Asylums: A Defence." 143 (1895): 307-15.
        Confirms the need for and procedures in private shelters for the insane. See #2560 and #2561.

2564   Steeves, G. Walter. "An Anomaly in Our Sanitation." 143 (1895): 667-74.
        Commands stricter standards for plumbers.

2565   Haweis, M.E. "Cattle Ships and Abattoirs." 143 (1895): 678-85.
        Rants that citizens are consuming meat from cattled diseased or butchered in filth.

2566   Shrubsole, O.A. "The Practicability of Vegetarianism." 145 (1896): 312-20.
        Maximizes merits of vegetarianism. See #866.

2567   Nathan, Walter. "The Influence of Stomach upon Mind." 146 (1896): 185-90.
        Dictates how and when to eat for physical and mental vigor.

2568   Cassidy, James [Edith Mary Story]. "Girl-Life in Ilford Village Homes." 146 (1896): 194-204.
        Spotlights refuges for girls ailing usually because of parental indigency or laxity.

2569   Bayley, E.H. "Nationalising the Lifeboat Service." 147 (1897): 120-27.
        Chides lifeboat service for its inability to save those in ship accidents.

2570   Corbet, W.J., M.P. "Lunacy Reform." 147 (1897): 200-10.
        Concludes from data that insanity is rising.

2571   James, Dr. Prosser. "Men as Nurses." 147 (1897): 309-10.
        Would recruit men for nursing.

2572   Herzfeld, A.G. "The Drink Evil and Its Cure." 147 (1897): 408-28.
        Presents assets and liabilities of drinking alcohol.

2573 Ethelmer, Ellis [Benjamin W. Elmy]. "The Contagious Diseases Acts: A Warning." 147 (1897): 477-83.
Comprehends that the Contagious Diseases Acts do not stifle venereal disease. See #2595.

2574 Corbet, W.J. "Is the Increase of Insanity Real or Only 'Apparent'?" 147 (1897): 539-50.
Insists that insanity had accelerated in rebuttal to the *Fortnightly Review*, #869. See #808, #854, #867, #2558, and #2576.

2575 "The Vaccination Question." 147 (1897): 634-44.
Partisan of vaccination discounts dirt as the root of smallpox.

2576 Corbet, W.J. "Plain Speaking about Lunacy." 148 (1897): 117-25.
Returns to opinions in #2558 and #2574 with a gloss on eugenics. See #854.

2577 "The Salisbury Treatment in England." 148 (1897): 208-16.
Peers at the prescription of Dr. J.H. Salisbury for beef and hot water to protect vitality.

2578 Wilson, Herbert W.A. "The Moral Influence of the Trained Nurse." 148 (1897): 320-35.
Contends that nurses, flattered as professionals, perform tolerably but have little sympathy for or sway over patients.

2579 Irwin, Margaret Hardinge. "The Problem of Home Work." 148 (1897): 541-57.
Groans that jobs undertaken in unsanitary domiciles endanger personal and public health.

2580 Crofts, H. Baptist. "Victorian Medicine: Its Status and Development." 148 (1897): 568-97.
Would intellectualize medicine by penning its history and defining diseases more rigorously.

2581 Haguch. "Comments on the Report of the Commissioners in Lunacy and the Swing of the Pendulum." 148 (1897): 672-81.
Admits that expensive insane asylums have not yielded more cures than those with more modest budgets.

2582 Wilson, Mona. "Employers' Liability and Workmen's Compensation." 149 (1898): 194-203.
Linchpin is the concept of strict liability in Workman's Compensation Act, 1897.

2583 X. "The New Lunacy Bill." 149 (1898): 493-98.
Comments on clauses in insanity legislation regarding asylum staff norms and salary.

2584 Dixie, Florence. " 'The True Science of Living': The New Gospel of Health." 150 (1898): 463-70.
Associates unhealthiness and obesity.

2585   Lloyd, Walter. "Sanitation and Small-Pox." 150 (1898): 548-60.
       Would suppress smallpox by vaccination, hygiene, sewerage, and
       pure water and air.

2586   Haguch. "The Fifty-Second Annual Report of the Commissioners
       in Lunacy." 150 (1898): 588-90.
       Compresses titled report on causes of and recovery from insanity
       and conditions in asylums.

2587   Leftwitch, Ralph W., M.D. "The Fallacies of Amateur Medicine."
       151 (1899): 70-74.
       Warns that those other than doctors, even nurses, do not have the
       knowledge or instruments to diagnose and treat illness and of the
       risks of taking another person's prescription.

2588   Buckland, A.W. "Remedies for Snake-Bite: Scientific and
       Empiric." 151 (1899): 182-96.
       Mirrors how different cultures tend snakebite.

2589   Foard, Isabella. "The Power of Heredity." 151 (1899): 538-53.
       Connects many afflictions to heredity.

2590   Haguch. "A Plea for Additional Commissioners in Lunacy." 151
       (1899): 615-19.
       Wants more and more medically prepared commissioners because
       the insane and asylums have multiplied since the 1850s.

2591   F. "The New Lunacy Bill and Its Pension Clauses." 151 (1899):
       663-66.
       Lingers over statutory provisions for officers of insane asylums.

2592   Hunter, A.S. "Vaccination and Dr. Garrett-Anderson." 151 (1899):
       699-703.
       Response to a letter, by Elizabeth Garrett Anderson in *The Times*,
       would extinguish smallpox by sanitation, not vaccination. See
       #2593.

2593   Observer. "Hydropathy and Small-Pox." 152 (1899): 101-03.
       Confutes #2592 with evidence that bathing does not stop smallpox.

2594   Haughton, E., M.D., B.A., T.C.D., Etc. "Fallacies of the
       Inoculators." 152 (1899): 214-20, 471-74; with a letter by James
       R. Williamson: 219.
       Scorns vaccination for smallpox.

2595   Ethelmer, Ellis [Benjamin W. Elmy]. "Contagious Diseases Acts."
       152 (1899): 249-60.
       Favors repeal of named acts because they had not diminished
       venereal diseases. See #2573 and #2597.

2596   "The Contagious Diseases Acts (Women)." 152 (1899): 397-443.
       Inventories symptoms and range of and remedies for venereal
       diseases. See #2597.

2597 "Do the Contagious Diseases Acts Succeed?" 152 (1899): 488-509, 608-27; 153 (1900): 135-58.
Concurs with #2595.

2598 Moque, Alice Lee. "An Educated Maternity." 153 (1900): 53-60.
Lobbies for physical training to improve female health.

2599 Linden, Simeon. " 'The Invalid Abroad': Sketches of Invalid Life in the High Alps." 153 (1900): 85-96.
Stereotypes the behavior of invalids when journeying outside the kingdom.

2600 *"Health's Improvement."* 153 (1900): 209-14.
Chats about ideas on diet of Thomas Muffet, a sixteenth-century doctor.

2601 Belderson, S.W. "Factory Acts and State Employees." 154 (1900): 177-81.
Would apply laws on wellness of industrial workers to their compatriots in government, chiefly postal clerks.

2602 Trobridge, George. "The Murder of Sleep." 154 (1900): 298-302.
Conjectures that diseases of the nerves increase as sleep, interrupted by night noises of civilization, decrease.

2603 Johnson, Maurice L. "Microbes: Are They Inherently Pathogenic?" 154 (1900): 325-33.
Correlates incidence of epidemic disease and microbes.

2604 Macnamara, N.C. "The Human Brain in Relation to Education." 154 (1900): 634-40.
Indicates how illness modified brain function.

AUTHOR INDEX

SUBJECT INDEX

alcohol, 139, 375, 376, 377, 482,
639, 700, 721, 782, 1127, 1470,
1667, 1704, 1773, 2028, 2472,
2572; adulterated, 166, 609,
668, 1135, 1183, 1241, 1313; as
anesthetic, 1432, 2483; as food,
224, 490, 492, 2226, 2483;
harmlessness of, 118, 270, 304,
811, 1549, 1553, 1758, 1761,
2402, 2474; legislation, 252,
270, 290, 368, 568, 668, 700,
937, 1549, 2475; as remedy, 58,
252, 490, 492, 567, 626, 628,
633, 1241, 1396, 1555, 1591,
1783, 2140; and tobacco, 494.
See also beer, wine
alcohol, harms of, 231, 258, 290,
368, 397, 424, 442, 479, 490,
492, 568, 579, 655, 694, 710,
719, 829, 937, 1015, 1208,
1326, 1385, 1482, 1491, 1495,
1498, 1499, 1502, 1507, 1605,
1757, 1763, 2371, 2531, 2553
alcoholism, 244, 366, 1176, 1485,
1491, 1494, 1496, 1843, 1993,
2184, 2226, 2363, 2529; and
asylums, 1431, 1436, 1617,
1838; and crime, 859; and
heredity, 534, 1517, 1519; and
insanity, 869, 1445, 1481, 1517,
1519; and poverty, 327, 505,
579, 694, 1445, 1517, 1519,
1965, 2409; and suicide, 1947
allergies, 1258, 1950
alternative medicine. *See*
homeopathy, hydropathy,
hypnosis, quackery, remedies
ambulances, 219, 1862
amnesia, 134, 1175. *See also*
memory
anatomy, 44, 498, 878, 1314,
1332, 1350, 1352, 1994, 2105,
2112, 2414, 2424, 2434. *See
also* specific structures
anemia, 286, 1123
anesthetics, 717, 1390, 1432,

1872, 2025, 2502. *See also*
alcohol, chloroform, drugs,
ether, nitrous oxide
aneurism, 2414
antiseptics, 1124, 1724, 1822,
1848, 1872. *See also*
disinfectants, surgery
anxiety. *See* stress
apothecaries. *See* pharmacists
astringents, 2020
athletics. *See* sports
Australia, 1468
Austria, 604, 2359

bacteria, 225, 454, 456, 458, 781,
1090, 1104, 1111, 1118, 1119,
1120, 1392, 1399, 1819, 1849,
1861, 1901, 2551. *See also*
microbes
bacteriology, 473, 1400. *See also*
Louis Pasteur
baldness. *See* hair
bathing. *See* hydropathy, hygiene
beards. *See* hair
beer, 118, 166, 194, 668, 1183
Belgium, 518, 1433, 2022, 2214
benefit societies. *See* insurance, of
the poor
blood, 274, 275, 277, 658, 716,
913, 1138, 1159, 1177, 1224,
1377, 1608, 1843, 2163. *See
also* anemia
body growth, 477. *See also*
dwarfism, gigantism
body temperature, 277, 1235. *See
also* fevers
Bohemia, 1575
brain, 267, 271, 333, 477, 485,
569, 572, 574, 584, 616, 701,
745, 753, 761, 771, 1311, 1361,
1370, 1417, 1426, 1432, 1434,
1514, 1550, 1635, 1709, 2159,
2211, 2489, 2550; and gender,
1906, 2410; and race, 2322. *See
also* nerves, nervous system,
phrenology

smallpox, vaccine (*continued*),
1701, 1724, 1731, 1732, 1744,
1863, 1948, 1969, 1986, 2069,
2095, 2110, 2171, 2523, 2533,
2534, 2575, 2585, 2592, 2594
snakebite. *See* accidents
somnambulism, 116, 204, 205,
1169, 1216
Spain, 790
spas, 287, 604, 790, 887, 905,
1575, 1775, 1930, 2124, 2181.
See also health resorts,
hydropathy, water, mineral
speech impaired, 240. *See also*
hearing impaired
Spencer, Herbert, 566, 2550
sports, 302, 344, 516, 638, 943,
1056, 1393, 1711; cycling, 107,
189, 309, 460, 850, 852, 1073,
1379, 1545, 1613, 1614, 1753,
1859; football, 222, 464, 1844;
gymnastics, 87, 172, 548, 1056,
1559; rowing, 302, 516, 1056;
swimming, 11, 1056, 1942,
2054. *See also* women's
stomach, 1560, 1624, 1643, 2567.
See also digestion, gastritis
stress, 124, 292, 361, 394, 409,
479, 482, 591, 635, 1169, 1455,
1723, 1783, 1788, 1904, 1958,
2401
suffocation, 276, 1162. *See also*
fires
suicide, 137, 199, 295, 388, 394,
430, 1340, 1907, 1947, 2054,
2478. *See also* death
superstition, 74. *See also*
remedies, folk
surgeons, 143, 555, 587, 845, 927,
1014, 1243, 1412, 1489, 1543,
2142, 2419, 2442, 2480. *See
also* doctors
surgery, 44, 129, 274, 435, 563,
646, 648, 717, 726, 847, 1124,
1581, 1582, 1584, 1585, 1587,
1693, 1710, 1724, 1848, 1872,

2376, 2514. *See also* anesthetics
Switzerland, 180, 308, 740, 2599
syphilis, 412, 1571, 2469, 2493.
See also venereal diseases

tea, 145, 265, 269, 1181, 1204,
1773, 2221
teeth, 161, 993, 1138, 1622, 1669,
1903, 2047; false, 2344
tetanus, 168, 855, 1104, 1402
thorn apple, 264, 269
throat, 136
tobacco, 57, 264, 269, 270, 424,
494, 623, 627, 655, 1181, 1182,
1470, 1493, 1650, 1704, 1771,
1873, 1983, 2026, 2030, 2213,
2350, 2412, 2531
trance, 832
trauma, 591, 1175, 1388, 1433
trichinosis, 2012
tuberculosis, 80, 176, 180, 423,
716, 736, 747, 848, 851, 870,
1320, 1468, 1644, 1724, 1802,
1812, 1819, 1821, 1879, 1889,
1892, 1894, 1895, 1905, 2077,
2085, 2294, 2304, 2335, 2455
tumor, 648
twins, 117, 958
typhoid fever, 624, 1392, 1446,
1615, 1697, 1706, 1742, 1816
typhus, 31, 41, 251, 510, 547, 615,
624, 650, 663, 907, 1240, 1333,
1697, 1999, 2004, 2239, 2417

unconsciousness, 207, 780, 1361.
See also anesthetics, sleep,
trance
United States, 879, 936, 1436,
1462, 1652, 1862, 2227, 2506
university students, 943, 2506
urinary stones, 664

vaccines, 473, 1397, 1822. *See
also* specific diseases
vegetarianism, 203, 866, 868, 953,
1239, 1386, 1755, 1825, 1882,

1887, 2052, 2472, 2507, 2526, 2566
venereal diseases, 332, 763, 1366, 1367, 1483, 1520, 2222, 2382, 2495, 2496, 2498, 2511, 2520, 2573, 2595, 2596, 2597. *See also* syphilis
ventilation. *See* air
vinegar, 1773
vision, 220, 646, 703, 724, 995, 998, 1268, 1420, 1548, 1743, 1848, 1918, 1921, 2007, 2119, 2151, 2256, 2328, 2403, 2557; specialists, 220, 965, 2403. *See also* cataract, color blindness, ophthalmia
vision impaired, 172, 200, 506, 635, 930, 990, 1053, 1112, 1268, 1346, 1490, 1536, 1548, 1556, 2172, 2299, 2459; education of, 111, 149, 531, 699, 730, 822, 1038, 1184, 1252, 1323, 1405, 1476, 1490, 1574, 2172, 2195, 2227, 2274, 2283, 2328, 2338; employment of, 506, 1025, 1031, 1323, 1405
vivisection, 67, 362, 365, 390, 392, 393, 408, 581, 734, 770, 774, 777, 779, 793, 794, 796, 797, 799, 800, 855, 955, 962, 1440, 1453, 1522, 1523, 1524, 1525, 1671, 1674, 1726, 1727, 1728, 1729, 1730, 1832, 1834, 2487, 2507, 2546
vomiting, 1173

Wales: copperworkers, 2384; doctor, 2400; insane, 1164; miners, 140, 1055
water, 258, 272, 341, 997, 1133, 1224, 1328, 1622, 1646, 1663; fountains, 1347; purification, 12, 751, 839, 1165, 1194, 2033. *See also* hydropathy, hygiene, sanitation
water, and government, 433, 547,

921, 935, 1194, 1330, 1336, 1474, 1615, 2171, 2378
water, London, 11, 33, 251, 340, 433, 461, 462, 463, 693, 712, 810, 828, 839, 883, 895, 900, 904, 920, 935, 964, 969, 970, 1006, 1042, 1156, 1158, 1187, 1195, 1210, 1317, 1318, 1454, 1610, 1628, 1659, 1660, 1663, 1823, 1891, 1893, 1917, 2014, 2152, 2171, 2180, 2197, 2377, 2378, 2426, 2439, 2460, 2494
water, mineral, 194, 283, 1111, 1118, 1773, 2061. *See also* spas
water, polluted, 251, 252, 322, 340, 433, 441, 463, 559, 632, 693, 712, 732, 772, 828, 839, 883, 895, 900, 904, 912, 920, 921, 935, 942, 948, 969, 970, 1006, 1041, 1042, 1075, 1087, 1111, 1142, 1158, 1187, 1195, 1210, 1219, 1275, 1316, 1317, 1318, 1325, 1359, 1392, 1418, 1422, 1446, 1454, 1628, 1659, 1660, 1681, 1742, 1751, 1830, 1917, 1951, 2004, 2014, 2016, 2071, 2141, 2152, 2224, 2361, 2367, 2377, 2378, 2439, 2460, 2470, 2494, 2518
water, pure, 218, 461, 462, 810, 964, 1244, 1259, 1347, 1374, 1378, 1474, 1687, 2094, 2180, 2426, 2585
water, supply of, 33, 225, 322, 325, 433, 463, 559, 693, 712, 751, 839, 904, 1156, 1187, 1256, 1259, 1267, 1336, 1374, 1418, 1474, 1610, 1659, 1823, 1891, 1893, 1945, 2014, 2071, 2094, 2171, 2180, 2197, 2494
wine, 118, 145, 626, 628, 1135, 1241, 1313
women: abused, 2332, 2382, 2568; compared to men, 83, 768, 769, 853, 1799, 1813, 1906, 2368, 2410, 2506;

E.M. Palmegiano, Ph.D., J.D., is professor of history and director of Faculty Research and Sponsored Programs at Saint Peter's College (NJ). She is First Vice President and President-elect of the American Journalism Historians Association. Professor Palmegiano specializes in studies of the Victorian press. Her previous books are *Crime in Victorian Britain: An Annotated Bibliography from Nineteenth-Century Magazines* (1993); *The British Empire in the Victorian Press, 1832-1867: A Bibliography* (1987); and *Women and British Periodicals: A Bibliography* (1976).